Contents

PART TWO: GYNAECOLOGY

PROGRESS IN
OBSTETRICS AND
GYNAECOLOGY

PROGRESS IN OBSTETRICS AND GYNAECOLOGY

Contents of Volume 9

PROGRESS IN OBSTETRICS AND GYNAECOLOGY
Volume Ten

EDITED BY

JOHN STUDD MD FRCOG

Consultant Gynaecologist,
Chelsea and Westminster Hospital,
London, UK

CHURCHILL LIVINGSTONE
EDINBURGH LONDON MADRID MELBOURNE NEW YORK AND TOKYO 1993

CHURCHILL LIVINGSTONE
Medical Division of Longman Group UK Limited

Distributed in the United States of America by
Churchill Livingstone Inc., 650 Avenue of the Americas, New York,
N.Y. 10011, and by associated companies, branches and
representatives throughout the world.

First published 1993
  Reprinted 1994

ISBN 0-443-04754-5

ISSN 0 261-0140

British Library Cataloguing in Publication Data
A catalogue record for this book is available from the British Library

Library of Congress Cataloging in Publication Data
is available

Contributors

Lindsey D. Allan MD FRCP
Professor in Fetal Cardiology, Guy's Hospital, London, UK

Philip Baker BMedSci BM BS MRCOG DM
Registrar, Department of Obstetrics and Gynaecology, Addenbrookes
Hospital, Cambridge; *Formerly* British Heart Foundation Clinical
Research Fellow, Nottingham University, UK

Alison Bigrigg BM FRCS (Ed) MRCOG
Lecturer, Department of Obstetrics and Gynaecology, University
Hospital of Wales, Cardiff, UK

I. I. Bolaji MRCOG
Clinical Research Fellow, University College Hospital, Galway, Ireland

Fiona Broughton Pipkin MA DPhil
Professor of Perinatal Physiology, University of Nottingham,
Nottingham, UK

James Browning FRCS MRCOG
Lecturer in Obstetrics and Gynaecology, University of Bristol, Bristol, UK

Linda Cardozo MD FRCOG
Consultant Obstetrician and Gynaecologist, King's College Hospital,
London, UK

Jonathan Carter MB BS FRACOG
Clinical Instructor, Division of Gynecologic Oncology, University of
Minnesota, Minneapolis, Minnesota, USA

Frank A. Chervenak MD
Director of Obstetrics and Maternal-Fetal Medicine, The New York
Hospital-Cornell Medical Center, New York, USA

Elizabeth A. Conover MS
Coordinator, Nebraska Teratogen Project; Genetic Counsellor, Meyer
Rehabilitation Institute, University of Nebraska Medical Center, Omaha,
Nebraska, USA

D. Keith Edmonds MB ChB FRCOG FRACOG
Consultant Gynaecologist, Queen Charlotte's and Chelsea Hospital,
London, UK

Nicholas M. Fisk PhD FRACOG MRCOG DDU
Professor of Obstetrics and Gynaecology, Institute of Obstetrics and
Gynaecology, Queen Charlotte's Hospital, London, UK

Harold Gee MD MRCOG
Senior Lecturer in Obstetrics and Gynaecology, Department of Fetal
Medicine, University of Birmingham, Birmingham, UK

Martin L. Gimovsky MD
Associate Professor, Department of Obstetrics and Gynaecology, Tufts
University School of Medicine; Associate Chairman, Department of
Obstetrics and Gynaecology, and Director of Education, Baystate
Medical Center, Massachusetts, USA

Malcolm Griffiths MB BS MRCOG
Senior Registrar, Department of Obstetrics and Gynaecology, Royal
Berkshire Hospital, Reading, Berkshire, UK

Richard C. Henshaw MB ChB MRCOG
Lecturer, and Honorary Senior Registrar, Department of Obstetrics and
Gynaecology, University of Aberdeen, Aberdeen, UK

Pam Johnson MRCGP MRCOG
Lecturer/Senior Registrar, Department of Obstetrics, St Helier Hospital,
Carshalton, Surrey; *Formerly* Research Registrar, Fetal Medicine Unit,
Guy's Hospital, London, UK

Margaret Johnson MD MRCP
Consultant Physician, Department of Thoracic Medicine, Royal Free
Hospital, London, UK

C. J. Kelleher MBBS BSC
Research Fellow, Department of Obstetrics and Gynaecology, King's
College Hospital, London, UK

Ronnie Lamont BSc MD MRCOG
Consultant in Obstetrics and Gynaecology, Northwick Park Hospital;
Honorary Senior Lecturer, Institute of Obstetrics and Gynaecology,
Hammersmith and Queen Charlotte's Hospitals, London, UK

Frank Lawton MD MRCOG
Consultant Gynaecologist, King's College Hospital, London, UK

Darryl J. Maxwell MRCOG MRACOG
Director, Fetal Medicine Unit, Guy's Hospital, London, UK

Laurence B. McCullough PhD
Professor of Medicine and Community Medicine, Center for Ethics,
Medicine and Public Issues, Baylor College of Medicine, Houston,
Texas, USA

Late **Fergus P. Meehan** MAO FRCOG MSc(Oxon)
Formerly Director of Clinical Research Unit, Department of Obstetrics
and Gynaecology, University College Hospital, Galway, Ireland

J. Newton MRCS FRCOG
Professor, and Head, Academic Department of Obstetrics and
Gynaecology, University of Birmingham, Birmingham, UK

S. G. Norman BSc BM BS BMedSci PhD MRCOG
Senior Registrar in Obstetrics and Gynaecology, King's College Hospital,
London, UK

John P. O'Grady MD
Professor, Department of Obstetrics and Gynaecology, Tufts University
School of Medicine; Chief, Maternal-Fetal Medicine, Baystate Medical
Center, Massachusetts, USA

Karl S. J. Oláh MB ChB MRCOG
Clinical Research Fellow, Department of Fetal Medicine, Birmingham
Maternity Hospital, Birmingham, UK

Joseph Onwude MB BS MRCOG
Senior Registrar, Department of Obstetrics and Gynaecology, St James's
University Hospital, Leeds, UK

Nagy M. Rafla MB MOG MRCOG
Consultant Obstetrician and Gynaecologist, Kent and Canterbury
Hospital, Canterbury, Kent, UK

Raj Rai BSc MB BS
Senior House Officer, Neonatal Unit, St Thomas' Hospital; *Formerly*
Honorary Research Fellow, UMDS, Department of Obstetrics and
Gynaecology, St Thomas' Hospital, London, UK

William F. Rayburn MD
John W. Records Professor, and Director, Division of Maternal-Fetal
Medicine, Department of Obstetrics and Gynecology, University of
Oklahoma Health Sciences Center, Oklahoma City, Oklahoma, USA

C. W. G. Redman MB BChir FRCP
Clinical Reader, Nuffield Department of Obstetrics and Gynaecology,
John Radcliffe Hospital, Oxford, UK

Philip W. Reginald MD MRCOG
Consultant, Department of Obstetrics and Gynaecology, Wexham Park
Hospital, Slough, Berkshire, UK

Ian L. Sargent BSc PhD
Lecturer, University of Oxford, and Nuffield Department of Obstetrics
and Gynaecology, John Radcliffe Hospital, Oxford, UK

John H. Shepherd FRCS MRCOG FACOG
Consultant Gynaecological Oncology Surgeon, St Bartholomew's
Hospital and Royal Marsden Hospital, London, UK

Shirish S. Sheth MD FACS FICS FCPS FICOG FAMS
Honorary Professor, King Edward Memorial Hospital, and Seth G. S.
Medical College, Bombay, India

Jane Siddall-Allum MB BS MRCOG
Lecturer, Department of Obstetrics and Gynaecology, St Mary's Hospital
Medical School, London; *Formerly* Registrar in Obstetrics and
Gynaecology, Wexham Park Hospital, Slough, Berkshire, UK

John Studd MD FRCOG
Consultant Obstetrician and Gynaecologist, King's College Hospital, and
Dulwich Hospital, London, UK

A. A. Templeton MD FRCOG
Regius Professor of Obstetrics and Gynaecology, University of Aberdeen,
Aberdeen, UK

K. F. Tham MB BS MMED MRCOG
Gynaecological Oncology Fellow/Senior Registrar, Gynaecological
Oncology Unit, St Bartholomew's Hospital and Royal Marsden Hospital,
London, UK

Jim Thornton MD MRCOG DTM & H
Senior Lecturer, and Honorary Consultant, Department of Obstetrics
and Gynaecology, University of Leeds, Leeds, UK

Leo B. Twiggs BS MD
Professor, and Head, Department of Obstetrics and Gynecology, and
Medical Director, Women's Cancer Center, University of Minnesota
Health Center, Minneapolis, Minnesota, USA

Martin McD. Usherwood MB BS FRCOG
Consultant in Obstetrics and Gynaecology, Aylesbury Vale Health
Authority, Stoke Mandeville Hospital, Aylesbury, Buckinghamshire, UK

Eboo Versi MA DPhil(Oxon) MB BChir MRCOG
Senior Lecturer, and Honorary Consultant, UMDS Department of
Obstetrics and Gynaecology, St Thomas' Hospital, London, UK

Swee Choo Yeoh MBBS MMed(O&G) MRCOG DPhil
Senior Lecturer, and Consultant, Department of Obstetrics and
Gynaecology, National University of Singapore, Singapore

PART ONE

Obstetrics

1. An ethical framework for obstetric practice

F. A. Chervenak   L. B. McCullough

Obstetric practice has developed specialized concepts to address the scientific and clinical dimensions of patient care. These concepts are adequate for many areas of clinical concern, but permit only implicit consideration of the physician's ethical obligations, i.e. what the physician ought to do or not do, because it is the right or correct thing to do or not do. We use 'ethical' here to distinguish such obligations from legal obligations, i.e. what one ought to do or not do because the law requires or forbids it. In obstetric ethics, ethical obligations are analyzed in terms of ethical principles. Adding the concepts and language of ethical analysis to the concepts and language of obstetric practice makes it possible for the physician to identify ethical obligations and to identify and manage conflicts between ethical obligations in patient care. The purpose of this chapter is to describe, in ethical concepts, a framework in terms of which the physician's ethical obligations in obstetric practice can be understood in concrete, clinical terms. In particular, we describe four types of ethical conflict in obstetric practice and illustrate them with clinical examples.

THE ETHICAL PRINCIPLES OF BENEFICENCE AND RESPECT FOR AUTONOMY

The ethical principles of beneficence and respect for autonomy, when applied in clinical practice, generate ethical obligations directing the physician to protect and promote the patient's interests.[1] Beneficence requires the physician to assess, objectively and rigorously, available diagnostic and therapeutic options and to implement those that protect and promote the interests of the patient by securing for the patient the greater balance of goods over harms. On this model of clinical judgment the physician evaluates the interests of the patient from medicine's perspective. The principle of beneficence must be balanced in clinical judgment by the principle of respect for autonomy. This principle obligates the physician to acknowledge that the patient, too, has a perspective on her interests, which perspective is based on her values and beliefs. This model of clinical judgment asserts that the patient possesses the freedom to choose alternatives based on her values and beliefs. The physician is therefore obligated to elicit and act on the value-based preferences of patients. Before application in particular circumstances, these two ethical principles are equally strong or weighty.[1] As a matter of ethical theory, both generate serious ethical obligations, which explain why ethical conflict can occur in clinical practice.

Protecting and promoting the interests of the pregnant woman and the interests of the fetus, when the fetus is a patient,[2] are the basic goals or purposes of obstetric care. These goals are the basis on which the principles of respect for autonomy and beneficence are applied in obstetric practice. These principles, in turn, generate ethical obligations to the pregnant woman and fetus. Figure 1.1 illustrates how these obligations work toward goals of protecting and promoting maternal and fetal interests.

Both autonomy-based and beneficence-based obligations of the physician protect and promote maternal interests. The pregnant woman can identify and express value-based preferences and obstetric practice has accumulated considerable experience about beneficence-based management strategies that protect and promote maternal health.

The fetus cannot have a perspective on its interests. Because of its insufficiently developed central nervous system the fetus has no values or beliefs that are necessary for an individual to have his or her own perspective on his or her own best interests. Hence, there can be no autonomy-based obligations to the fetus. Fetal interests in obstetric practice must, therefore, be understood in terms of the principle of beneficence, which grounds ethical obligations to the fetus. Because beneficence and respect for autonomy are theoretically equally weighted principles, beneficence-based obligations to the fetus must be regarded as serious obligations.

The pregnant woman has beneficence-based obligations to the fetus when the fetus is a patient,[2] in a pregnancy being taken to term because she is its ethical, though not for that reason alone necessarily legal, fiduciary. She is expected to protect and promote the fetal patient's interests and, by

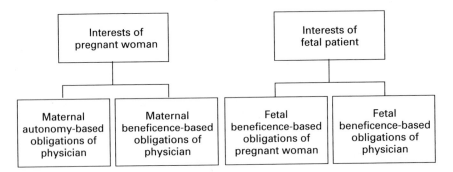

Fig. 1.1 Ethical obligations in obstetrical care. Modified from Chervenak & McCullough.[3]

doing so, those of the child the fetus will become. From medicine's perspective, the goods to be sought for the child the fetus will become and therefore for the fetal patient are prevention of disease, handicapping conditions, and premature death as well as the cure or management of disease, handicapping conditions, pain, and suffering.[1]

It seems appropriate to refer to the fetus as a patient in pregnancies being taken to term.[4,5] In terms of this framework the viable fetus is a patient, because it is capable of surviving ex utero to become a child.[2] Before viability, however, the fetus becomes a patient only as a result of the pregnant woman's decision to take a pregnancy to term.[2] Abortion before viability is consistent with either the physician's or the pregnant woman's possible beneficence-based obligations to the fetus, because before viability such obligations cannot exist independently of the pregnant woman's decision about whether to go to term. It is a fundamental feature of obstetric ethics that, before viability, no pregnant woman is ethically obligated to the fetus to regard it as a patient. Her decision to confer or withhold such status is entirely a function of her own autonomy.[2]

In pregnancies being taken to term, the ethical obligations of a physician to a pregnant woman and her fetus almost always work in concert because the physician and the woman most often mutually agree on a plan of management that will best serve both maternal and fetal interests. However, because autonomy-based and beneficence-based obligations to the fetal patient are theoretically equally strong or weighty, conflicts among these ethical obligations can occur in obstetric practice.

CONFLICTS AMONG ETHICAL OBLIGATIONS

These conflicts can be divided into four groups:

1. Conflicts between maternal autonomy-based obligations of the physician and maternal beneficence-based obligations of the physician
2. Conflicts between fetal beneficence-based obligations of the pregnant woman and fetal beneficence-based obligations of the physician.
3. Conflicts between maternal autonomy-based obligations of the physician and fetal beneficence-based obligations of the physician.
4. Conflicts between maternal beneficence-based obligations and fetal beneficence-based obligations of the physician[3] (Fig. 1.1).

Conflicts between maternal autonomy-based and beneficence-based obligations of the physician

Meaningful communication between the physician and the pregnant woman in the form of patient education and eliciting the pregnant woman's values and beliefs and her value-based preferences are essential for a positive synergism between autonomy-based and beneficence-based obligations to her and prevention of potential ethical conflicts.[6] A patient who is well-informed about her pregnancy and options for management has a greater capacity for autonomous decision-making. The physician who is knowledgeable about the patient's values and preferences is in a better position to work with the pregnant woman to identify a management plan that would be consistent with her perspective on her interests.

Sometimes, the pregnant woman and her physician identify conflicting management strategies to serve the woman's interests. A patient who is a Jehovah's Witness, for example, may refuse the administration of life-saving blood products during cesarean delivery because accepting this intervention could jeopardize her eternal salvation; the obstetrician may assess that such refusal would jeopardize her earthly existence.[7] A young woman in her first pregnancy may insist that she have a tubal ligation at the time she has a cesarean delivery because she is certain of her choice and does not desire the risk of a second operation; the physician may believe that such a procedure would lead to possibly irreversible damage to her reproductive capabilities. In such cases the physician confronts a conflict between his or her beneficence-based obligations to the pregnant woman, i.e. to carry out the management plan that, from medicine's perspective, protects and promotes the interests of the pregnant woman, and autonomy-based obligations to the pregnant woman, i.e. to implement the management plan that the patient, on the basis of a voluntary and informed choice, has determined to be in her interests.

In some circumstances, autonomy-based obligations to the pregnant woman justifiably override beneficence-based obligations to her, especially when the basic beliefs and values of the woman are at stake. It would be a form of unjustified paternalism to override an autonomous decision that is based on such serious matters in a woman's life as her religious beliefs and convictions or her self-determination regarding her reproductive capabilities. Either of these would constitute an assault on her autonomy. It is important to appreciate that fulfilling such autonomy-based obligations does not obliterate all beneficence-based obligations to her. The physician is still obligated under beneficence to provide all forms of medical support other than blood products to a Jehovah's Witness who refuses them and to offer to help the patient with a tubal ligation to obtain subsequent tubal reanastomosis if she so desires.

In some cases, beneficence-based obligations justifiably override autonomy-based obligations. This can occur when a woman's decisions are significantly reduced in their autonomy, e.g. if there is a seriously reduced ability on her part to understand choices and make voluntary decisions, or when immediate action in an emergency situation is necessary to preserve her health or life. In such circumstances, the physician may be justified in acting in a way that is contrary to what the woman may indicate. A woman in her first pregnancy in labor warrants analgesia and emotional support to help her manage pain. To accede to the infrequent demand for cesarean delivery, when this same woman is in considerable labor pain and is very frightened as a consequence, however, would violate beneficence-based obligations to protect maternal health. Because such a request probably does not reflect her basic values and beliefs, autonomy-based obligations are diminished. Moreover, less risky forms of pain relief, e.g. epidural anesthesia, are warranted by beneficence and so cesarean delivery for pain relief is not justified on beneficence-based grounds. Although a woman may strongly desire a low transverse cesarean delivery to permit vaginal delivery in subsequent pregnancies, intraoperatively the physician may realize that because of a poorly developed lower uterine segment, a vertical uterine incision is necessary to avoid injury to the uterine vessels. Time constraints may not permit the physician to obtain informed consent for such an incision. Thus, in some cases, a woman's preferences are justifiably overridden in favor of beneficence-based obligations.

In both cases, ethically informed clinical judgment concludes that potential goods (avoidance of cesarean section, avoidance of possible hysterectomy) outweigh potential harms (maternal discomfort and psychic stress, the necessity of future cesarean sections) of non-intervention in the first case and intervention in the second. In all cases in which beneficence-based obligations to the woman justifiably take precedence, there is always an autonomy-based obligation to explain later to the woman what was done and why it was done. This is one important sense in which respect for autonomy helps to prevent dehumanized obstetric care and unwarranted paternalism.

Conflicts between fetal beneficence-based obligations of the pregnant woman and of the physician

Usually the pregnant woman and the physician will be in agreement on the plan of management that provides the greatest balance of fetal goods over harms. However, there is the potential for conflict in matters concerning the diagnosis or management of fetal disorders because the woman and the physician may have well-founded but conflicting views about what is in the interests of the fetal patient and the child it will become.

Such conflicts can occur in the context of fetal diagnosis and therapy. For example, invasive fetal therapy to place a vesiculoamniotic shunt to alleviate fetal urethral obstruction involves uncertainty about risks of morbidity and mortality due to the underlying condition, the efficacy of the therapy to correct the defect, and the risks of morbidity and mortality during and after the intervention. The physician and the pregnant woman in their analyses of the interests of the fetus may evaluate these matters differently. In such cases, there may be a genuine dilemma, i.e. the necessity to choose between two courses of action with substantial ethical justification. At the present time the authors believe that there can be no decisive resolution of the dilemma surrounding experimental invasive fetal therapy until these levels of uncertainty are reduced. That is, the pregnant woman is reasonable to hold that beneficence-based obligations, on her part and the physician's, to perform experimental interventions in such cases are minimal. Thus, to respect a woman's decision concerning experimental, invasive therapies generally is an acceptable way to manage these uncertainties, because no major beneficence-based obligations to the fetus are violated by doing so. This parallels the general ethical rule in pediatrics that parents are not obligated to consent to using their child as a research subject.

Conflicts between maternal autonomy-based and fetal beneficence-based obligations of the physician

Conflicts between maternal autonomy-based obligations and fetal beneficence-based obligations are probably the most common and challenging ethical conflicts in obstetric practice. It is especially important that beneficence-based obligations be determined on a careful, objective, and rigorous assessment of the goods and harms of a management strategy, so that the fetus's interests can be established on systematic and, therefore, reliable grounds. These obligations include such routine matters in obstetric care as providing education about the effects on the fetus of maternal cigarette, alcohol, and drug use and compassionate attempts to modify such maternal behaviors by repeated emphasis on the potential ill-effects on the fetus.

In some situations, the fetal patient can benefit from maternal bed rest, hospitalization, or extended fetal heart rate monitoring. In addition, certain drugs administered to the pregnant woman, such as tocolytic agents to prevent premature birth, insulin to prevent macrosomia, digoxin to correct supraventricular tachycardia, or a steroid preparation to induce lung maturity may provide clear benefit to the fetal patient. Thus, it is evident that for optimal fetal outcome in some pregnancies maternal participation in designing and implementing the obstetric plan, with subsequent restriction on maternal autonomy, is necessary.

When this cooperation is not present, conflicts between autonomy-based obligations to the pregnant woman and beneficence-based obligations to the fetal patient can arise. The physician should, as a first-line strategy, attempt to discharge fetal beneficence-based obligations by respectfully, but vigorously, attempting to persuade the woman to accept the required restrictions or treatment.[6]

This sort of ethical conflict becomes difficult to resolve when more invasive procedures are needed for fetal diagnosis or management, such as amniocentesis to determine lung maturity, intrauterine blood transfusion for erythroblastosis, or cesarean section in the event of well-documented fetal distress. This is because a woman may determine that the risks to her wellbeing are not worth taking, even though the fetus is expected to benefit from the proposed intervention.

We propose the following guidelines to negotiate this ethical conflict. The greater likelihood that a particular intervention will result in a clearly substantial benefit for the fetus, i.e. a significant decrease in morbidity and mortality, the stronger are the beneficence-based obligations to the fetus. This guideline is based on the moral logic of beneficence-based obligations, namely, to produce a greater balance of goods over harms. The greater the likelihood that the fetus will be at a substantial risk from the intervention, e.g. increased morbidity and mortality, the weaker are fetal beneficence-based obligations, again as a matter of the moral logic of beneficence-based obligations. The greater the risk of harms to the woman, i.e. increase in morbidity and mortality, the stronger the maternal autonomy-based obligations in those cases in which the woman refuses the intervention. This is because fiduciary obligations of the pregnant woman to the fetus do not obligate her to accept any and all risks, especially those that she or her physician regard as serious, far-reaching, and irreversible. These guidelines permit fetal diagnosis and treatment, in the authors' view, when the risks to the fetus are minimal, the potential benefit for the fetus is substantial, and the risks to the woman are those she should reasonably accept on behalf of her fetus, i.e. they are not serious, far-reaching, or irreversible.[3]

Because the outlook for fetal anencephaly is universally dismal, beneficence-based obligations to such a fetus are non-existent, and termination of pregnancy, even in the third trimester, is a justified alternative on beneficence-based grounds.[8] By contrast, if maternal brain death were to occur, autonomy-based obligations to her no longer exist and fetal beneficence-based obligations move to the fore, thus possibly justifying sustaining maternal biologic life until fetal maturity,[9] if there are reliable reasons to think that this is what the pregnant woman would have wanted. While the two previous paradigms are useful in considering extreme cases, obstetric practice presents more challenging ethical conflicts, such as whether to perform a cesarean delivery for a breech presentation at 24–25 weeks of gestation or whether to use experimental vesiculoamniotic shunting in the management of fetal urethral obstruction. In both instances, the benefits to the fetus of the obstetric intervention would be unclear because the fetus of 24–25 weeks' gestation may not survive any mode of delivery[10] and because further clinical studies are necessary before it can be reliably concluded that vesiculoamniotic shunting provides a clearly substantial benefit to the fetus.[11]

By contrast, if intrapartum fetal monitoring reveals severe bradycardia, which is subsequently not responsive to prolonged conservative measures, the beneficence-based obligation to perform a cesarean delivery to preserve fetal life and avoid morbidity and handicapping conditions associated with asphyxic brain damage can become compelling enough to justify overriding maternal autonomy-based obligations that are generated by her refusal of the procedure.

There are significant clinical dimensions of implementing such a conclusion. Respect for autonomy in such cases requires the physician again to adopt the first-line strategy of attempting to persuade the woman to permit the procedure, by informing her that cesarean delivery is indeed necessary to save her fetus's/child's life and to avoid potentially serious handicapping conditions, should the fetus survive vaginal delivery. A more coercive approach, e.g. threatening to seek or actually seeking a court order, may in very restricted circumstances be morally justifiable. However, this is a matter of considerable controversy in the literature.[12–14] Consideration of this very serious compromise of maternal autonomy requires the physician to be able to show that the benefit to the fetus of such action is clear and overwhelming and the woman should be accorded respect and compassion, not degradation. Because remedies short of legal action, e.g. vigorous persuasion, involve fewer negative consequences for the physician–patient relationship and maternal–infant bonding,[15] the authors believe that these and other remedies of preventive ethics[6] are far more preferable than resorting to court orders because these strategies respect the woman's autonomy while acknowledging beneficence-based obligations to the fetus and because court orders may not be forthcoming in all cases.[3]

Conflicts between maternal and fetal beneficence-based obligations of the physician

Ethical conflicts can exist between maternal and fetal beneficence-based obligations. The most difficult of these involves putting one party at great risk of substantial morbidity and mortality to avoid great risk of similarly grave consequences for the other. These ethical conflicts can sometimes be agonizing in obstetric practice. Maternal malignancy or abdominal ectopic gestation may necessitate termination of a wanted pregnancy as the only reliable means to save the woman's life. In other cases, potentially fetotoxic drugs, such as diphenylhydantoin, may be needed to prevent serious maternal disorders such as seizures. The resolution of these sorts of conflicts presents the physician and pregnant woman with tragic choices. This is because there is no clearly convincing ethical argument in obstetric ethical theory or general philosophical ethical theory that the woman's life is more important than that of the fetal patient or that one form of serious morbidity and handicap in the pregnant woman is more grave than morbidity and handicap in the fetal patient. The authors believe that to respect the pregnant woman's decisions is an acceptable course in these tragic cases, because of the negative consequences for her and for the integrity of the patient–physician relationship of failing to do so.

CONCLUSION

When physicians confront ethical conflicts in obstetric practice, successful clinical management of such conflicts requires identification of the component ethical obligations of the conflict and rigorous judgment about the relative weight or priority of those obligations.[3] This process requires thorough documentation and objective assessment of the interests of the pregnant woman and fetal patient. An ethically justified decision is consistent with what can be shown to be the weightiest obligations as the result of ethical analysis and argument. At times, however, there is no clear resolution: the competing obligations appear to be of equal weight. It should be recognized that reasonable and conscientious people determine the weight of moral obligations differently from others. In such cases, the strategies of preventive ethics should be the physician's main response.[6]

REFERENCES

1. Beauchamp T L, McCullough L B. Medical ethics: the moral responsibilities of physicians. Englewood Cliffs, N J: Prentice-Hall, 1984; pp 22–51.
2. Chervenak F A, McCullough L B. Does obstetric ethics have any role in the obstetricians's response to the abortion controversy? Am J Obstet Gynecol 1990; 163: 1425
3. Chervenak F A, McCullough L B. Perinatal ethics. A practical method of analysis of obligations to mother and fetus. Obstet Gynecol 1985; 66: 442
4. Pritchard J A, MacDonald P C. Williams obstetrics. 16th ed. New York: Appleton-Century-Crofts, 1980: p vii
5. Harrison M R, Golbus M S, Filly R A. The unborn patient. New York: Grune & Stratton, 1984
6. Chervenak F A, McCullough L B. Clinical guides to preventing ethical conflicts between pregnant women and their physicians. Am J Obstet Gynecol 1990; 162: 303
7. Jewett J F. Report from the Committee on Maternal Welfare: Total exsanguination. N Engl J Med 1981; 305: 1218
8. Chervenak F A, Farley M A, Walter L et al. When is termination of pregnancy during the third trimester morally justifiable? N Engl J Med 1984; 310: 501
9. Dillon W P, Lee R V, Tronolone M J et al. Life support and maternal brain death during pregnancy. JAMA 1982; 248: 1089
10. Hack M, Fanaroff A A. How small is too small? Considerations in evaluating the outcome of the tiny infant. Clinics Perinatol 1988; 15: 773
11. Manning F, Harrison M R, Rodeck C et al. Catheter shunts for fetal hydronephrosis and hydrocephalus. Report of the International Fetal Surgery Registry. N Engl J Med 1986; 315: 336
12. Annas G J. Protecting the liberty of pregnant patients. N Engl J Med 1987; 316: 1213
13. Nelson L J, Milliken N. Compelled medical treatment of pregnant women. Life, liberty, and law in conflict. JAMA 1988; 259: 1060
14. Chervenak F A, McCullough L B. Justified limits on refusing intervention. Hast Cent Report 1991; 21: 12
15. Engelhardt H T Jr. Current controversies in obstetrics: wrongful life and forced fetal surgical procedures. Am J Obstet Gynecol 1986; 151: 313

2. Prenatal diagnosis

J. G. Thornton   J. L. Onwude

Obstetricians offering prenatal diagnosis or screening bear a heavy responsibility. Not only may diagnostic errors result in loss of normal pregnancies or the avoidable birth of handicapped children, but the decision to offer testing itself may be harmful. Failure to offer testing restricts women's choice but offering testing may cause anxiety, and directly or indirectly lead to the miscarriage of normal pregnancies. The dilemma is unavoidable, but obstetricians must be aware of the main tests available so that they can make informed decisions about screening, and counsel their patients accordingly.

Although many fetal conditions are potentially detectable, only a relatively small number are sufficiently common for screening to be worthwhile. These include Down's syndrome and other chromosomal aneuploidies, neural tube defects (NTDs), and in selected populations, the haemoglobinopathies and Tay–Sachs disease. Screening for cystic fibrosis (CF), the commonest single-gene disorder in Caucasian populations, is being evaluated in a number of centres and screening for fragile-X carriers is theoretically possible and may be the next major development.

Clinicians will only test for other rare diseases if there is a relevant family history and in such cases specialist genetic advice should be sought. Nevertheless, some single-gene disorders are common enough for every obstetrician to need to keep up to date. Such conditions include the haemoglobinopathies, sickle cell disease and thalassaemia, CF, muscular dystrophy and fragile-X syndrome. There have been a number of developments in CF screening over the last few years, culminating in the cloning of the gene[1] and the DNA mutations associated with fragile-X have recently been described.[2]

This chapter is aimed at enabling obstetricians to keep up to date with developments in this rapidly evolving field. Firstly we describe developments in the screening and diagnosis of NTD and Down's syndrome. Secondly, we will discuss prenatal diagnosis of the single-gene disorders including CF, haemoglobinopathies, Duchenne muscular dystrophy and fragile-X syndrome.

13

SCREENING TESTS FOR PRENATAL DIAGNOSIS

The distinction between screening and diagnostic tests is often spurious since most tests will be used in both ways in different patients. Nevertheless, some tests are usually applied to relatively large low-risk populations and will be described here as screening tests. They include serological screening for Down's syndrome and NTDs, and ultrasound examination.

Neural tube defects

NTDs (spina bifida, anencephaly and encephalocele) are the most common severe congenital abnormalities detected at birth, with a rate of over 2 per 1000 births in some areas.[3] Only congenital heart disease is more common. The incidence of NTD varies geographically and between races and in many countries seems to be falling over time. Good recent data are hard to come by since there is some evidence that terminations for NTDs are under-reported.[4] The incidence is higher in the UK than the USA and within the UK it is more common towards the North and West. Excluding anencephaly, a reasonable estimate for the UK would be 1 per 1000 births in the South East rising to 2–4 per 1000 births in South Wales and Northern Ireland. In the USA some populations may have a risk as low as 1 in 10 000 births.[5]

A positive family history is associated with a greatly increased risk. With one previous affected child, older reports had indicated a recurrence risk of 5% but recent figures are lower and probably reflect the temporal downward population risk. A reasonable estimate after one affected child in the UK is 2%.[3] The risk for women with spina bifida themselves is 3–4%.[6]

There are two methods of screening — measurement of maternal serum alpha-fetoprotein (MSAFP) and high-resolution ultrasound scanning.

Maternal serum alpha-fetoprotein

MSAFP is raised in pregnancies where the fetus has an open NTD. The levels rise with increasing gestational age, so it is usually measured between 15 and 17 weeks, with values related to gestation. Results are expressed as multiples of the median (MoM) for unaffected pregnancies at that gestation. MoM rather than centiles or ratios to the mean were chosen early in the screening programme in the 1970s because laboratories with small experience can produce a stable median relatively easily. Pregnancies affected with open NTD on average have a MSAFP of 4 MoM.[7] Amniocentesis (see below) has been usually offered to women with levels over a certain cut-off, typically 2.0 or 2.5 MoM.

A previous article in this series[8] has described the effectiveness of

MSAFP screening in population terms. If the prior incidence of NTD is 1 in 1000, then performing amniocentesis on all cases over a cut-off MSAFP level of 2.5 MoM will result in a false-positive rate of approximately 3% and a detection rate of approximately 80%. Overall, of pregnancies with MSAFP greater than 2.5 MoM, 1 in 50 will have an NTD; that is, 50 amniocenteses will need to be performed to detect one NTD.

The calculations for an individual with a raised level of MSAFP are rather different since they depend both on the individual's prior risk (or more correctly, the prior odds) and on the exact level of MSAFP. For each level of MSAFP, a likelihood ratio for NTD is calculated from the ratio of the height of the population distributions in affected and unaffected pregnancies (Fig. 2.1). In the example shown in Figure 2.1 a patient with MSAFP of 3 MoM has a likelihood ratio for NTD of $a:u$. The individual's posterior odds are the product of the prior odds and likelihood ratio:

$$\text{Prior odds} * \text{likelihood ratio} = \text{posterior odds}$$

This is Bayes' theorem. It is used for calculating individual risks for any condition given a particular test result and taking into account prior risks. Tables of individual risks have been published.[5] The top line of each triple in Table 2.1 is the same as the risks given by Adams et al[5] and indicates the risks of an affected fetus for a range of prior risks and levels of MSAFP. It

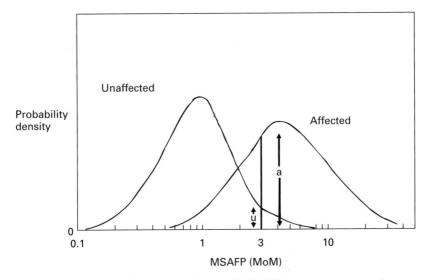

Fig. 2.1 Probability distribution for the levels of (MSAFP) expressed as maternal serum alpha-fetoprotein multiples of the median (MoM) in pregnancies unaffected and affected by open spina bifida. The height of the probability density for affected pregnancies (a) and for unaffected pregnancies (u) at 3 MoM is indicated. The ratio $a:u$ is the likelihood ratio for an affected pregnancy at 3 MoM.

Table 2.1 Risks of ventral wall defects (VWD) and open spina bifida (OSB) for a range of prior incidences of OSB and a range of levels of alpha-fetoprotein (AFP)

AFP MoM	VWD only	Prior incidence of OSB per 1000								
		0.1	0.2	0.4	0.8	1.0	2.0	3.5	5.0	25.0
2.0	3600.0	18 000.0	9000.0	4500.0	2300.0	1800.0	900.0	510.0	360.0	71.0
	11 000.0	**56 000.0**	**28 000.0**	**14 000.0**	**6900.0**	**5600.0**	**2800.0**	**1600.0**	**1100.0**	**220.0**
	35 000.0	170 000.0	86 000.0	43 000.0	21 000.0	17 000.0	8600.0	4900.0	3400.0	670.0
2.5	1500.0	4700.0	2400.0	1200.0	590.0	470.0	240.0	140.0	95.0	19.0
	4500.0	**15 000.0**	**7300.0**	**3600.0**	**1800.0**	**1500.0**	**730.0**	**420.0**	**290.0**	**58.0**
	14 000.0	45 000.0	22 000.0	11 000.0	5600.0	4500.0	2200.0	1300.0	890.0	180.0
3.0	590.0	1500.0	740.0	370.0	190.0	150.0	75.0	43.0	31.0	6.8
	1800.0	**4600.0**	**2300.0**	**1100.0**	**570.0**	**460.0**	**230.0**	**130.0**	**92.0**	**19.0**
	5600.0	14 000.0	7000.0	3500.0	1800.0	1400.0	700.0	400.0	280.0	56.0
3.5	250.0	530.0	270.0	130.0	68.0	54.0	28.0	16.0	12.0	3.1
	760.0	**1600.0**	**820.0**	**410.0**	**210.0**	**170.0**	**83.0**	**48.0**	**34.0**	**7.4**
	2300.0	5100.0	2500.0	1300.0	630.0	510.0	250.0	150.0	100.0	21.0
4.0	110.0	210.0	110.0	54.0	28.0	22.0	12.0	7.1	5.2	1.8
	330.0	**660.0**	**330.0**	**160.0**	**83.0**	**66.0**	**34.0**	**20.0**	**14.0**	**3.6**
	1000.0	2000.0	1000.0	510.0	250.0	200.0	100.0	59.0	41.0	8.9
4.5	50.0	93.0	47.0	24.0	13.0	10.0	5.6	3.6	2.8	1.4
	150.0	**280.0**	**140.0**	**72.0**	**36.0**	**29.0**	**15.0**	**9.1**	**6.7**	**2.1**
	460.0	880.0	440.0	220.0	110.0	88.0	45.0	26.0	18.0	4.4
5.0	24.0	44.0	22.0	12.0	6.3	5.3	3.1	2.2	1.9	1.2
	72.0	**130.0**	**67.0**	**34.0**	**17.0**	**14.0**	**7.6**	**4.7**	**3.6**	**1.5**
	220.0	410.0	200.0	100.0	52.0	42.0	21.0	13.0	9.1	2.6

Three risks are given. The top figure of each triple, in small type, indicates the risk if a dating scan only has been performed, excluding anencephaly and multiple pregnancy. The bottom figure of each triple, in small type, indicates the risk after a negative ultrasound examination of 90% sensitivity, assuming that the scan is independent of AFP. The middle figure, in bold type, represents our best estimate of the true risk, assuming the scan information is partially dependent on the level of AFP.

can be seen that for any given level of MSAFP (say 3 MoM), the risk for a woman with a previous affected child (prior risk 25 per 1000) is much greater than a woman without an affected child (prior risk 1 per 1000).

Even if ultrasound examination is not available, the decision to perform amniocentesis should be individualized. Many hospitals have recently dropped MSAFP screening for NTD because of the availability of high-resolution ultrasound (see below) but since MSAFP is part of many schemes for Down's screening, doctors still need to interpret raised levels.

High-resolution ultrasound for NTD screening

The sensitivity of ultrasound for anencephaly is near 100% and for open spina bifida between 60 and 96%.[9–11] Whether the higher figures can be achieved in routine practice for low-risk women has not yet been documented, although in a recent randomized trial of routine ultrasound only 50% of major malformations were detected at screening.[12]

To achieve maximum sensitivity ultrasound should be performed at 18–20 weeks. Besides examination of the spine itself the cranial anatomy may also give a clue to the existence of a spina bifida if mild hydrocephalus, frontal flattening (the lemon sign) or posterior displacement of the cerebellum due to the Arnold–Chiari malformation (the banana sign) are detected.[13]

A combination of MSAFP screening to alert the ultrasonographer combined with detailed scanning if the risks are raised may achieve the best discrimination but has not been tried in practice. Nevertheless the interpretation of MSAFP in the light of ultrasound information has been practised informally by many obstetricians. The posterior odds after MSAFP measurement can be used as new prior odds and multiplied by the likelihood ratio of NTD after a negative scan, given a reasonable estimate of ultrasound sensitivity. A conservative estimate for a good ultrasonographer alerted to the raised MSAFP would be a sensitivity of 90%. If we assume a false-positive rate of 5%, this gives a likelihood ratio (LR) for a negative scan of (specificity/1–sensitivity) = 95/10 = 9.5. However a simple application of Bayes' theorem as described above is not justified since it is likely that the tests are not independent. That is, both MSAFP and ultrasound are better at detecting the larger defects. We therefore make a necessarily arbitrary adjustment to account for non-independence and have done this in Table 2.1 by raising the LR of a negative scan to the power 0.5.

In Table 2.1, the lowest risk figure for each triple is the risk assuming the ultrasound scan and MSAFP were independent and the middle figure in bold type is the risk after adjustment for non-independence. This middle figure is the best estimate given current knowledge. It will be seen that the range of posterior risks is wide, so that the decision to offer amniocentesis after raised MSAFP and a negative ultrasound scan should also be

Table 2.2   Risk of Down's syndrome at the time of amniocentesis and at the expected date of delivery (EDD)

At amniocentesis			At EDD	
Age (completed years)	Affected pregnancies	Risk*	Age† (years and decimals)	Risk
35	19	1:285	35.95	1:348
36	35	1:174	36.95	1:276
37	47	1:146	37.95	1:216
38	64	1:122	38.95	1:168
39	84	1:91	39.95	1:130
40	88	1:80	40.95	1:99
41	70	1:67	41.95	1:75
42	69	1:45	42.95	1:57
43	62	1:30	43.95	1:43
44	30	1:33	44.95	1:32
45	23	1:21	45.95	1:24
46	19	1:11	46.95	1:18

* From Table 2 in Ferguson-Smith & Yates.[15]
† Age at amniocentesis in completed years plus 0.5 (average age in decimals) plus 0.45 (average interval from amniocentesis). From Table 4.2 in Cuckle & Wald.[16]

individualized. Expanded tables and a full description of the mathematics have been published.[14]

CHROMOSOMAL ANEUPLOIDIES

The rate of many chromosomal abnormalities varies with maternal age to the extent that age alone has long been used as a screening test.

Down's syndrome

One in 900 live births is affected with Down's syndrome in England and Wales. The risk increases with rising maternal age so that in round figures it is 1 in 1000 at age 30, 1 in 400 at 35, 1 in 200 at 38, 1 in 100 at 41 and 1 in 50 at 43.

Table 2.2 is a more detailed table based on combined results from eight studies.[15,16] Two points should be noted. Firstly, the risk is based on the woman's age at the expected date of delivery, which will be 6 months or so more than her age at booking. Secondly, the risk is of Down's syndrome at birth. Since affected fetuses have a high rate of spontaneous miscarriage and stillbirth, the risk at the time of amniocentesis is about 23% higher.

Other chromosome abnormalities

With the possible exception of Turner's syndrome, the risks of other chromosome abnormalities also rise with maternal age. The total risk of other abnormalities, excluding balanced translocation, is roughly equal to the mother's age-related risk of Down's syndrome. It is doubtful whether it is worth screening for these other abnormalities in their own right since they are lethal (+18, +13), associated with only mild abnormality (XXX, XXY, XYY, XO), or it is very difficult to predict the ultimate outcome (marker chromosomes and mosaics). Nevertheless, patients contemplating amniocentesis or chorion villus biopsy should be warned about the possibility of detection of these other abnormalities.

Family history

If a mother has had a previous affected child the risk in a subsequent pregnancy is increased. The precise risk depends on whether the affected pregnancy ended in live birth or miscarriage, whether the child had non-disjunction (the common form) or translocation, and if the latter, whether either parent is a balanced translocation carrier. If a Down's pregnancy went to term and both parents have a normal karyotype, the risk of recurrence is 0.34% above the age-specific risk. The risks with translocation carriers are complex and depend on the exact type of translocation so that expert advice should be sought. However, for the commonest 14/21 balanced translocation the risk is approximately 10% if the mother is the carrier, and 2% if the father. In the absence of a parental balanced translocation the existence of more remote relatives with Down's syndrome does not affect the age-specific risk.

SCREENING TESTS FOR DOWN'S SYNDROME

Traditionally maternal age supplemented by family history has been the main screening test for Down's syndrome and clinics have offered amniocentesis to women over a cut-off age around 35–38 years. This is not very sensitive since only 35% of Down's births occur to women aged over 35 years. A number of serological tests have been recommended for screening since Merkatz et al[17] made the key observation that MSAFP was lower in Down's affected pregnancies than controls.

Maternal serum alpha-fetoprotein

In contrast to NTD, the levels of MSAFP are lower in Down's affected pregnancies than controls. Like the risks of NTD, the posterior odds must take into account not only the level of MSAFP but also the prior odds, which are related to maternal age and whether the mother has had a previous affected child. Bayes' theorem is used and tables have been published.[4]

Triple test

There are a number of other serological markers for Down's syndrome, including low unconjugated oestriol (E_3 affected 0.7 the median of controls) and raised human chorionic gonadotrophin (hCG affected 2.08 the median of controls).[18-20] Since MSAFP, human chorionic gonadotrophin and oestriol appear each to give some independent predictive information, they have been combined with maternal age into a single screening test, the triple test.[21] This has increased screening efficiency with a detection rate of 60% for a false-positive rate of 5%. The triple test is already available in a number of centres and has proved practicable and acceptable to patients.[22] The most recent serological marker of Down's to be used for risk revision has been the urea-resistant neutrophil alkaline phosphotase (URNAP).[23] Used alone this test has been claimed to have a detection rate of 79% for a false-positive rate of 5%. Unfortunately it is a labour-intensive assay and experience with it is still limited.

DIAGNOSTIC TESTS FOR FETAL ABNORMALITY

Chorion villus biopsy

Chorion villus biopsy is performed between 8 and 14 weeks' gestation although there is, in practice, no upper limit if the abdominal route is used. Under ultrasound control, a special cannula is passed through the cervix into the chorion frondosum or a needle is inserted through the abdomen. Historically, the cervical route was developed first[24,25] but the abdominal route has become progressively more popular.[26,27] Only local anaesthesia is needed. For karyotyping, it is possible to obtain a direct chromosome spread within 24 hours — a service which is much appreciated by patients. Early diagnosis permits termination, if indicated, to be performed before movements have been felt and by the less traumatic suction method.

There has been no randomized trial comparing chorion villus biopsy with no procedure, but two trials have compared it with amniocentesis. The Medical Research Council trial of 1991[28] was larger and had a more complete follow-up. Chorion villus biopsy was associated with an excess risk of spontaneous miscarriage (3%), termination for abnormality (0.5%) and late fetal loss (0.5%), leading to an overall increased loss rate of 4% compared to amniocentesis. There was also a relatively high risk of mosaicism detected on chorionic villus samples. This led to a high rate of later amniocentesis/fetal blood sampling to decide whether it was confined to the placenta.

A report of four cases of oromandibular limb hypoplasia syndrome after chorionic villus sampling[29] was followed by reports of three further cases. Such reports may be chance associations but further support for this being a genuine — albeit rare — side-effect came from a case control study of chorionic villus sampling frequency in pregnancies resulting in fetuses with transverse limb defects in general, identified from a birth defects register.[30] Since most such cases have resulted after chorionic villus sampling at less than 9 weeks' gestation, many centres now defer the procedure until after that time unless there is a strong reason for a particularly early diagnosis.

There has been one randomized trial comparing transabdominal with transcervical chorionic villus sampling and both appeared to have the same rate of miscarriage.[31]

Amniocentesis

This is normally performed between 16 and 20 weeks' gestation with the aim of obtaining fetal cells for karyotyping or DNA analysis or to measure amniotic alpha-fetoprotein and cholinesterase to detect NTD. It used to be performed either without ultrasound examination at all, or after ultrasonic identification and marking of a pool of liquor, but without ultrasound during the procedure. A better method is to insert the needle under direct ultrasound control. This reassures the mother and is good practice for more complicated needling procedures. A 22-gauge spinal needle is used and local infiltration is unnecessary; it often causes more pain than the actual procedure. A pool of liquor and a convenient approach avoiding both the placenta and fetus are identified by ultrasound. Without changing the plane of the transducer it is moved slightly to one side and steadied by an assistant. After cleaning the skin over the entry point, the needle is inserted in the plane of the ultrasound image. By angling the transducer slightly it is possible to visualize the needle in the subcutaneous tissue before it enters the uterus. This is the time to adjust the needle direction to avoid the fetus and placenta and to follow exactly the line intended. When the needle is in the amniotic cavity 10–20 ml of fluid is aspirated. Anti-D immunoglobulin (250 i.u.) is given if the mother is Rh-negative.

The major risk is of miscarriage. Three non-randomized trials in the 1970s[32–34] suggested that the risk was of the order of 0.5% and many obstetricians felt this was a high estimate since in those trials blind aspiration had been performed for many cases. However in 1986, a large randomized and methodologically superior study[35] indicated that the excess risk of miscarriage was 1%. Although that report originally indicated that a relatively large 18-gauge needle had been used, which might have caused a high rate of miscarriage, the authors later corrected themselves and stated that a 20-gauge needle had been used.

Other side-effects include an increase in respiratory distress syndrome at birth and minor postural forms of talipes.[36] A recent controlled follow-up study of amniocentesis has also indicated a raised rate of middle ear infections and ear drum abnormalities.[37]

Early amniocentesis at 8–15 weeks' gestation is a recent development. Karyotyping success rate ranges between 68 and 100% when performed between 8 and 14 weeks' gestation.[38,39] The risks of early amniocentesis have not yet been compared in a randomized trial with either chorionic villus sampling or late amniocentesis.

Single-gene disorders

The risks of recurrence of single-gene defects depend both on the mode of inheritance and on the relationship of affected family members. It is sometimes claimed that the division into recessive and dominant modes of inheritance is arbitrary since in such cases as sickle cell disease and thalassaemia, there are phenotypic effects visible in the heterozygotes as well as homozygotes. The answer is that the terms recessive and dominant apply to the phenotype rather than the gene. A rare phenotype transmitted through several sucessive generations in a family without consanguinity, which affects both males and females, and is transmitted by both sexes and from male to male, is considered autosomal dominant. Autosomal recessive inheritance describes a rare phenotype which affects brothers and sisters with normal parents but in a situation where there is consanguinity.[40] According to this definition there are 558 autosomal recessive, 934 autosomal dominant and 115 X-linked confirmed single-gene phenotypes. In addition, there are 710 autosomal recessive, 893 autosomal dominant and 128 X-linked single-gene phenotypes where the genetic loci are not confirmed.[40]

Recessive inheritance

We will select CF as the paradigm recessive condition in Caucasians. CF has an incidence in the UK of approximately 1 in 2000 births, and affected children suffer from perinatal intestinal obstruction (meconium ileus), intestinal malabsorption causing failure to thrive, and recurrent lung infections leading to bronchiectasis, respiratory failure and death in the second or third decade. The phenotype is variable, with girls doing rather worse than boys and a small number of individuals having a relatively benign course. Treatment involves surgical relief of meconium obstruction in the neonatal period, enzyme supplements to improve absorption and regular chest physiotherapy and antibiotics to prevent pulmonary infection. Life expectancy is increasing with modern treatment and some individuals have borne children of their own. Despite this, most parents who had an affected child in the past elected to have no more children, and more recently, with the availability of prenatal diagnosis, have opted for the selective termination of affected fetuses.

Cystic fibrosis

Since CF is inherited as an autosomal recessive condition, most cases will occur to parents with no relevant family history. One in 22 people in the UK are asymptomatic carriers. The chances of two such carriers mating, assuming no consanguinity, is 1 in 484. One in four of the children of such matings will be homozygous for the CF gene and affected; two will be heterozygous carriers and one will be unaffected. The CF gene has been cloned[1] and a number of different mutations have been identified. Many of these mutations affect only a small number of families but three account for 80% of mutant alleles in most Caucasian populations.[41] The commonest single mutation is a three-base deletion named F_{508} which accounts for 70% of alleles in the UK and North America but somewhat less (48%) in Southern Europe.[42] Heterozygote screening of couples without a family history of CF is thus possible. It is uncertain at present when such screening should be undertaken and whether it will cause more harm than good.

Possible methods of screening

Screening could be offered to young people before marriage, after marriage or in the antenatal period. If screening of individuals before marriage is performed, it gives the individual heterozygotes the maximum possible reproductive options. They may select a homozygous negative partner, opt not to reproduce, or avail themselves of prenatal diagnostic tests. If couples are tested when the woman is already pregnant, the minimum number of tests will be performed but the only options left for couples who discover they are both carriers is whether or not to undergo prenatal diagnosis and termination of affected pregnancies. Individuals could be screened and their partners only tested if they screen positive or couples could be screened as a unit. If couples are screened as a unit, the testers need to decide whether to report couples with one carrier member as screen-positive or negative.

Furthermore those couples in which one parent carries a mutation but the other does not may suffer significant anxiety, since no specific prenatal test can be offered. Their numbers will depend on whether all partners are screened or whether men are only tested if the woman has already been found to be a carrier. Their risk of an affected child will be higher than the general population because the negative partner may still carry an unidentified mutation. For example, with no family history, a carrier rate of 1 : 22 and 80% of mutations detectable, the risk would be 1 in 494.[41] An advantage would be that affected partners may inform their siblings who may wish heterozygote testing. It has been recently recommended[43] that partners should be tested together and couples with one mutation heterozygote informed only that they are at low risk of an affected child, without any numeric risk being specified. This would involve deliberately withholding information, and runs against the principles of non-directive genetic counselling and respect of autonomy. It would restrict the freedom of mutation-negative partners of carriers to undergo retesting for new mutations in a later pregnancy.

Parents with a family history

If the parents already have an affected child the risk of recurrence for any recessive condition is 1 in 4 whatever the population carrier rate. However if the index case is only related to one parent (for example, a sibling, nephew or niece, or one parent has had an affected child but now has a new partner), the risk is very low, reflecting the low population carrier rate for most recessive disorders. The exceptions to this rule are the most common genetic conditions such as CF, sickle cell disease, thalassaemia and Tay–Sachs disease, with high carrier frequencies.

If one parent has a sibling affected with CF, the risk of an affected child is 1 in 132 (Fig. 2.2). In this family, testing both parents for the F_{508} mutation will considerably affect the risk. If the mother is mutation-negative, her carrier risk drops to $2/3 * 0.3 = 2/9$ and if the father is negative, his carrier risk drops to 1 in 66. The risk of an affected child is then 1 in 880. If both were found to carry the mutation, the risk would be 1 in 4 but prenatal diagnosis would be possible. If only one was a mutation carrier, exclusion testing would be possible. This would involve testing the fetus for the identified mutation. If negative, the child cannot be affected and the parents can be reassured. If it is mutation-positive, the fetus has definitely inherited one copy of the gene and will be affected if it also receives the abnormal gene from the other parent. Imagine that the father and the fetus in Figure 2.2 were mutation-positive but the mother mutation-negative. The mother has a 2/9 prior risk of carrying an un-identified mutation and the fetus a 1 in 9 posterior risk of inheriting this and being affected. The parents may opt to terminate the pregnancy at this risk.

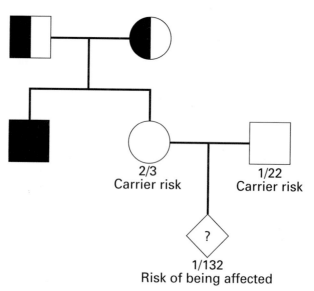

Fig. 2.2   The prior risk of an affected child when one parent has a sibling affected with cystic fibrosis.

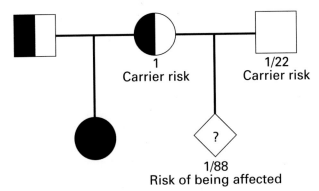

Fig. 2.3 The prior risk of an affected child when one parent has a child affected with cystic fibrosis and remarries.

Figure 2.3 shows the prior risks if one parent has had an affected child and remarried and Figure 2.4 if one parent's sibling has had an affected child. For diseases such as CF where carrier detection is possible, it is in these situations where it may be worthwhile.

Haemoglobinopathies

The thalassaemias and sickle cell disease are considered together for two reasons. They are extremely common and they have been understood at

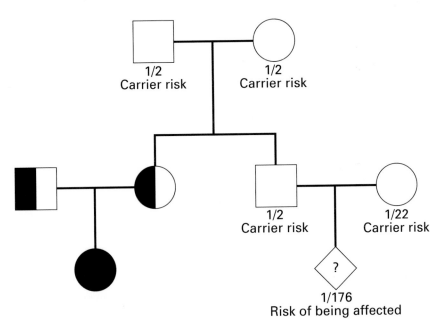

Fig. 2.4 The prior risk of an affected child when one parent's sibling has had a child affected with cystic fibrosis.

a molecular (protein and DNA) level for longer than other genetic conditions.

Sickle cell disease

African, Indian, Mediterranean and Middle Eastern people are at risk of sickle cell disease with carrier rates of up to 25% in some regions. Heterozygotes have little disability and have prospered during the period of human evolution because they have a relative resistance to malaria. The homozygous phenotype is variable with some infants dying in childhood after a series of painful crises, and others following a milder course compatible with successful reproduction.

Prenatal screening for sickle cell disease depends first on screening women from at-risk populations with haemoglobin electrophoresis. The partners of carriers are then offered testing and if they also are carriers, fetal testing may be offered. All cases of sickle cell disease reported are due to the same mutation and DNA diagnosis is therefore always possible using a chorion villus biopsy or amniocentesis sample. In the UK, all prenatal testing for haemoglobinopathies is performed in a single supra-regional laboratory in Oxford.

Screening programmes in the UK have had relatively little impact for a number of reasons. Firstly if testing is only initiated in pregnancy, there may be little time to complete it in time for termination. Secondly, the variable course of homozygous disease makes counselling difficult. Finally, until recently, efforts to publicize the service have been sporadic, leaving at-risk populations confused.

Thalassaemias

Fetuses affected with homozygous alpha-thalassaemia are hydropic in utero and are stillborn or die soon after birth. If a hydropic fetus is detected on ultrasound, termination can be offered but otherwise prenatal diagnosis is of little importance.

Beta-thalassaemia is a more important cause of childhood disease and geographically occurs in a broad band from the Mediterranean to the Middle East and South East Asia. Carrier rates are as high as 1 in 7 in Cyprus. Heterozygotes are almost symptomless. Homozygotes have defective synthesis of beta haemoglobin chains. They are healthy at birth since fetal haemoglobin (HbF) is produced normally but anaemia develops in early childhood following the onset of production of adult haemoglobin (HbA). Regular blood transfusion prolongs life, but causes iron overload which requires treatment with iron chelating agents — a major ordeal for young children and their families. Bone marrow transplantation offers the possibility of cure but carries its own risks.

Screening by haemoglobin electrophoresis in antenatal clinics is possible. If both parents are carriers then diagnosis by identification of a DNA mutation is possible in almost all cases using chorionic villus sampling or amniocentesis samples. A scheme for identification of individuals who are thalassaemia carriers was described in an earlier volume in this series.[44]

Tay–Sachs disease

Tay–Sachs disease (G_{m2-} gangliosidosis) is rare among Caucasians but among Ashkenazi Jews the carrier rate may be as high as 1 in 30. Screening of such high-risk groups for carrier status is possible by measurement of hexosaminidase A in leukocytes or serum. With prenatal testing of pregnancies at risk, the incidence of Tay–Sachs disease among American Ashkenazi Jews has decreased by 95% since 1970.[45] Such programmes are available to people of Jewish extraction in most regions of the UK and eligible patients should be referred to the regional clinical genetics service.

Dominant inheritance

In general the risk of an affected child is 1 in 2 if one parent is affected and zero (or more precisely, the population mutation rate) if both parents are healthy. Difficulties arise firstly in diseases with late onset, such as Huntington's chorea, where a parent at risk may have children before the age at which the disease usually manifests. Secondly, when there is variable penetrance, such as in myotonic dystrophy, a mildly affected mother may bear a severely affected child. Counselling, carrier testing and prenatal diagnosis in both these disorders is fraught with difficulties and is a task for experts.

X-linked inheritance

The two most important diseases in this group are Duchenne muscular dystrophy and haemophilia. Typically a carrier woman at risk of bearing an affected child will be identified because she has an affected brother or has borne an affected child. We saw above how the prior risk of an affected child, if the mother has a brother affected with CF, was 1 in 132 (Fig. 2.2). In contrast, if the mother has one brother affected with Duchenne muscular dystrophy, the prior risk of an affected child is 1 in 6 (Fig. 2.5). The prior risk is only 1 in 6 and not 1 in 4 because we take account of the possibility that the affected brother had a new mutation. This is the reason why even the generalist obstetrician should know the inheritance pattern of common diseases. The woman with the CF brother may or may not be offered genetic counselling. The woman with a Duchenne muscular dystrophy brother must be offered it.

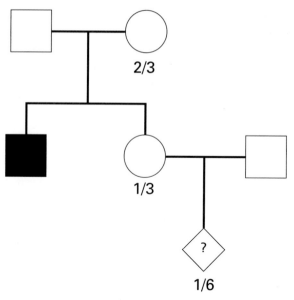

Fig. 2.5   The prior risk of an affected child when the mother has a brother affected with Duchenne muscular dystrophy.

Fragile-X syndrome

This is the second commonest single cause of mental retardation in males, with a birth frequency of 0.4–0.8/1000 males[46,47] Affected males have mild phenotypic abnormalities, macro-orchidism, typical facies with high forehead, prominent lower jaw, large ears and mental retardation, usually in the moderate to severely retarded range. Almost all affected males and most carrier females show a fragile site on the X chromosome at q27.3 when cells are cultured in folate-deficient medium.

Fragile-X differs from typical X-linked diseases in that some females are affected, albeit usually mildly, and normal transmitting males occur. Moreover the risk of a transmitting female having a retarded child is greater if the transmitting female is herself affected. Daughters of affected females are more likely to be affected themselves than carrier daughters of normal transmitting males.

In 1991 it was discovered that a trinucleotide (CCG) repeat sequence at the fragile site was greatly amplified in affected males and fragile site-positive females. A lower level of amplification was also present in transmitting males and fragile site-negative female carriers.[2,48] It has been suggested that inheritance of these unstable DNA repeat sequences explains the observed behaviour of the clinical disease.[48] Identification of these mutations offers the possibility of improved methods of prenatal diagnosis and population screening.

Traditionally women identified to be at risk of producing a child with the fragile-X syndrome were offered chorionic villus sampling or fetal blood sampling with cell culture to identify the fragile site in fetal cells. Fragile sites are less easily demonstrated on chorionic villus samples than fetal blood so negative chorionic villus sampling results needed fetal blood confirmation. If the fetus was female with a fragile site it was not possible to predict the degree, if any, of handicap and many parents opted for abortion.[49]

Identification of the DNA repeat sequence is now possible using restriction enzymes and Southern blot analysis with specific probes. It should allow confirmation of the diagnosis in chorionic villus specimens. If, as is suggested, there is a relation between the level of amplification of the repeat sequence and degree of mental impairment, then prognosis may be predicted more accurately. Finally, since techniques for testing for repeat sequences are likely to become technically much easier than cytogenetic analysis, they ultimately open up the possibility of population screening for fragile-X carriers.

REFERENCES

1. Kerem B, Rommens J M, Buchanan J A et al. Identification of the cystic fibrosis gene: genetic analysis. Science 1989; 245: 1073–1080
2. Yu S, Kremer E, Pritchard M et al. The fragile-X genotype is characterized by an unstable region of DNA. Science 1991; 252: 1179–1181
3. MacFarlane A, Mugford M. Birth counts. Statistics of pregnancy and childbirth. London: Her Majesty's Stationery Office, 1984: 260
4. Cuckle H S, Wald N J, Thompson S. Estimating a woman's risk of having a pregnancy associated with Down's syndrome using her age and serum alpha-fetoprotein level. Br J Obstet Gynaecol 1987; 94: 387–402
5. Adams M J Jr, Windham G C, James L M et al. Clinical interpretation of maternal serum alpha-fetoprotein concentrations. Am J Obstet Gynecol 1984; 148: 241–254
6. Carter CO, Evans K. Children of adult survivors with spina bifida cystica. Lancet 1973; ii: 924–926
7. United Kingdom collaborative study of alpha-fetoprotein in relation to neural tube defects: maternal serum alpha-fetoprotein measurement in antenatal screening for anencephaly and spina bifida in early pregnancy. Lancet 1977; i: 1323–1332
8. Bennett M J. The value of alpha-fetoprotein screening programmes. In: Studd J, ed. Progress in obstetrics and gynaecology. Edinburgh: Churchill Livingstone, 1981: 18–29
9. Robinson H P, Hood V D, Adam A H et al. Diagnostic ultrasound: early detection of fetal neural tube defects. Obstet Gynecol 1980; 56: 705–710
10. Roberts C J, Hibbard B M, Roberts E E, Evans K T, Laurence K M, Robertson I B. Diagnostic effectiveness of ultrasound in detection of neural tube defects — the South Wales experience of 2509 scans (1977–1982) in high risk mothers. Lancet 1983; ii: 1068–1069
11. Sabbagha R E, Sheikh Z, Tamura R K et al. Predictive value, sensitivity and specificity of ultrasonic targeted imaging for fetal anomalies in gravid women at high risk of birth defects. Am J Obstet Gynecol 1985; 152: 822–827
12. Saari-Kemppainen A, Karjalainen O, Ylostalo P, Heinonen O P. Ultrasound screening and perinatal mortality. Controlled trial of systematic one stage screening in pregnancy. Lancet 1990; 336: 387–391
13. Van de Hof M C, Nicolaides K H, Campbell J, Campbell S. Evaluation of the lemon and banana signs in one hundred and thirty fetuses with open spina bifida. Am J Obstet Gynecol 1990; 162: 322–327
14. Thornton J G, Lilford R J, Newcombe R G. Tables for estimation of individual risks of

fetal neural tube and ventral wall defects incorporating prior probability of maternal serum alpha-fetoprotein levels and ultrasonographic examination results. Am J Obstet Gynecol 1991; 164: 154–160

15. Ferguson-Smith M A, Yates J R W. Maternal age specific rates for chromosome aberrations and factors influencing them: report of a collaborative European study on 52 965 amniocenteses. Prenat Diagn 1984; 4: 5–44

16. Cuckle H S, Wald N J. Screening for Down's syndrome. In: Lilford R J, ed. Prenatal diagnosis and prognosis. London: Butterworths, 1990: 67–92

17. Merkatz I R, Nitowsky H M, Macri J N, Johnson W E. An association between low MSAFP and fetal chromosomal abnormalities. Am J Obstet Gynecol 1984; 148: 886–894

18. Wald N J, Cuckle H S, Densem J W et al. Maternal serum unconjugated oestriol as an antenatal screening test for Down's syndrome. Br J Obstet Gynaecol 1988; 95: 334–341

19. Canick J A, Knight G J, Palomaki G E, Haddow J E, Cuckle H S, Wald N J. Low second trimester maternal serum unconjugated oestriol in pregnancies with Down's syndrome. Br J Obstet Gynaecol 1988; 95: 330–333

20. Norgaard-Pedersen B, Larsen S O, Arends J, Svenstrup B, Tabor A. Maternal serum markers in screening for Down's syndrome. Clin Genet 1990; 37: 35–43

21. Wald N J, Cuckle H S, Densem J W et al. Maternal serum screening for Down's syndrome in early pregnancy. Br Med J 1988; 297: 883–887

22. Thornton J G, Cartmill R S V, Williams J, Holding S, Lilford R J. Clinical experience with the triple test for Down's syndrome screening. J Perinat Med 1991; 19: 151–154

23. Cuckle H S, Wald N J, Goodburn S F, Sneddon J, Amess J A L, Dunn S C. Measurement of activity of urea resistant neutrophil alkaline phosphatase as an antenatal screening test for Down's syndrome. Br Med J 1990; 301: 1024–1026

24. Tietung Hospital of Ansham Iron and Steel Company. Fetal sex prediction by sex chromatin of chorionic villi cells during early pregnancy. Chin Med J 1975; 2: 41–45

25. Kazy Z, Rozovsky I S, Bakharev V A. Chorion biopsy in early pregnancy: a method of early prenatal diagnosis for inherited disorders. Prenat Diagn 1982; 2: 39–45

26. Maxwell D J, Lilford R J, Czepulkowski B, Heaton D, Coleman D. Transabdominal chorionic villus sampling. Lancet 1986; i: 123–126

27. Lilford R J, Irving H C, Linton G, Mason M K. Transabdominal chorionic villus biopsy: 100 consecutive cases. Lancet 1987; i: 1415–1416

28. MRC working party on the evaluation of chorionic villus sampling: Medical Research Council European trial of chorionic villus sampling. Lancet 1991; 337: 1491–1499

29. Firth H V, Boyd P A, Chamberlain P, Mackenzie I Z, Lindenbaum R H, Huson S M. Severe limb abnormalities after chorionic villus sampling at 56–66 days gestation. Lancet 1991; 337: 762–763

30. Mastroiacovo P, Cavalcanti D P. Limb reduction defects and chorionic villus sampling. Lancet 1991; 337: 1091

31. Brambati B, Terzian E, Tognoni G. Randomised clinical trial of transabdominal versus transcervical chorionic villus sampling methods. Prenat Diagn 1991; 11: 285–293

32. MRC working party on amniocentesis. An assessment of the hazards of amniocentesis. Br J Obstet Gynaecol 1976; 59: 1–5

33. NICHD National Registry for Amniocentesis Study Group. Midtrimester amniocentesis for prenatal diagnosis-safety and accuracy. JAMA 1976; 236: 1471–1476

34. Simpson N E, Dallaire L, Miller J R et al. Prenatal diagnosis of genetic disease in Canada: report of a collaborative study. Can Med Assoc J 1976; 115: 739–746

35. Tabor A, Madsen M, Obel E B et al. Randomised controlled trial of genetic amniocentesis in 4606 low-risk women. Lancet 1986; i: 1287–1293

36. Hislop A, Fairweather D. Amniocentesis and lung growth: an animal experiment with clinical implications. Lancet 1982; ii: 1271–1272

37. Finegan J-A K, Quarrington B J, Hughes H E et al. Child outcome following mid-trimester amniocentesis: development, behaviour and physical status at age 4 years. Br J Obstet Gynaecol 1990; 97: 32–40

38. Rooney De, McLachlan N, Smith J et al. Early amniocentesis: a cytogenetic evaluation. Br Med J 1989; 229: 25

39. Nevin J, Nevin N C, Dornan J C, Sim D, Armstrong M J. Early amniocentesis: experience of 222 consecutive patients, 1987–1988. Prenat Diagn 1990; 10: 79–83

40. McKusick V A. Mendelian inheritance in man. 6th ed. Baltimore, Md: Johns Hopkins University Press, 1983

41. Lemna W K, Feldman G L, Kerem B et al. Mutation analysis for heterozygote detection and prenatal diagnosis of cystic fibrosis. N Engl J Med 1990; 322: 291–296
42. Estiville X, Chillon M, Casals T et al. F_{508} gene deletion in Southern Europe. Lancet 1989; ii: 1404
43. Vassart G, Cochaux P, Abramowicz M. Cystic fibrosis screening. Nature 1990; 343: 586
44. Letsky E A. Anaemia in obstetrics. In: Studd J, ed. Progress in obstetrics and gynaecology, volume 6. Edinburgh: Churchill Livingstone, 1987: 23–58
45. Kaback M M. Heterozygote screening. In: Emery A E H, Rimoni D, eds. Principles and practice of medical genetics. Edinburgh: Churchill Livingstone, 1990
46. Gustavson K M, Blomquist H K, Holmgrem G. Prevalence of the fragile-X syndrome in mentally retarded children in a Swedish county. J Med Genet 1986; 23: 581–587
47. Webb T, Bundey S, Thake A, Todd J. The frequency of the fragile-X chromosome among school children in Coventry. J Med Genet 1986; 23: 396–399
48. Sutherland G R, Haan E A, Kremer E. Heredictary unstable DNA: a new explanation for some old genetic questions? Lancet 1991; 338: 289–292
49. Webb T. Prenatal diagnosis of the Fragile-X syndrome. In: Drife J O, Donnai D, eds. Antenatal diagnosis of fetal abnormalities. London: Springer-Verlag, 1991: 169–179

3. Non-immune hydrops fetalis

P. Johnson   L. D. Allan   D. J. Maxwell

Fetal non-immune hydrops is an uncommon but important condition accounting for a disproportionate 3% of overall perinatal mortality.[1] As with all cases involving fetal malformation, the reason for occurrence, prognosis and risk of recurrence constitute fundamental information necessary to the proper counselling of parents. The need to provide these details combined with recent advances in prenatal investigation has focused attention on the merits of early detection, full investigation and individualized management. In selected cases, appropriate therapy has become available.

Many cases of non-immune hydrops are referred to tertiary centres for investigation. However, it is essential for all obstetricians who may be involved in the counselling and management of the patients to have a clear understanding of the condition, its pathogenesis, associations and prognosis and to be aware of the benefits of accurate and complete investigation of the fetus, mother and, at times, father. This chapter will deal specifically with these issues and seek to provide an appropriate protocol for the management of affected pregnancies.

DEFINITION

Hydrops fetalis has been recognized for over 100 years.[2] However, non-immune hydrops was first described by Potter[3] who differentiated between the hydrops associated with Rhesus immunization and that where the histological evidence of erythroblastosis was absent. She emphasized the need for the differentiation as the prognosis for future pregnancies with and without erythroblastosis is very different.

Not surprisingly, there are a number of definitions of hydrops fetalis, and the employment of these varying definitions makes comparisons between publications on the subject difficult. Many workers have employed definitions such as 'pathological increase in fluid accumulations in serous cavities and/or oedema of soft tissues'.[4] This includes isolated effusions, which may or may not be precursors of full hydrops.[5-7] An alternative definition of this condition was provided by Mahony et al in 1984: 'generalised skin thickening of >5mm and/or two or more of the following — placental enlargement, pericardial effusion, pleural effusion and ascites'.[8]

For the purpose of this chapter, we feel that the most satisfactory definition is: 'the presence of excess extracellular fluid in two or more sites, without any identifiable circulating antibody to red blood cell antigens'.[9]

INCIDENCE

Estimates of incidence vary widely, depending on the definition employed and whether prenatal or paediatric data are considered. Table 3.1 shows estimates of incidence from some of the larger published series. With an incidence of 1 : 2000–1 : 3000, most obstetric units will see at least one case of hydrops per year. As our ability to diagnose the condition prenatally improves, the overall incidence could be expected to increase. However, Hutchison et al in 1982[12] commented that the incidence had not changed over two decades — although this was before high-resolution ultrasound was widely available. The high frequency with which non-immune hydrops is associated with fetal and neonatal loss is one reason why interest in the subject has grown despite a stable incidence over recent years. A fall in the incidence of Rhesus immunization over the past 20 years has further served to focus the attention on non-immune hydrops.

PERINATAL MORBIDITY AND MORTALITY

Published series carry widely varying loss rates for this condition, depending upon the source of data (Table 3.2). In the presence of a structural abnormality, the mortality from hydrops approaches 100%.[17] However, in a series of cases identified from paediatric records,[13] 50% of babies survived. This series is inevitably biased towards those fetuses with an underlying good prognosis, as many of the poorest cases die in utero and would therefore not be included in data collected from neonatal intensive care unit records. However, it serves to underline the differences between the experience of those involved in prenatal care and our paediatric colleagues. We must be aware of the need constantly to adjust our thinking to take into account new knowledge, in particular the emergence of fetal therapy for some underlying conditions. Successful treatment depends upon knowledge of the pathogenesis and aetiology,

Table 3.1 Incidence of non-immune hydrops fetalis

Incidence	Authors
1 : 2566	Maidman et al (1980)[10]
1 : 3538	MaCafee et al (1970)[11]
1 : 3748	Hutchison et al (1982)[12]

Table 3.2   Quoted mortality rates in non-immune hydrops fetalis

Authors	Mortality rate	%
Etches & Lemons (1979)[13]	11/22	50
Carlton et al (1989)[14]	35/52	67
Mahony et al (1984)[8]	18/27	67
Watson & Campbell (1986)[15]	29/38	76
Holzgreve et al (1985)[5]	84/103	82
MaCafee et al (1970)[11]	27/33	82
Kleinman et al (1982)[16]	11/13	85
Castillo et al (1986)[17]	20/21	95
Hutchison et al (1982)[12]	60/61	98

and the possibility of prenatal treatment has provided the incentive for further research.

RECENT ADVANCES

The cornerstone of recent advances in the management of non-immune hydrops is the more widespread availability of high-resolution ultrasound in primary referring centres. Combined with this, there has been an increasing appreciation of the multiplicity of underlying causes and a willingness to refer to more specialized centres for detailed investigation.

Full investigation within a specialist centre frequently involves Doppler ultrasound examination and fetal blood sampling. Normal fetal biochemical and haematological indices are available at all gestations. The appreciation of parvovirus as a highly fetotoxic agent[18] has led to its addition to the basic virology screen performed on both fetus and mother.

The rapid expansion of data available regarding fetal welfare has allowed the appropriate selection of those fetuses suitable for intrauterine therapy. This includes the ultrasound-guided drainage of serous collections as well as transplacental and direct fetal drug administration.

In our own laboratory, estimation of fetal cardiac size and direct measurement of umbilical venous pressure at the time of fetal blood sampling has improved our assessment of fetal cardiac function.[19]

PATHOGENESIS

Non-immune hydrops has been recognized as an end-result from an array of disorders of the fetus, umbilical cord and placenta that lead to deranged fluid homeostasis.[17] The fetal disease can involve a wide range of organ systems, and it therefore seems unreasonable to argue for a common mechanism as responsible for the signs of hydrops in all cases regardless of aetiology.

There are currently three main hypotheses for the pathophysiological mechanism underlying hydrops:

1. Anaemia.
2. Cardiac failure.
3. Reduction in osmotic pressure (hypoproteinaemia).

Whatever the underlying cause, it is likely that a combination of these mechanisms can occur in any particular fetus. Before invasive fetal investigation was available, the only data accessible to workers in the field were derived from postnatal and postmortem material. While amniocentesis allows the diagnosis of certain underlying conditions, examination of fetal blood gives far more information. Initially, blood was obtained at fetoscopic blood sampling,[20] but is now obtained by ultrasound-guided fetal blood sampling.

Anaemia

Hydrops is known to occur in association with fetal anaemia secondary to Rhesus immunization, alpha-thalassaemia, fetomaternal haemorrhage etc. If anaemia were the single direct cause, its effect would be to cause high-output cardiac failure. Evidence to support this includes elevation of umbilical venous pressure in Rhesus-immunized, anaemic hydropic fetuses[21] and in anaemic fetuses from other causes.[19] However, there is also direct evidence that hypoproteinaemia occurs in fetuses which are anaemic and hydropic.[20,22] Anaemia is also often associated with hypoxia and acidosis, which may predispose to epithelial damage in capillaries and thereby allow the loss of fluid from the intravascular compartment into the extravascular space.

The elevation of umbilical venous pressure in anaemic fetuses could be directly due to portal hypertension rather than elevation of central venous pressure. Portal hypertension is thought to arise in severely affected fetuses with Rhesus haemolytic anaemia due to hypertrophy of hepatic erythropoietic tissue.[20,23] This could lead to impairment of the synthetic function of hepatic cells with resultant hypoproteinaemia. Therefore, although anaemia is frequently associated with hydrops, the exact mechanism of the development of hydrops remains unclear.

Cardiac failure

Cardiac failure is believed to be the commonest mechanism by which fetal hydrops develops.[24] In postnatal life it is associated with cardiomegaly and elevation of central venous pressure. The cardinal sign of fetal cardiac failure is an increase in cardiac size, which can be assessed by measurement of the cardiothoracic ratio.[25] Fetal venous pressure can be measured at the time of fetal blood sampling and the elevation of these clinical parameters in fetal hydrops[19] strongly supports cardiac failure as one of the main mechanisms.

Disorders of cardiac function associated with hydrops include cardio-myopathies, tachyarrhythmias and bradycardias, particularly congenital heart block. There are many types of structural heart disease associated with fetal cardiac failure, for example, obstructive left-heart disease, Ebstein's anomaly and atrial isomerism.[16,26–29] Extracardiac causes of cardiac failure include anaemia and hypoproteinaemia.

Elevation of fetal venous pressure has been shown to reduce lymph flow, which may be a major contributor to the development of hydrops in the presence of cardiac failure.[30] Furthermore, cardiac failure can be success-fully treated in utero. It therefore becomes essential to assess cardiac function in the investigation of non-immune hydrops, in order to identify those in whom therapy may be appropriate. However, the presence of a structural cardiac defect does not mean that cardiac failure is the sole cause of associated hydrops,[31] as other mechanisms may be active.

Reduced osmotic pressure

Hypoproteinaemia with subsequent reduction in osmotic pressure is the favoured mechanism involved in the pathogenesis of hydrops fetalis. Hydrops secondary to hypoproteinaemia may arise in a number of condi-tions, including anaemia[20] and congenital nephrosis,[32] and this is supported by postnatal data.[23] Even with pure 'output failure' secondary to paroxysmal atrial tachycardia, hypoproteinaemia was present in two of three hydropic fetuses tested.[33] However, whether hypoproteinaemia always precedes the onset of hydrops is not clear. In our own series, hypoproteinaemia was present in each fetus with ascites that was tested (unpublished data). However, the protein content of the ascitic fluid is higher than the serum protein, so the hypoproteinaemia may be the result of loss of protein from the circulation, rather than the cause.

Others

Although there is evidence to support all these theories, and those suggesting alternatives such as hypomobility and impaired lymphatic drainage,[6] it is most likely that the genesis of hydrops varies with the underlying abnormality. It is difficult to implicate any of the three main mechanisms as the sole cause of hydrops in, for example, multiple pterygium syndrome, skeletal dysplasias and chromosomal abnormalities.

Obstruction of venous return has been suggested as a mechanism responsible for the development of hydrops in the presence of a space-occupying lesion in the thorax, e.g. congenital cystic adenomatoid malformation of the lung or congenital diaphragmatic hernia. Impaired lymphatic drainage may be responsible for the development of hydrops, particularly in association with cystic hygromata, in karyotypic abnor-malities (45XO and 47+21) and where connective tissue malformation is apparent (skeletal dysplasias etc.). Cessation of lymph flow in the thoracic duct leads to generalized oedema, and this may be an additional mechanism exerting its effect in the generation of hydrops in fetal heart failure.[30]

DETECTION AND DIAGNOSIS

The diagnosis of non-immune hydrops is almost always made prenatally by ultrasound examination of the fetus, which in many areas is routine for all pregnancies. In addition to routine scanning, often between 16 and 20 weeks' gestation, ultrasound examination of the fetus is employed in the investigation of maternal complications of pregnancy, many of which are associated with hydrops. Of the cases seen in the Fetal Medicine Unit at Guy's, 45% were diagnosed at the routine booking scan with gestational ages from 14 to 24 weeks. The remainder were diagnosed during ultrasound examination for a variety of indications, including polyhydramnios, abnormal fetal heart rate and reduced fetal movements.

The demonstration of gross hydrops is straightforward using ultrasound. It may, however, be more difficult to visualize small pericardial and pleural effusions. Although the diagnosis of hydrops is usually obvious, confusion can arise with conditions such as cystic hygroma and intra-abdominal cysts.[5] As with many other fetal conditions, hydrops is dynamic and both isolated effusions and full hydrops have been documented as being temporary,[15,27,34] particularly in association with fetal cardiac dysrhythmias. In addition, isolated effusions are known to progress to full hydrops in some cases and repeat ultrasound examination is essential for complete assessment of the fetus. Accurate documentation of scan findings is crucial if the disease process is to be understood.

ASSOCIATED CONDITIONS

Non-immune hydrops is associated with a large number of both fetal and maternal conditions. In some cases there is an obvious causal link to the condition, though in others, the relationship is less clear. In one series, 48% of the fetuses with non-immune hydrops had a structural abnormality[35] while many others have metabolic, haematological and infectious disorders.

Maternal

When not detected by routine ultrasound examination, the diagnosis of non-immune hydrops is frequently made during the investigation of maternal complications of pregnancy, many of which often occur in the presence of hydrops. These maternal complications are so common in pregnancies complicated by fetal hydrops that Hutchison et al[12] estimated

Table 3.3   Maternal complications in non-immune hydrops fetalis

Authors	Polyhydramnios %	PET %	Anaemia %	PPH %	Perm labour %
MaCafee et al (1970)[11]	75	42	10		
Hutchison et al (1982)[12]	75	29	45	64	
Mahony et al (1984)[8]	48				
Holzgreve et al (1985)[5]	50	11	3	4	
Castillo et al (1986)[17]	43	14			19
Gough et al (1986)[36]	60	19		16	19

PET = Pre-eclampsia; PPH = postpartum haemorrhage; Prem labour = premature labour.

that 80% of cases of non-immune hydrops would be detected by investigation of maternal complications alone.

The frequency with which these maternal complications occur is relatively constant through all the published series (Table 3.3). Polyhydramnios is the commonest complication. Problems with the third stage are also common and should be anticipated. In the series of Gough et al,[36] 5 of 31 patients required manual removal of the placenta, with 2 of these having significant postpartum haemorrhage, as did 3 others. All associated complications can occur at any gestation. With the increased risk of pre-eclampsia and premature labour it is easy to appreciate that non-immune hydrops is not without significant maternal morbidity.

Polyhydramnios and premature labour are often associated with each other. The mechanism for the development of polyhydramnios in non-immune hydrops is unclear but it may be associated with the underlying cause, for example diaphragmatic hernia and congenital cystic adenomatoid malformation of the lung, both conditions where fetal swallowing may be obstructed. It is not a universal finding; oligohydramnios is present in some cases.

Fetal

Driscoll published a list of 20 associated fetal diseases in 1966.[37] This list now exceeds 100 and the reader is recommended to Machin's excellent review on the subject.[6] Twenty years ago an underlying diagnosis was only achieved in 60–70% of cases but we can now expect to establish a cause in 80–85%. This has led to a marked decrease in the number of idiopathic cases over the last 10 years, and this decrease should continue with thorough investigation of all cases.

In our own experience in the Fetal Medicine Unit at Guy's Hospital, shown in Table 3.4, abnormalities of the fetal cardiovascular system were the underlying pathology in 15/45 cases. This is a higher proportion than in most other series and reflects the inevitable bias in our referred population due to the presence of the department of Fetal Echocardiography at Guy's. However, in most series, abnormalities of the

Table 3.4 Fetal hydrops seen at Guy's from 1 August 1989 to 31 July 1991

Congenital heart disease	
Supraventricular tachycardia, normal heart	9
Supraventricular tachycardia, structural heart abnormality	2
Complete heart block	2
Sinus bradycardia	2
Total	15
Anaemia	
Twin–twin transfusion	2
Fetomaternal haemorrhage	1
Unexplained	2
Total	5
Infection	
Parvovirus	6
Rubella	1
Total	7
Karyotype anomaly	4
Multiple pterygium syndrome	2
Apert's syndrome	1
Placental haemangioma	1
Renal abnormality	1
Meconium peritonitis	1
Congenital chylothorax	1
Idiopathic	
Normal investigation and postmortem	2
Normal investigation, no postmortem	4
Resolved, alive and well	1
Total	7
Total referred 47	
1 Rhesus immunization, 1 full follow-up not available	
Total for analysis 45	

cardiovascular system are the single largest group of underlying pathologies in non-immune hydrops (Table 3.5).

Chromosomal anomalies are the second largest group in all series. The abnormalities vary from the trisomies to much more subtle karyotype defects. The fact that this is the second largest group underlines the need to karyotype a fetus with non-immune hydrops, particularly when subtle chromosome rearrangements are considered, as these may be due to a parental translocation which would markedly alter the chances of a similar abnormality recurring — essential information when counselling.

Over the past 20 years, the proportion of cases with the 'idiopathic' label has fallen. This is entirely due to fetal investigation. In our own series, 15% of cases had no cause found, although in all of these investigation was incomplete.

Intrauterine viral infections are well-recognized as causes of hydrops. The commonest infections in the past have been rubella, toxoplasmosis

Table 3.5 Non-immune hydrops underlying diagnosis

Authors	CVS	Chrom	Pulm	Renal	Twins	Idiopathic
MaCafee et al (1970)[11]	3/33	2/33	3/33	2/33	6/33	13/33
Etches & Lemons (1979)[13]	3/22		2/22	1/22		7/22
Hutchison et al (1982)[12]	5/61	3/61	3/61	2/61		23/61
Keeling et al (1983)[24]	17/50	2/50		3/50		8/50
Holzgreve et al (1985)[5]	21/103	16/103	6/103	3/103		16/103
Allan et al (1986)[26]	21/48	3/48	1/48	2/48		15/48
Castillo et al (1986)[17]	7/21	2/21				
Gough et al (1986)[36]	13/31			22/31		
Warsof et al (1986)[38]	20%	16%				
Watson & Campbell (1986)[15]	4/38	9/38	3/38	2/38		12/38
Fish et al (1987)[4]	61/421	45/421	17/421	16/421	44/421	125/421
Jauniaux et al (1990)[39]	99/298	10/298	60/298	4/298		
	121/600	94/600	26/600	14/600		93/600
Ruiz Villaespesa et al (1990)[40]	16/59	3/59		3/59	7/59	8/59
Holzgreve (1991)[41]	29/128	19/128	10/128	5/128	11/128	

CVS = Cardiovascular; Chrom = chromosomal abnormality;
Pulm = pulmonary.

and cytomegalovirus. Human parvovirus B19 was described in 1975.[42] It is known to cause fetal infection[43] and has also been shown to be one of the underlying infectious agents in non-immune hydrops.[18] This agent may have been responsible for many of the cases where no cause was found prior to the isolation of the virus. Fetal infection with parvovirus results in anaemia, which is potentially treatable,[44] and myocarditis.[45] Diagnosis of intrauterine infections depends on the identification of immunoglobulin M in the fetal circulation and presence of viral DNA in fetal tissues.

INVESTIGATION

Examination of the fetus begins with a detailed ultrasound scan, including echocardiography and Doppler blood flow studies. The sites and degree of fluid collection and skin oedema are accurately documented and recorded on videotape, which makes monitoring of progress clearer. It is difficult to ascertain the cause of hydrops from the sites of fluid collection alone. However, Saltzman et al[46] published a study where certain sites were more frequently associated with some pathologies than others. Liquor volume is assessed, and a four-quadrant column measured.[47] If liquor is reduced, the depth of the largest pocket is measured. The placenta is examined for thickness and echogenicity.

All fetal anatomy is carefully examined. Structural abnormalities of all systems have been recorded in association with hydrops, and the strong correlation with skeletal dysplasias means that all long bones, hands, feet, digits and thoracic skeleton as well as skull shape must be examined.

The value of B and M mode echocardiography cannot be over-stressed.[16,26,48] Subtle structural and functional abnormalities of the heart are often associated with hydrops, and these may not be detected on four-chamber screening. Repeat assessment may be necessary in the case of intermittent dysrhythmias, sometimes necessitating admission for prolonged monitoring of the fetal heart rate. Standard fetal heart rate monitors will not recognize tachycardias above 220 beats/min. Failure to obtain an adequate record may be the first indication of an intermittent tachycardia.

Fetal blood sampling is central to the adequate investigation of non-immune hydrops. Blood can be obtained from a variety of sites including the placental insertion of the umbilical cord, the fetal insertion, intra-hepatic vein and heart. The risk of fetal loss following a blood sampling is generally quoted as 1–2%.[49] In our own experience, we have recognized that the number of losses following the procedure varies with the under-lying pathology. Fetuses with hydrops are 'sick', and blood analysis often reveals severe anaemia and hypoxia or acidosis. Spontaneous losses are high and it is therefore not surprising that pregnancy loss is high following fetal blood sampling in the investigation of hydrops. In a series of 268 blood samplings, the loss rate in structurally normal fetuses was 1.3%, whereas in the hydrops group 25% of the pregnancies were lost within 2 weeks of the procedure, which directly reflects the initial poor fetal condition.[50] This is important in counselling parents before commencing investigations. Once intrauterine death or spontaneous miscarriage has occurred, the likelihood of obtaining satisfactory genetic, haematological, biochemical and viral results diminishes. If an underlying cause has not been identified, we are unable to answer the main questions asked by the parents: why did it happen, and will it happen again? Our experience is that over 90% of patients will accept the invasive procedure offered. We are confident that the risk of the procedure is outweighed by the value of the knowledge gained from the investigations performed.

Fetal blood may be examined for a number of parameters. In all cases, full blood count, karyotype, blood gas analysis, virology and biochemical evaluation, including plasma protein, are performed. In the presence of a family history of metabolic disease, various enzymes may be investigated. The volume of blood required for all these tests is small (approximately 2 ml). However, particularly at early gestations, the volume of blood must be kept to a minimum, and it is reasonable to limit investigations to those thought to be most useful in the light of ultrasound findings. Whilst karyotyping can be performed using liquor or chorionic villi, adequate biochemical and haematological information can only be obtained if fetal blood is available. Viral studies, including the demonstration of viral DNA,[51] can be performed on other fetal tissue, but blood sampling gives a quicker result.

At Guy's, we measure the pressure in the blood vessel entered using a fluid-filled system which attaches to the hub of the needle.[52] We have found that the umbilical venous pressure is elevated in cases with cardio-megaly, implying that cardiac failure is the underlying cause.[19] This is particularly important when therapy for heart failure is considered. In addition, we found that the survival in those fetuses with cardiac failure (5 of 8) was better than those with no evidence of cardiac failure (none of 4).

Results from fetal blood sampling can be available rapidly. Blood gas, biochemistry and full blood count results are available within a few minutes. The fetal karyotype can be ready within 72 hours. The viral studies are generally available within 7 days.

The protocol for investigation of cases of non-immune hydrops fetalis referred to the Fetal Medicine Unit at Guy's is outlined in Table 3.6. This protocol has been developed since the unit was opened in August 1988. Many of the maternal investigations will have been performed when the woman booked for antenatal care, and may not need repeating. Some, for example autoantibody screen, will not be appropriate in every case.

While this is an outline of our management protocol, it is obviously adapted to suit individual cases. In many instances, there are clues to the underlying cause which are immediately evident. Many of the techniques used in our investigation of non-immune hydrops are limited to specialist centres. However, there are useful investigations which can be performed at the time of initial diagnosis at the local unit. We believe that all cases of non-immune hydrops should be referred to a unit where facilities exist for detailed anomaly scans, including echocardiography and fetal blood sampling.

PROGNOSIS

Whilst successful therapy can be administered in some cases of non-immune hydrops, the majority of cases are still associated with a poor prognosis. In many instances, this is due to the underlying cause of the hydrops, which may be a lethal chromosomal or structural anomaly. However, in order to identify those cases where a good outcome may be anticipated, with or without prenatal therapy, appropriate prenatal investigations must be performed. In addition, even if a poor outcome is expected, information is gained prenatally which may not be available after delivery.

MANAGEMENT

The management of cases of non-immune hydrops is multidisciplinary. Once the diagnosis has been confirmed and the underlying pathology identified, it is essential for all involved in the patient's care to discuss the management options with the patient. A large number of our patients travel a considerable distance, and it is important to consider this aspect in planning further management.

Depending upon the gestational age at diagnosis and the underlying abnormality, termination of pregnancy is an option frequently chosen by

Table 3.6 Protocol for the investigation and management of non-immune hydrops

---

Maternal
History
    Age, parity, gestation
    Previous scan findings in this pregnancy
    Past medical and obstetric history
    Family history, e.g. metabolic disorders etc.
    Recent infections and contacts
    Fetal activity

Investigations
    Blood group and antibodies
    Full blood count (± electrophoresis)
    Kleihauer-Betke stain
    Viral screen
        Toxoplasma
        Cytomegalovirus
        Rubella
        Parvovirus
    Syphilis serology
    Oral glucose tolerance test
    Autoantibody screen, e.g. anti Ro

Fetal
Detailed anomaly scan including skeletal survey

Echocardiography

Assessment of liquor volume and placenta

Doppler blood flow studies
    Umbilical artery
    Middle cerebral artery
    Descending aorta
    Ductus venosus

Fetal blood sample
    Full blood count
    Blood group and Coombs test
    Karyotype
    Blood gases
    Serum protein and albumin
    Viral screen
        Toxoplasma
        Cytomegalovirus
        Rubella
        Parvovirus

Drainage procedures
    Enzymology
    Pleural effusions
    Ascites
    Polyhydramnios (fluid aspirated sent for biochemistry and cytology)

---

parents. This is usually performed at the referring hospital. It is important to stress the need for postmortem examination in all cases, both to the parents and referring obstetrician. Even with a prenatal diagnosis made on ultrasound, and possibly confirmed by blood tests, a postmortem examination serves to confirm or refute the diagnosis and may afford extra information. It is even more important where a prenatal diagnosis of the underlying cause has not been made. If parents refuse postmortem, photographs and an X-ray are extremely valuable. These investigations should be performed by the pathologist rather than a junior member of the obstetrics team. Postmortem examination is also important following an intrauterine death or spontaneous miscarriage.

There are a number of therapeutic options available in some cases of non-immune hydrops. However, it is essential that as much information as possible is gathered before considering therapy to avoid inappropriate intervention. Therapy should only be commenced in the light of a firm diagnosis and understanding of the precise condition being treated, e.g. cardiac failure. It is ideal to wait until the fetal karyotype is available, but circumstances may dictate that initial therapy should be commenced before all results are known, for example intrauterine transfusion for fetal anaemia.

Prenatal therapy falls into three main areas:

1. Transplacental drug therapy.
2. Direct fetal drug therapy.
3. Invasive procedures.

Transplacental drug therapy

The main conditions which respond to this therapeutic approach are the fetal dysrhythmias, particularly supraventricular tachycardias. It is essential that the rhythm disturbance is accurately diagnosed in a referral centre before treatment is commenced. Inappropriate administration of anti-arrhythmic agents carries risks for the mother as well as the fetus. Once the type of dysrhythmia has been identified, antiarrhythmic agents may be administered to the mother, with careful monitoring of her electro-cardiogram and blood levels. Drugs used in this approach include digoxin, verapamil, amiodarone and flecainide.[26,53-55] Treatment needs to be tailored to each individual case[56] and careful monitoring is essential. It is possible to check fetal blood levels of the therapeutic agent in cases where response is poor. Once rhythm control is achieved, resolution of fetal hydrops is often slow and may take weeks rather than days.

Direct fetal drug therapy

Maternal administration of drugs may be ineffective because of maternal metabolism, maternal side-effects and variable passage across the placenta, particularly in the presence of hydrops.[57] In such cases, direct fetal therapy can be attempted using the intraperitoneal, intramuscular or intravascular routes.[45,53]

Invasive procedures

Alternative therapeutic options include blood and albumin transfusions and drainage of fluid collections. Intrauterine blood transfusions have been employed in the management of Rhesus haemolytic disease for many years. Transfusions were initially intraperitoneal but are generally now intravenous, employing the umbilical vein or intrahepatic vein.[22,58] Intra-uterine transfusion has been successfully employed in the treatment of a fetus infected with parvovirus,[44] and workers in Japan have had some success with the administration of intraperitoneal albumin in cases of 'idiopathic' non-immune hydrops.[59]

Drainage procedures

The presence of large pleural effusions can cause pulmonary hypoplasia, which is the commonest cause of death in neonates with hydrops.[60] If such fluid collections are drained in utero, the progression of the pulmonary damage may be halted. Fluid collections may be aspirated under ultra-sound control, or chronically drained by the insertion of a pigtail catheter. Successful attempts to drain pleural effusions with good outcome have been reported.[61,62] We have drained both pleural and ascitic fluid in a number of cases of non-immune hydrops, with variable success. The drainage of ascites prior to delivery reduces the difficulties encountered in resuscitation, and improves ventilation of the newborn by reducing the splinting of the diaphragm that ascites can cause.[63] In cases of hydrops secondary to supraventricular tachycardias, it is our practice to drain ascites once control of the rhythm has been achieved if spontaneous reso-lution does not occur. However, it is our experience that if such drainage procedures are performed within 1 week of control of the tachyarrhythmia, the ascites will always recur. Therefore, we delay drainage until the fetus has remained in sinus rhythm for at least a week.

All invasive procedures carry an inherent risk of fetal demise or pre-mature labour. Therapeutic procedures also carry the risk of salvaging a severely compromised fetus with the possible result of a live but severely handicapped baby. This is of particular importance where there is evi-dence of hypoxia or acidosis, which commonly accompany fetal anaemia and hydrops. The long-term effects of metabolic compromise at early gestations are unclear, and one must remain aware of the potentially catastrophic consequences of therapeutic intervention at all costs. As knowledge increases so also will the ability to tailor therapeutic inter-vention to appropriate cases with a greater likelihood of long-term survival.

OBSTETRIC MANAGEMENT

The obstetric management of cases complicated by non-immune hydrops is rarely straightforward. There is often a great temptation to deliver such a sick fetus before term. This should be avoided. The problems of prematurity are greatly increased when the neonate has pleural effusions and ascites which make resuscitation extremely difficult. The primary consideration should be to define the underlying cause, which will clarify whether fetal therapy is possible.

The common maternal complications must also be considered. Polyhydramnios is a condition which is common and causes severe maternal symptoms in some cases. There are two therapeutic options which have been tried with varying success: maternal administration of indomethacin and amniocentesis. Neither of these methods are proven, although drainage of liquor will often provide symptomatic relief and may also improve fetal oxygenation.[64] It can also make delivery easier.

There is no evidence that mode of delivery has a marked effect on outcome. However, in our unit, delivery of such babies will often be planned in order to ensure that an appropriate intensive care cot and paediatric services are available. For this reason, many such cases are delivered by elective caesarean section. It is our practice to perform drainage procedures of liquor and ascites immediately before delivery. This makes the delivery easier and less traumatic for fetus and mother, and facilitates resuscitation.

The high incidence of third-stage complications must not be overlooked. Blood should be taken for group and save during labour, and access to maternal circulation established.

It is essential that the paediatric team are aware of the nature of the fetal problem before delivery, as resuscitation is often difficult and adequate senior assistance must be available.

CONCLUSIONS

Non-immune hydrops fetalis remains a condition for which a guarded prognosis at best is appropriate. With such a high fetal loss rate, it is essential that all information that can be obtained in order to make a correct diagnosis is sought while the pregnancy is ongoing, and that postmortem examination is performed if at all possible. Our main responsibility is to the parents of an affected fetus, and we must do all we can in order to offer them the most accurate prognosis, appropriate management and be able to answer their questions when the pregnancy outcome is known.

The modern investigation and management of non-immune hydrops is a demanding area in which to work, providing diagnostic, pathophysiological and therapeutic challenges. Although the ability to perform full investigation of all cases does not lie within the scope of the facilities available in the district general hospital, referral to an appropriate centre is easily arranged.

ACKNOWLEDGEMENTS

Pam Johnson and Lindsey Allan are grateful to the British Heart Foundation for their financial support. The authors thank Jo Motteram for her assistance in the preparation of this manuscript.

REFERENCES

1. Andersen H M, Drew J H, Beischer N A, Hutchison A A, Fortune D W. Non-immune hydrops fetalis: changing contribution to perinatal mortality. Br J Obstet Gynaecol 1983; 90: 636–639
2. Ballantyne J W. The diseases of the fetus. Edinburgh: Oliver and Boyd, 1892
3. Potter E L. Universal edema of the fetus unassociated with erythroblastosis. Am J Obstet 1943; 46: 130–134
4. Fish W, Golichowski A, Lemons J A. Hydrops fetalis. Indiana Med 1987; 80: 1150–1157
5. Holzgreve W, Holzgreve B, Curry C J R. Nonimmune hydrops fetalis: diagnosis and management. Semin Perinatol 1985; 9: 52–67
6. Machin G A. Hydrops revisited: literature review of 1414 cases published in the 1980s. Am J Med Genet 1989; 34: 366–390
7. Okamura K, Takahashi T, Akagi K et al. Three cases of fetal ascites with successful outcome and seven year evaluation of NIHF. Tohuku J Exp Med 1988; 155: 335–342
8. Mahony B S, Filly R A, Callen P W, Chinn D H, Golbus M S. Severe nonimmune hydrops fetalis: sonographic evaluation. Radiology 1984; 151: 757–761
9. Romero R, Pilu G, Jeanty P, Ghidini A, Hobbins J G. (eds) Prenatal diagnosis of congenital anomalies. Connecticut: Appleton Lange, 1988
10. Maidman J E, Yeager C, Anderson V et al. Prenatal diagnosis and management of nonimmunologic hydrops fetalis. Obstet Gynecol 1980; 56: 571–576
11. MaCafee C A J, Fortune D W, Beischer N A. Non immunological hydrops fetalis. J Obstet Gynaecol Br Commonwlth 1970; 77: 226–237
12. Hutchison A A, Drew J H, Yu V Y H, Williams M L, Fortune D, Beischer N A. Nonimmunologic hydrops fetalis: a review of 61 cases. Obstet Gynecol 1982; 59: 347–352
13. Etches P C, Lemons J A. Nonimmune hydrops fetalis: report of 22 cases including three siblings. Pediatrics 1979; 64: 326–332
14. Carlton D P, MacGillivray B C, Schreiber M D. Nonimmune hydrops fetalis: a multidisciplinary approach. Clin Perinatol 1989; 16: 839–851
15. Watson J, Campbell S. Antenatal evaluation and management in nonimmune hydrops fetalis. Obstet Gynecol 1986; 67: 589–593
16. Kleinman C S, Donnerstein R L, DeVore G R et al. Fetal echocardiography for evaluation of in utero congestive cardiac failure. N Engl J Med 1982; 306: 568–575
17. Castillo R A, Devoe L D, Hadi H A, Martin S, Geist D. Nonimmune hydrops fetalis: clinical experience and factors related to a poor outcome. Am J Obstet Gynecol 1986; 155: 812–816
18. Brown T, Anand A, Ritchie L D, Clewley J P, Reid T M S. Intrauterine parvovirus infection associated with hydrops fetalis. Lancet 1984; ii: 1033–1034
19. Johnson P, Sharland G, Allan L D, Tynan M, Maxwell D J. Umbilical venous pressure in nonimmune hydrops fetalis: correlation with cardiac size. Am J Obstet Gynecol 1992 (in press)
20. Nicolaides K H, Rodeck C H, Lange I et al. Fetoscopy in the assessment of unexplained fetal hydrops. Br J Obstet Gynaecol 1985; 92: 671–679
21. Weiner C P, Heilskov J, Pelzer G, Grant S, Wenstrom K, Williamson R A. Normal

values for human umbilical venous and amniotic fluid pressures and their alteration by fetal disease. Am J Obstet Gynecol 1989; 161: 714–717

22. Grannum P A T, Copel J A, Moya F R et al. The reversal of hydrops fetalis by intravascular intrauterine transfusion in severe isoimmune fetal anemia. Am J Obstet Gynecol 1988; 158: 914–919

23. Phibbs R H, Johnson P, Tooley W H. Cardiorespiratory status of erythroblastotic newborn infants II: blood volume, hematocrit, and serum albumin concentration in relation to hydrops fetalis. Pediatrics 1974; 53: 13–23

24. Keeling J W, Gough D J, Iliff P. The pathology of non-Rhesus hydrops. Diagn Histopathol 1983; 6: 89–111

25. Paladini D, Chita S K, Allan L D. Prenatal measurement of cardiothoracic ratio in evaluation of heart disease. Arch Dis Child 1990; 65: 20–23

26. Allan L D, Crawford D C, Sheridan R, Chapman M G. Aetiology of non-immune hydrops: the value of echocardiography. Br J Obstet Gynaecol 1986; 93: 223–225

27. Harlass F E, Duff P, Brady K, Read J. Hydrops fetalis and premature closure of the ductus arteriosus: a review. Obstet Gynecol Surv 1989; 44: 541–543

28. Ramzin M S, Napflin S. Transient intrauterine supraventricular tachycardia associated with transient hydrops fetalis: case report. Br J Obstet Gynaecol 1982; 89: 965–966

29. Wolfson D J, Pepkowitz S H, van de Velde R, Fishbein M C. Primary endocardial fibroelastosis associated with hydrops fetalis in a premature infant. Am Heart J 1990; 120: 708–711

30. Brace R A. Effects of outflow pressure on fetal lymph flow. Am J Obstet Gynecol 1989; 160: 494–497

31. McFadden D E, Taylor G P. Cardiac abnormalities and nonimmune hydrops fetalis: a coincidental, not causal, relationship. Pediatr Pathol 1989; 9: 11–17

32. Fleischer A C, Shah D M, Jeanty P, Sacks G A, Boehm F H. Hydrops fetalis. Clin Diagn Ultrasound 1989; 25: 283–306

33. Harkavy KL. Aetiology of hydrops fetalis. Arch Dis Child 1977; 52: 338

34. Mueller-Heubach E, Mazer J. Sonographically documented disappearance of fetal ascites. Obstet Gynecol 1983; 61: 253–257

35. Beischer N A, Fortune D W, Macafee J. Nonimmunologic hydrops fetalis and congenital abnormalities. Obstet Gynecol 1971; 38: 86–95

36. Gough J D, Keeling J W, Castle B, Iliff P J. The obstetric management of non-immunological hydrops. Br J Obstet Gynaecol 1986; 93: 226–234

37. Driscoll S D. Current concepts: hydrops fetalis. N Engl J Med 1966; 275: 1432–1434

38. Warsof S L, Nicolaides K H, Rodeck C. Immune and non-immune hydrops. Clin Obstet Gynecol 1986; 29: 533–542

39. Jauniaux E, Van Maldergem L, De Munter C, Moscoso G, Gillerot Y. Nonimmune hydrops fetalis associated with genetic abnormalities. Obstet Gynecol 1990; 75: 568–572

40. Ruiz Villaespesa A, Suarez Mier M P, Lopez Ferrer P, Alvarez Baleriola I, Rodriguez Gonzalez J I. Nonimmunologic hydrops fetalis: an etiopathogenetic approach through the postmortem study of 59 patients. Am J Med Genet 1990; 35: 274–279

41. Holzgreve W. The fetus with nonimmune hydrops. In: Harrison M R, Golbus M S, Filly R A, eds. The unborn patient — prenatal diagnosis and treatment. Philadelphia: W B Saunders, 1991

42. Cossart Y E, Field A M, Cant B, Widdows D. Parvovirus-like particles in human sera. Lancet 1975; i: 72–73

43. Knott P D, Welply G A C, Anderson M J. Serologically proved intrauterine infection with parvovirus. Br Med J 1984; 289: 1660

44. Soothill P. Intrauterine blood transfusion for non-immune hydrops fetalis due to parvovirus B19 infection. Lancet 1990; 336: 121–122

45. Naides S J, Weiner C P. Antenatal diagnosis and palliative treatment of non-immune hydrops secondary to fetal parvovirus B19 infection. Prenat Diagn 1989; 9: 105–114

46. Saltzman D H, Frigoletto F D, Harlow B L, Barss V A, Benacerraf B R. Sonographic evaluation of hydrops fetalis. Obstet Gynecol 1989; 74: 106–111

47. Phelan J P, Ock Ahn M, Vernon Smith C, Rutherford S E, Anderson E. Amniotic fluid index measurements during pregnancy. J Reprod Med 1987 32: 601–604

48. Platt L D, DeVore G R. In utero diagnosis of hydrops fetalis: ultrasound methods. Clin Perinatol 1982; 9: 627–636
49. Daffos F, Capella-Pavlovsky M, Forestier F. Fetal blood sampling during pregnancy with use of a needle guided by ultrasound: a study of 606 consecutive cases. Am J Obstet Gynecol 1985; 153: 654–660
50. Maxwell D J, Johnson P, Hurley P, Neales K, Allan L D, Knott P. Pregnancy loss after fetal blood sampling — an evaluation in relation to indication. Br J Obstet Gynaecol 1991; 98: 892–897
51. Thurn J. Human parvovirus B19: historical and clinical Review. Rev Infect Dis 1988; 10: 1005–1011
52. Johnson P, Maxwell D J. Fetal intracardiac pressures. Contemp Rev Obstet Gynaecol 1990; 2: 141–144
53. Maxwell D J, Crawford D C, Curry P V M, Tynan M J, Allan L D. Obstetric importance, diagnosis and management of fetal tachycardias. Br Med J 1988; 297: 107–110
54. Gembruch U, Manz M, Bald R et al. Repeated intravascular treatment with amiodarone in a fetus with refractory supraventricular tachycardia and hydrops fetalis. Am Heart J 1989; 118: 1335–1338
55. Harrigan J T, Kangos J J, Sikka A et al. Successful treatment of fetal congestive heart failure secondary to tachycardia. N Engl J Med 1981; 304: 1527–1529
56. Kleinman C S, Copel J A. Direct fetal therapy for cardiac arrhythmias: who, what, when, where, why and how? Ultrasound Obstet Gynecol 1991; 1: 158–160
57. Hansmann M, Gembruch U, Bald R, Manz M, Redel D A. Fetal tachyarrhythmias: transplacental and direct treatment of the fetus — a report of 60 cases. Ultrasound Obstet Gynecol 1991; 1: 162–170
58. Nicolini U, Santolaya J, Ojo E et al. The fetal intrahepatic vein as an alternative to cord needling for prenatal diagnosis and therapy. Prenat Diagn 1988, 8: 665–671
59. Shimokawa H, Hara K, Malda H, Mujamoto S, Korjanagi T, Nakano H. Intrauterine treatment of idiopathic hydrops fetalis. J Perinat Med 1988; 16: 133–138
60. Keeling J W. Fetal hydrops. In: Keeling J, ed. Fetal and neonatal pathology. Berlin: Springer Verlag, 1987
61. Benacerraf B R, Frigoletto F D. In utero treatment of a fetus with diaphragmatic hernia complicated by hydrops. Am J Obstet Gynecol 1986; 155: 817–818
62. Schmidt W, Harms E, Wolf D. Successful prenatal treatment of non-immune hydrops fetalis due to congenital chylothorax: case report. Br J Obstet Gynaecol 1985; 92: 685–687
63. Bell S G. Nonimmune hydrops fetalis. Neonat Netw 1988; 7: 15–27
64. Fisk N M, Tannirandorn Y, Nicolini U, Talbert D G, Rodeck C H. Amniotic pressure in disorders of amniotic fluid volume. Obstet Gynecol 1990; 76: 210–214

4. Fetal cells in maternal blood and their use in non-invasive prenatal diagnosis

S. C. Yeoh   I. Sargent   C. Redman

Inherited gene disorders place heavy burdens on worldwide health services. With recent advances in molecular biology, many of these may now be detected in the antenatal period. Several techniques have been developed to obtain small but relatively pure samples of nucleated fetal cells which are required for genetic diagnoses. However, all current procedures necessitate sampling from the pregnancy sac and this has several inherent disadvantages. Of these, fetal loss and infection are perhaps the most consistent disadvantages. Accordingly, significant benefits may be derived from the development of non-invasive methods of prenatal diagnosis.

CURRENT TECHNIQUES OF FETAL CELL ISOLATION

These are summarized in Table 4.1. Fetal fibroblasts may be isolated and cultured from the liquor amnii in the early part of the second trimester of pregnancy. However, in a randomized study by Tabor et al,[1] amniocentesis was clearly associated with a 1% increase in the abortion rate. Other reported complications have included amnionitis in the mother, and respiratory distress and postural deformities in the neonate.[2] In addition, diagnostic errors have been reported, and these have been attributed to

Table 4.1 Current techniques of fetal cell sampling and their drawbacks

Technique	Drawbacks
Amniocentesis	Second-trimester procedure Miscarriage rate increased by about 1% Diagnostic errors due to culture of maternal cells and chromosomal pseudomosaicism arising in culture
Chorionic villus sampling (CVS)	Overall fetal loss rate 3–5% Subsequent amniocentesis rate as high as 10% (to complete prenatal diagnosis) Diagnostic errors due to maternal cell contamination and chromosomal mosaicism limited to trophoblasts
Fetal blood sampling (FBS)	Miscarriage rate 5% Preterm delivery rate 15% Amniotic fluid leak

chromosomal pseudomosaicism arising in culture[3-6] and maternal cell contamination.[7]

An alternative source of nucleated fetal cells is the early placenta which may be sampled from as early as the eighth to ninth weeks of gestation. Although the overall fetal loss rate after first-trimester chorionic villus sampling (CVS) was reported to be between 3 and 5%,[8] the procedure-related loss may be as low as 0.6%.[9] However, as many as a tenth of all patients who had CVS subsequently required amniocentesis in the second trimester to confirm or complete the prenatal diagnostic procedure.[10]

Chromosomal mosaicism confined only to placental cells[11] has been ascribed to postzygotic non-disjunction in the cytotrophoblast.[12] This has given false-positive results and chromosome complement inconsistencies between chorionic villi and fetus have become well-recognized.[9,10] Conversely, contamination of chorionic villi with maternal cells has led to false-negative results.[13]

Fetal blood may be sampled by fetoscopy and ultrasound-guided needling of the cord in the second trimester. Following fetoscopy, fetal losses averaging 5% and preterm delivery rates of 15% may be expected.[14] Ultrasound-guided needling has lower morbidity and a fetal loss rate of 1.5%, without appreciable increase in preterm delivery or amniotic fluid leakage, has been reported.[15]

With micromanipulation techniques, cells may be sampled from embryos for preimplantation genetic diagnosis. This idea is appealing since, if only 'good' embryos were to be replaced, then, distressing pregnancy termination would not be necessary. Animal experiments have shown that cells can be taken from embryos and blastocysts without impairing their development. Successful pregnancies have been achieved with such embryos[16,17] and prenatal diagnosis of Lesch–Nyhan syndrome[16] and beta-thalassaemia[18] have been reported using mouse embryos.

Using micromanipulated human blastomeres, it has been possible to differentiate males from females.[19] However, widespread application in humans will be limited by the high costs and relatively low success rates of in vitro fertilization.[20] Moreover, embryo biopsy is potentially teratogenic, given the discordance of fetal malformations amongst monozygotic twins.[21]

FETOMATERNAL CELL TRAFFIC — DOES IT OCCUR?

If nucleated fetal cells could be isolated from maternal peripheral blood, their DNA could be utilized for non-invasive prenatal genetic diagnosis. Theoretically, such techniques have several advantages (Table 4.2). These methods could be applied in the first trimester of pregnancy, would be without risk of miscarriage, and should be easy to repeat and thus amenable to population screening. To be uniformly feasible, however, nucleated fetal cells would have to traffic to the maternal circulation soon after

Table 4.2   Advantages of non-invasive prenatal diagnosis

Applicable in the first trimester of pregnancy
Without risk of miscarriage or injury to fetus
Without risk of maternal infection
Simple to repeat
Amenable to population screening

Table 4.3   Early evidence presented to support the contention that fetal cells circulate in the maternal peripheral blood

Fetal cell type	Evidence
Erythrocytes	Development of maternal anti-Rhesus antibodies in Rhesus-negative mothers
	Kleihauer-Betke technique
Leukocytes	Detection of anti-HLA antibodies directed against paternally inherited fetal HLA
	Presence of male (fetal-derived) chromosomes in maternal blood
Trophoblasts	Large multinucleated cells (syncytiotrophoblasts by morphology) in maternal uterine vein blood and lung tissue

HLA= Human leukocyte antigen.

implantation, and would have to do so consistently and in sufficient numbers. In the following section, the early evidence presented to support the notion that nucleated fetal cells circulate in the maternal blood is examined. These relatively simple techniques are summarized in Table 4.3.

Erythrocytes

Rhesus (Rh)-positive fetal erythrocytes bearing Rh(D) antigens gain entry into Rh-negative Rh(d) maternal blood, to induce an immunological response in the mother, recognized clinically as Rhesus isoimmunization. In general, erythroblastosis fetalis manifests in second and higher-order pregnancies because larger transplacental haemorrhages, the commonest cause of sensitization, occur at delivery. However, Rhesus isoimmunization is also seen in primigravidae[22,23] where spontaneous fetomaternal haemorrhages may follow natural anatomical breaks which have been observed in the placental barrier.[24]

In the Kleihauer-Betke technique, acid elution of adult haemoglobin (HbA) from adult erythrocytes renders them 'ghosted' and unstainable. Larger fetal erythrocytes which contain fetal haemoglobin (HbF) are resistant to such treatment and remain clearly stained. With this technique, fetal erythrocytes have been detected in maternal peripheral blood samples from as early as 8 weeks' gestation.[25]

Unfortunately, using this and newer techniques, it has not been possible to quantify fetomaternal haemorrhage accurately. Any fetal erythrocytes exhibiting antigens distinct from those of the mother will meet with rapid destruction by maternal immune defences. For example, it has been shown that ABO-incompatibility between mother and baby affords protection against Rhesus isoimmunization.[25] However, even in ABO-compatible pregnancies, only 16% of at-risk mothers ever develop Rhesus isoimmunization,[26] perhaps because 50% of Rh(d) individuals do not mount an antibody response to a small Rh(D) challenge.[27] This could also suggest that fetomaternal haemorrhage is not an invariable event in pregnancy.

Leukocytes

Neither the syncytiotrophoblast nor the cytotrophoblast expresses paternally derived HLA-A, B or DR antigens.[28–31] In contrast, fetal leukocytes have been shown to express polymorphic HLA class I and class II antigens from as early as 12 weeks' gestation.[32] During pregnancy, primiparae may develop anti-human leukocyte antigen (HLA) antibodies which are directed against paternal HLA antigens inherited by the offspring.[33,34] Thus, it may be deduced that maternal immune reactions occurred in response to fetal leukocytes which found their way into the maternal blood.

Identification of Y chromosome-containing cells is one method by which male cells of presumptive fetal origin can be distinguished from maternal female cells. Accordingly, conventional karyotyping[35–37] and quinacrine Y chromosome fluorescence[38–40] have been used to identify embolic fetal leukocytes.

In conventional karyotyping, lymphocytes are stimulated to divide with a mitogen and the cell cycle is arrested in metaphase by the addition of colchicine. Chromosome spreads, stained with Giemsa, are painstakingly examined under high magnification. Quinacrine binds to nuclear chromatin in interphase and metaphase to give brilliant fluorescence of band Yq12 on the long arm of the Y chromosome. In contrast to conventional karyotyping, large numbers of cells may be rapidly screened. However, only a proportion (between 30 and 50%) of interphase male leukocytes exhibit fluorescence.[41,42] In addition, fluorescence of autosomes[43] and absence of fluorescence in lymphocytes taken from normal males[44,45] are acknowledged sources of error.

With conventional karyotyping, male 46,XY mitoses in maternal blood samples were detected from as early as the eighth week of gestation.[46] These mitoses were probably derived from fetal lymphocytes because of their morphology and response to mitogens. Although cytotrophoblasts can divide and differentiate, neither they nor syncytiotrophoblasts, terminally differentiated cells, respond to mitogens.[47]

The proportion of presumed fetal 46,XY to maternal 46,XX mitoses ranged from 0.17%[37] to 0.43%.[35] These figures were higher than expected when compared to reported estimates of fetomaternal haemorrhage in Rhesus isoimmunization (0.4–1.0 ml). In vitro studies suggest that the inconsistencies could be attributed to inhibition of maternal cell division by fetal cells.[48,49] If correct, this phenomenon would cause an apparent increase in the proportion of fetal mitoses. However, the proportion of fetal white cells used in these in vitro experiments was considerably higher when compared to estimates for the in vivo situation.

All studies were flawed by false positives variously attributed to the presence of an abnormal fifth small acrocentric chromosome,[50] autosomal fluorescence and previous male pregnancies. The last is implausible since prolonged survival of semiallogenic lymphocytes over several years is improbable. Another important discrepancy was the failure to demonstrate Y fluorescence in metaphase chromosomes of those in whom interphase lymphocytes were positive for Y chromatin.[40,51]

As with red cells, fetal white cell traffic may be erratic since only 20–40% of multiparae develop anti-HLA antibodies[52,53]. The invariable presence of false negatives in the karyotyping and quinacrine fluorescence studies supports this notion.

Trophoblasts

Placentation gives rise to two major areas of intimate fetomaternal contact. In the intervillous spaces, syncytiotrophoblasts and 'buds' of syncytium[54] are bathed by maternal blood. Cytotrophoblasts mingle directly with maternal tissues by invasion of the decidua and myometrium to form the interstitial cytotrophoblast, and the spiral arteries to form the endovascular cytotrophoblast. As a result, any cells which become detached from the trophoblast layer may simply pass into the maternal circulation.

Large multinucleated cells which resembled syncytiotrophoblasts have been identified in maternal blood sampled from the broad ligament veins, ovarian veins and inferior vena cavae, from 18 weeks' gestation.[54] These cells may be carried to the lungs via the inferior vena cava where they may become trapped within pulmonary capillaries and eventually destroyed. Cells which resembled syncytiotrophoblasts have been identified in lung sections of 44% of women dying in pregnancy but curiously, inflammatory changes were absent.[55] However, it is possible that a few trophoblasts may escape this net to reach the peripheral circulation, from where it has been claimed that they can be isolated and established in culture.[56,57]

Fetomaternal trophoblast traffic may be a normal pregnancy event influenced by a number of factors. Increased trophoblast deportation has been associated with advancing gestation, parturition, eclamptic convulsions and manual removal of the placenta.[54,55,58] Of interest is the association between trophoblast traffic and pre-eclampsia: more cells of presumed trophoblast origin have been found in the uterine venous blood of pre-eclamptic patients than in non-pre-eclamptic controls.[59,60] In some cases of pre-eclampsia, cytotrophoblasts have also been demonstrated in the maternal uterine venous blood.[60]

FLOW CYTOMETRY

In addition to monoclonal antibodies, two technological developments have encouraged renewed attempts to isolate and identify any nucleated fetal cells which may circulate in the maternal peripheral blood. Indeed, it has been shown that it is feasible to combine flow cytometry[61] and gene amplification by means of the polymerase chain reaction (PCR) for this purpose.[62]

Flow cytometry is a process by which individual cells may be rapidly characterized as they pass in a fluid stream through a measuring apparatus (Fig. 4.1). As many as 1000 cells may be individually examined in just 1 second. Cells are labelled in suspension with antibodies and red or green fluorescent tags. The labelled cells are then injected through a flow chamber which is designed to generate a fluid stream of single cells. As individual cells cross the path of a focused beam of monochromatic laser light, several pieces of information are generated.

The incident laser light stimulates the fluorochromes bound to the surface of the cells to emit red or green fluorescence which is then routed via a system of filters and mirrors to fluorescence detectors (or photo-multiplier tubes). Light is also deflected by the cells: two components of light scatter are generally analysed. These, termed forward angle light scatter and 90° light scatter, correlate well with the relative size and granularity of the cells.

Following amplification, the fluorescence and light scatter signals are digitized and the data subjected to computerized analyses. Populations of cells with specified attributes may then be defined with computer-derived gates, and their characteristics analysed using sophisticated software. In a

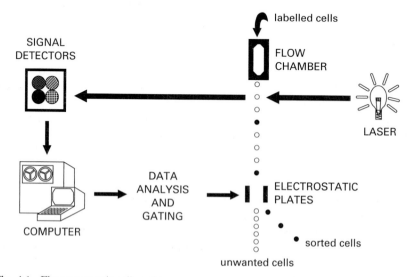

Fig. 4.1 Flow cytometric cell sorting.

simple example, the relative proportion of natural killer cells in a given sample of cells may be quickly and accurately derived.

Specified cells may be physically sorted on the basis of computerized gates set by the investigator. In this process, the fluid stream is rapidly oscillated by a piezoelectric crystal to break it into individual droplets, each of which may or may not contain a cell. When a droplet which contains a cell with the required features has been identified, an electrostatic charge is applied to it. The droplet is then deflected out of the main fluid stream by an electrical plate bearing the opposite electrical charge and collected. Uncharged droplets containing unwanted cells pass through into a waste reservoir (Fig. 4.1). In routine sorting, upwards of 20 000 000 cells may be individually examined in an hour and recovery rates of the desired cells range from 40 to 99%. Although the separated sample invariably contains some contaminating cells, purities in excess of 95% can be routinely achieved.

While flow cytometers have been used with considerable accuracy to separate cells which comprise as little as 5% of a mixed cell population,[61] their use in the detection and isolation of cells at lower frequencies (rare events) has not been well-documented.

Any fluorescent signals emanating from the rare cells (i.e. less than 1% of the cell population) will inevitably be overshadowed by background noise, if standard methods of immunofluorescence labelling are used. Therefore, if fetal cells are to be accurately separated from maternal ones, high signal-to-noise ratios are needed.[62] Factors by which this may be achieved include reduction of background noise, cellular autofluorescence and the use of brighter fluorochromes.[63] Repeated cycles of flow cytometric enrichment and cell culture have been used to purify rare cell clones with frequencies as low as $1:10^3–10^6$,[64–66] but this option would not be practical for sorting embolic fetal cells.

THE POLYMERASE CHAIN REACTION

To verify that any cells sorted from maternal blood are derived from the fetus, it is necessary to demonstrate that these contain fetal-specific DNA. Despite intensive enrichment procedures, only a few fetal cells heavily contaminated by maternal cells can be isolated from the maternal blood. Thus, routine methods of gene analysis, for example, Southern blot hybridization, were not possible.

The PCR is a technique whereby a specific fragment of DNA can be amplified as much as 10^8-fold in a matter of a few hours.[67–69] In addition to being a powerful research tool for DNA cloning and sequencing,[70–72] this procedure has widespread clinical applications. These include diagnosis of residual malignancies such as leukaemia and lymphoma[73–75] and the detection of carriers of phenylketonuria[76] and cystic fibrosis.[77,78] The PCR has also been applied in the prenatal diagnosis of several genetic disorders

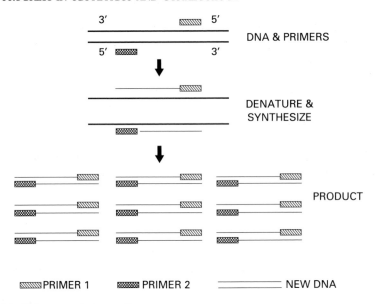

Fig. 4.2 Polymerase chain reaction.

and these include haemophilia A, beta-thalassaemia and sickle cell anaemia.[79-82] By facilitating selective amplification of minute amounts of fetal DNA present in the maternal blood, the PCR has made non-invasive prenatal diagnosis a feasible option.

Essentially, the PCR involves repeated cycles of DNA amplification. Each cycle comprises three steps: heat denaturation of DNA, strand annealing and enzymatic extension with a DNA polymerase enzyme (Fig. 4.2). Two synthetic oligonucleotide primers (short sequences of single-stranded DNA) are selected. These are designed such that they are complementary to regions which flank the fragment of interest, and to opposite strands of the target DNA. The primers are orientated so that their 3′ termini point towards each other. In the presence of a DNA polymerase enzyme, deoxyribonucleotide triphosphates (dNTPs) and appropriate reaction conditions, DNA synthesis proceeds between them in the 3′ to 5′ direction (Fig. 4.2).

In the first amplification cycle, the double-stranded DNA molecule is heat-denatured to produce two single-stranded templates. In the annealing phase which follows, the primers bind to their complementary sites on the DNA templates. Finally, in the extension phase, a new strand of DNA is synthesized by DNA polymerase from the 3′ end of each primer, such that the primer forms the 5′ terminus of the new strand.

Incorporation of the primers into their own extension products leads to selective enrichment of the target sequence which now lies between the 5′ termini of both primers. Since the extension products are themselves complementary to the primers, successive amplification cycles double the amount of DNA synthesized in the previous cycle, and exponential accumulation (2^n, where n is the number of amplification cycles) of the target fragment occurs.

The advent of a heat-resistant DNA polymerase, *Taq* polymerase, which is not destroyed by high temperatures, means that the enzyme does not have to be replenished after each denaturation step. This attribute has enabled automation of the PCR[69] with heating blocks specifically designed for this purpose.

Unfortunately, the exponential nature of the PCR reaction only extends as far as 25–30 amplification cycles, beyond which point increasing the number of cycles does not significantly increase the DNA yield.[68,69] There are several possible causes for this plateau: these include enzyme in-activation, renaturation between the products themselves and an excess of product-templates, with which complete enzyme polymerization is impossible within the allotted time.[83] Finally, *Taq* polymerase is not completely heat-stable, retaining only a third of its original activity after 15 PCR cycles.[84]

Even so, the PCR is a very sensitive technique and it has been used to detect specific DNA sequences from as little as 75 cells,[67] and even a single sperm.[85] Ironically, the exquisite sensitivity of the reaction also causes its major drawback since minute amounts of contaminant DNA will also be amplified. This is critically important when dealing with a very few cells[19,86] and strict observance of precautionary measures is vital.[87]

Obviously, errors which arise at an early stage of the PCR will be magnified to a greater degree than those which occur later. The effects of these errors may be reduced by the addition of a second level of specificity. These include hybridization of amplified sequences with internal oligo-nucleotide probes designed to recognize a specific sequence within the amplified DNA fragment.[88]

FETAL CELL ISOLATION FROM MATERNAL PERIPHERAL BLOOD

In this section, recent attempts to label a variety of fetal cells with monoclonal antibodies to distinguish and separate these from maternal cells are discussed. These studies are detailed in Table 4.4.

Erythrocytes

It has been suggested that flow cytometry may be used as an appropriate alternative to the Kleihauer-Betke technique to determine the proportion of fetal Rh(D) erythrocytes in the blood of Rh(d) postpartum women.[89,90] In these studies, polyclonal anti-Rh(D) antibodies were used and embolic fetal cells were detected in all at-risk patients. The frequency of fetal red cells ranged from $1 : 3.9 \times 10^3$ to $1 : 7.9 \times 10^4$ maternal erythrocytes, with a mean value of $1 : 1.4 \times 10^4$.[89]

Table 4.4   Isolation of fetal cells from maternal peripheral blood

Fetal cell type	Authors	Antibody specificity	Separation technique
Erythrocytes	Medearis et al (1984)[89] Nance et al (1989)[90]	Rh (D) PcAb	Flow cytometry
	Bianchi et al (1990)[91]	Transferrin receptor McAb	Flow cytometry
Leukocytes	Iverson et al (1981)[92]	HLA-A2 PcAb	Flow cytometry
	Yeoh (1990)[63]	Panel of anti-HLA McAbs	Flow cytometry
Trophoblasts	Covone et al (1984)[93] (1988),[94] Kozma et al (1986),[95] (1987),[96] Pool et al (1987),[97] Bertero et al (1988),[98] Adinolfi et al (1989)[99]	?Syncytiotrophoblast McAb	Flow cytometry
	Mueller et al (1990)[100]	Villous syncytiotrophoblast and non-villous cytotrophoblast	Immunomagnetic beads

PcAb = Polyclonal antibody; McAb = monoclonal antibody; HLA = human leukocyte antigen.

Nucleated fetal erythrocytes may be labelled with a monoclonal antibody against the transferrin receptor and separated by flow cytometric cell sorting.[91] Although this may be expected to have wider application than the Rhesus system, errors could arise because the transferrin antigen is also present on activated lymphocytes, some tumour cells and trophoblasts.

Leukocytes

Fetal and maternal leukocytes can be readily distinguished from each other on the basis of their HLA types. Isolation of fetal leukocytes from the maternal blood using flow cytometry would require prior knowledge of their HLA type. This may be predicted if those of the mother and father are known. For example, a father could be HLA-A2 positive (A2+) and the mother HLA-A2 negative (A2–). Therefore, the baby must inherit an HLA-A2 allele if the father is homozygous for HLA-A2 and has a one in two chance of inheriting it if the father is heterozygous. An antibody which identifies the HLA-A2 antigen could then be used to label any fetal A2+ leukocytes in the maternal peripheral blood.

Accordingly, fetal white cells have been labelled with a polyclonal antibody to HLA-A2[92] and a wider panel of anti-HLA monoclonal antibodies,[63] and sorted from maternal cells by flow cytometry. By using three monoclonal antibodies which identified common HLA antigens, 47% of mother–father pairs had appropriate HLA differences.[63] This figure may be improved with the use of a wider selection of anti-HLA antibodies.

The isolation of fetal leukocytes for prenatal diagnosis is appealing since these cells are a reliable source of genetic material. Unlike trophoblasts, chromosomal mosaicisms restricted to leukocytes have not been reported. However, the fetal HLA type would need to be known in advance and a large library of monoclonal antibodies would be necessary to explore all the possible combinations of differences between mother and fetus. Clearly, these requirements are impractical.

Trophoblasts

Several attempts to isolate trophoblasts from maternal blood by flow cytometry have been reported. In earlier work, three monoclonal antibodies were used: H315, which identifies syncytiotrophoblast,[101] H317 which labels syncytiotrophoblasts and cytotrophoblasts[101] and 18B/A5 which reacts with cytotrophoblast.[102]

Much interest was generated by the study of Covone et al[93] where trophoblasts were identified in the peripheral blood of pregnant women by labelling with H315. In further studies, cells identified by H315 and H317 were shown to be more numerous in uterine venous blood than in antecubital venous blood.[95,96] In contrast, cytotrophoblasts could not be detected with 18B/A5.[96]

However, it is now known that H315 does not label trophoblasts specifically and maternal leukocytes may adsorb shed H315 antigen. Thus, sorted H315+ cells did not bind antibodies for alternative trophoblast markers such as placental alkaline phosphatase and human chorionic gonadotrophin[97] and demonstrated maternal genes only.[94,98,99]

Newer monoclonal antibodies show promise. These include FDO161G and FDO66Q which react with a membrane surface protein of villous syncytiotrophoblasts and non-villous cytotrophoblast cells.[100] These antibodies have been successfully used in conjunction with immunomagnetic beads to isolate trophoblasts from peripheral blood samples obtained from 12 women in the first trimester and one woman in the third trimester of pregnancy.

FETAL GENE AMPLIFICATION

The PCR may be used to amplify fetal-specific gene sequences from sorted cells to show conclusively that some of these are derived from the fetus. Alternatively, the PCR may be directly employed to amplify fetal-specific DNA sequences from unenriched samples of maternal blood. The latter is an attractive alternative since preliminary enrichment procedures for the fetal cells may be omitted and quicker answers would be obtained.

In studies where an enrichment procedure was carried out (Table 4.5), fetal genes were identified from amongst the sorted cells by detection

Table 4.5   Amplification of fetal genes from maternal peripheral blood

Fetal gene sequence amplified	Authors	Preliminary enrichment for:
Multiple-copy Y chromosome	Adinolfi et al (1989)[99]	Syncytiotrophoblasts, and without enrichment
	Lo et al (1989)[103]	Nil
	Bianchi et al (1990)[91]	Nucleated erythrocytes
	Mueller et al (1990)[100]	Trophoblasts
Single-copy Y chromosome	Lo et al (1990)[104]	Nil
Hb Lepore-Boston	Camaschella et al (1990)[105]	Nil
Single-copy HLA-DR4	Yeoh et al (1991)[88]	Leukocytes

of multiple-copy DNA sequences believed to be specific for the Y chromosome.[91,100] Success or failure to detect the Y chromosome DNA sequence correlated well with attendant male or female pregnancies respectively. However, a few false positives and a larger number of false negatives were present in both reports.

In one study,[88] fetal DNA was positively identified by amplification of a single-copy gene, HLA-DR4. Here, HLA-A2 positive fetal leukocytes were isolated by flow cytometry from HLA-A2 negative maternal peripheral blood mononuclear cells obtained at 28 weeks' gestation. Following selective amplification of a paternally inherited fetal HLA-DR4 DNA sequence, the presence of the fetal cells was further verified by hybridization with a HLA-DR4 specific internal allele-specific oligonucleotide (ASO) gene probe.

In this report, the sensitivity of detection was one HLA-DR4 positive cell in 10^5 HLA-DR4 negative cells. However, fetal HLA-DR4 could not be detected in DNA prepared from unsorted maternal blood obtained at 28 and 32 weeks' gestation. Thus, in this study, the frequency of fetal: maternal cells in the maternal circulation was lower than $1:1 \times 10^5$. These results are in broad agreement with those of Adinolfi et al[99] who could detect $1:7 \times 10^4$ cells by selective DNA amplification of male sequences in mixtures of male and female cells, but could not amplify these male sequences from the peripheral blood DNA of mothers carrying male fetuses.

The sensitivity of the PCR may be increased to $1:10^7$ by using a dual amplification system with an additional pair of internal primers for a Y chromosome DNA sequence.[103] This has permitted successful direct amplification of fetal genes from unsorted maternal blood samples (Table 4.5). When results were assessed by gel electrophoresis, male cells were detected in DNA prepared from the blood of 12 mothers carrying male fetuses from as early as 9 weeks' gestation. Although male cells were not detected in the peripheral blood of 7 women bearing female fetuses, a false-positive was reported in a non-pregnant female negative control.

In this and other studies[19,99] where an identical set of primers had been used to amplify a 149 base pair Y chromosome specific repeat sequence,[106] verification by internal ASO probe hybridization was not carried out. Moreover, false positives may have arisen because the amplified fragment may not be specific for the Y chromosome.[107] However, when the PCR was applied to detect a presumably more specific single-copy Y chromosome DNA sequence, false positives and false negatives were also reported.[104]

More recently, the PCR has been successfully applied to detect the presence of paternally inherited haemoglobin (Hb) Lepore-Boston in the blood of mothers at risk of carrying fetuses with the Hb Lepore-Boston and beta-thalassaemia combination.[105]

CONCLUSION

At least three types of nucleated fetal cells may be separated from the maternal peripheral blood. Isolation of pure populations of fetal cells is desirable as these would be necessary to diagnose autosomal recessive inherited diseases, including some of the commonest gene disorders, e.g. beta-thalassaemia and cystic fibrosis. Contamination with maternal cells would not only give erroneous results but would also restrict prenatal diagnosis to autosomal dominant disorders where the mutant allele is derived from the father, e.g. Huntington's chorea.

Prenatal diagnosis in the first trimester is advantageous, principally because termination of affected pregnancies during this time is quicker, safer, simpler and psychologically less traumatic for the parents. But the first-trimester fetus has a very modest blood volume and the numbers of fetal cells which may pass into the maternal blood during this time would be expected to be considerably lower than in advanced pregnancy.

If embolic fetal leukocytes are to be routinely purified, their passage to the maternal circulation must occur predictably and in sufficient numbers. Since fetal leukocytes probably enter the maternal circulation as a result of episodic fetomaternal haemorrhages, it is likely that their number will vary from time to time in the same individual, as well as between individuals.

Although nucleated erythrocytes comprise 10% of erythroid cells in peripheral blood at 10 weeks' gestation, their proportion falls rapidly to 1% at 20 weeks and just 0.01% at term. Similarly, the reticulocyte count declines from about 40% at 10 weeks to 5–10% at 20 weeks and 3–10% at term.[108,109] Since the numbers of fetal erythrocytes which may be separated from maternal blood is low, that of nucleated red cells required for prenatal genetic diagnosis will be several orders of magnitude lower. Furthermore, it has not been established if gene material prepared from cells in which the nuclei are known to be either degenerate or degenerating may be reliably used for prenatal diagnosis.

A method based on detecting circulating trophoblasts would be more generally practical. These nucleated fetal cells carry trophoblast-specific markers which are common to all pregnancies, but are absent in adult cells.

Amplification of DNA prepared directly from unsorted maternal blood to detect fetal gene defects is an attractive alternative. Quicker answers would be obtained since enrichment may be omitted. However, heavy contamination of samples with maternal DNA would restrict the application to paternally inherited autosomal dominant diseases. Moreover, because the PCR is a very sensitive procedure, false-positive results remain an important disadvantage.

For non-invasive prenatal diagnosis to become a practical proposition, the techniques described would have to be developed further. Prenatal population screening of genetic defects requires that the techniques used are non-invasive, inexpensive, accurate and rapid. Further refinements in cell sorting, development of suitable trophoblast monoclonal antibodies and improvements in DNA amplification techniques will help make non-invasive prenatal diagnosis a reality.

REFERENCES

1. Tabor A, Philip J, Madsen M, Bang J, Obel E B, Norgaard-Pedersen B. Randomised controlled trial of genetic amniocentesis in 4606 low-risk women. Lancet 1986; i: 1287–1293
2. Medical Research Council. An assessment of the hazards of amniocentesis. Br J Obstet Gynaecol 1978; 85 (suppl 2): 1–16
3. Peakman D C, Moreton M F, Corn B J, Robinson A. Chromosomal mosaicism in amniotic fluid cell cultures. Am J Hum Genet 1979; 31: 149–155
4. Worton R G. Stern R. A Canadian collaborative study of mosaicism in amniotic fluid cell cultures. Prenat Diagn 1984; 4: 131–144
5. Bui T-H, Iselius L, Lindsten J. European collaborative study on prenatal diagnosis: mosaicism, pseudomosaicism and single abnormal cells in amniotic fluid cell cultures. Prenat Diagn 1984; 4: 145–162
6. Hsu Y L F, Perlis T E. United States survey on chromosome mosaicism and pseudomosaicism in prenatal diagnosis. Prenat Diagn 1984; 4: 97–130
7. Benn P A, Hsu L Y F. Maternal cell contamination of amniotic fluid cell cultures: results of a US nationwide survey. Am J Med Genet 1983; 15: 297–305
8. Ward R H T, Petrou M, Modell BM, Knott PD, Maxwell D, Hooker JG. Chorionic villus sampling in a high-risk population — 4 years' experience. Br Obstet Gynaecol 1988; 95: 1030–1035
9. Green J E, Dorfmann A, Jones S L, Bender S, Patton L, Schulman J D. Chorionic villus sampling: experience with an initial 940 cases. Obstet Gynecol 1988; 71: 208–212
10. Canadian Collaborative CVS-Amniocentesis Clinical Trial Group. Multicentre randomised clinical trial of chorion villus sampling and amniocentesis. Lancet 1989; i: 1–6
11. Kalousek D K, Dill F J. Chromosomal mosaicism confined to the placenta in human conceptions. Science 1983; 22: 665–667
12. Crane J P, Cheung S W. An embryogenic model to explain cytogenetic inconsistencies observed in chorionic villus versus fetal tissues. Prenat Diagn 1988; 8: 119–129
13. Old J M. Personal communication, 1990
14. Nicolaides K, Rodeck C H. Fetoscopy. Br J Hosp Med 1984; 396–405
15. Daffos F, Capella-Pavlovsky M, Forestier A. Fetal blood sampling via the umbilical cord using a needle guided by ultrasound. Prenat Diagn 1983; 3: 271–274
16. Monk M, Handyside A, Hardy K, Whittingham D. Preimplantation diagnosis of

deficiency of hypoxanthine phosphoribosyl transferase in a mouse model for Lesch–Nyhan syndrome. Lancet 1987; ii: 423–425

17. Summers P M, Campbell J M, Miller M W. Normal in-vivo development of marmoset monkey embryos after trophectoderm biopsy. Hum Reprod 1988; 3: 389–393

18. Holding C, Monk M. Diagnosis of ß thalassaemia by DNA amplification in single blastomeres from mouse preimplantation embryos. Lancet 1989; ii: 532–534

19. Handyside A H, Pattinson J K, Penketh R J A, Delhanty J D A, Winston R M L, Tuddenham E G D. Biopsy of human preimplantation embryos and sexing by DNA amplification. Lancet 1989; i: 347–349

20. Bartels D. High failure rates in in-vitro fertilization treatments. Med J Aust 1987; 147: 474–475

21. Järmulowicz M. Embryo biopsy. Lancet 1989; i: 547

22. Tovey L A D, Townley A, Stevenson B J, Taverner J. The Yorkshire antenatal anti-D immunoglobulin trial in primigravidae. Lancet 1983; ii: 244–246

23. Thornton J G. Page C, Foote G, Arthur G R, Tovey L A D, Scott J S. Efficacy and long term effects of antenatal prophylaxis with anti-D immunoglobulin. Br Med J 1989; 298: 1671–1673

24. Kline B S. Microscopic observations of the placental barrier in transplacental erythrocytotoxic anemia (erythroblastosis fetalis) and in normal pregnancy. Am J Obstet Gynecol 1948; 56: 226–237

25. Cohen F, Zuelzer W W, Gustafson D C, Evans M M. Mechanisms of isoimmunisation. I. The transplacental passage of fetal erythrocytes in homospecific pregnancies. Blood 1964; 23: 621–646

26. Bowman J M. Rhesus haemolytic disease. In: Wald N J, ed. Antenatal and neonatal screening. Oxford: Oxford University Press, 1984: pp 314–344

27. Mollison PL. The Rh blood group system. In: Mollison P L, Engelfriet C P, Contreras M. eds. Blood transfusion in clinical medicine. 8th ed. Oxford: Blackwell Scientific Publications, 1987: pp 328–372

28. Sunderland C A, Redman C W G, Stirrat G M. HLA A, B, C antigens are expressed on nonvillous trophoblast of the early human placenta. J Immunol 1981; 127: 2614–2615

29. Sunderland C A, Naiem M, Mason D Y, Redman C W G, Stirrat G M. The expression of major histocompatibility antigens by human chorionic villi. J Reprod Immunol 1981; 1: 323–331

30. Redman C W G, McMichael A J, Stirrat G M, Sunderland C A, Ting A. Class I major histocompatibility complex antigens on human extra-villous trophoblast. Immunology 1984; 52: 457–468

31. Ellis S A, Sargent I L, Redman C W G, McMichael A J. Evidence for a novel HLA antigen found on human extravillous trophoblast and a choriocarcinoma cell line. Immunology 1986; 59: 595–601

32. Adinolfi M. New and old aspects of the ontogeny of immune responses. In: Stern C M M, ed. Immunology of pregnancy and its disorders. London: Kluwer Academic Publishers, 1989; pp 33–59

33. Oh J H, Maclean L D. Comparative immunogenicity of HLA-A antigens: a study in primiparas. Tissue Antigens 1975; 5: 33-37

34. Tongio M M, Mayer S. Narrowing of feto-maternal immunization at time of delivery. Tissue Antigens 1977; 9: 174–176

35. Walknowska J, Conte F A, Grumbach M M. Practical and theoretical implications of fetal/maternal lymphocyte transfer. Lancet 1969; i: 1119–1122

36. de Grouchy J, Trebuchet C. Transfusion foeto-maternelle de lymphocytes sanquins et detection du sexe du foetus. Ann Genet 1971; 14: 133–137

37. Schindler A-M, Graf E, Martin-du-Pan R. Prenatal diagnosis of fetal lymphocytes in the maternal blood. Obstet Gynecol 1972; 40: 340–346

38. Schroder J, de la Chapelle A. Fetal lymphocytes in the maternal blood. Blood 1972; 39: 153–161

39. Grosset L, Barrelet V, Odartchenko N. Antenatal fetal sex determination from maternal blood during early pregnancy. Am J Obstet Gynecol 1974; 120: 60–63

40. Schroder J, Schroder E, Cann H M. Fetal cells in the maternal blood. Lack of response of fetal cells in the maternal blood to mitogens and mixed leukocyte culture. Hum Genet 1977; 38: 91–97

41. Pearson P L, Bobrow M, Vosa C G. Technique for identifying Y chromosomes in human interphase nuclei. Nature 1970; 226: 78–80
42. Schroder J. Transplacental passage of blood cells. J Med Genet 1975; 12: 230–242
43. Jonasson J A. Analysis and interpretation of human chromosome preparations. In: Rooney D E, Czepulkowski B H, eds. Human cytogenetics. A practical approach. Oxford: IRL Press, 1986: pp 85–134
44. Caspersson T, Zech L, Johansson C, Modest E J. Identification of human chromosomes by DNA-binding fluorescent agents. Chromosoma 1970; 30: 215–227
45. Polani P E, Mutton D E. Y-fluorescence of interphase nuclei especially circulating lymphocytes. Br Med J 1971; i: 138–142
46. Whang-Peng J, Leitin S, Harris C, Lee E, Sites J. The transplacental passage of fetal leucocytes into the maternal blood. Proc Soc Exp Biol Med 1973; 142: 50–53
47. Midgley A R, Pierce G B, Deneau G A, Gosling JRG. Morphogenesis of syncytiotrophoblast in vivo: an autoradiographic demonstration. Science 1963; 141: 349–350
48. Adinolfi M. Inhibition of mitosis of maternal lymphocytes by fetal cells. Lancet 1976; i: 97
49. Lawler S D, Ukaejiofo E O, Reeves B R. Interaction of maternal and neonatal cells in mixed-lymphocyte cultures. Lancet 1975; ii: 1185–1187
50. Jacobs P A, Smith P G. Practical and theoretical implications of fetal/maternal lymphocyte transfer. Lancet 1969; ii: 745
51. Adinolfi M C, Gorvette D P. The transfer of lymphocytes through the human placenta. In: Centaro A, Carretti N, eds. Immunology in obstetrics and gynaecology. (Proceedings of the 1st International Congress, Padua). Amsterdam: Excerpta Medica, 1973: pp 177–82
52. Burke J, Johansen K. The formation of HL-A antibodies in pregnancy. The antigenicity of aborted and term fetuses. J Obstet Gynaecol Br Commonwlth 1974; 81: 222–228
53. Skacel P O, Stacey T E, Tidmarsh C E F, Contreras M. Maternal alloimmunization to HLA, platelet and granulocyte-specific antigens during pregnancy: its influence on cord blood granulocyte and platelet counts. Br J Haematol 1989; 71: 119–123
54. Douglas G W, Thomas L, Carr M, Cullen N M, Morris R. Trophoblast in the circulating blood during pregnancy. Am J Obstet Gynecol 1959; 78: 960–969
55. Attwood H D, Park W W. Embolism to the lungs by trophoblast. J. Obstet Gynaecol Br Commonwlth 1961; 68: 611–617
56. Goodfellow C F, Taylor P V. Extraction and identification of trophoblast cells circulating in peripheral blood during pregnancy. Br J Obstet Gynaecol 1982; 89: 65–68
57. Goodfellow C F, Taylor P V, Jackson S. Culturing trophoblast from peripheral blood. Lancet 1984; ii: 1479
58. Roffman B Y, Simons M. Syncytial trophoblastic embolism associated with placenta increta and pre-eclampsia. Am J Obstet Gynecol 1969; 104: 1218–1220
59. Jäameri K E U, Koivuniemi A P, Carpen E O. Occurrence of trophoblasts in the blood of toxaemic patients. Gynaecologia 1965; 160: 315–320
60. Chua S, Wilkins T, Sargent I, Redman C. Trophoblast deportation in pre-eclamptic pregnancy. Br J Obstet Gynaecol 1991; 98: 973–979
61. Shapiro H M. Parameters and probes. In: Practical flow cytometry. 2nd ed. New York: Alan R Liss, 1988: pp115–165
62. Yeoh S C, Sargent I L, Redman C W G R, Thein S L. Detecting fetal cells in maternal circulation. Lancet 1989; ii: 869–870
63. Yeoh S C. The isolation and identification of fetal leucocytes in the maternal circulation. D Phil Thesis, Oxford University
64. Dangl J L, Herzenberg L A. Selection of hybridomas and hybridoma variants using the fluorescence activated cell sorter. J Immunol Methods 1982; 52: 1–14
65. Kavathas P, Herzenberg L A. Amplification of a gene coding for human T-cell differentiation antigen. Nature 1983; 306: 385–387
66. Johnston R N, Beverley S M, Schimke R T. Rapid spontaneous dihydrofolate reductase gene amplification shown by fluorescence-activated cell sorting. Proc Natl Acad Sci USA 1983; 80: 3711–3715
67. Saiki R K, Scharf S, Faloona F et al. Enzymatic amplification of β-globin genomic

sequences and restriction site analysis for diagnosis of sickle cell anemia. Science 1985; 230: 1350–1354

68. Saiki R K, Gyllensten U B, Erlich H A. The polymerase chain reaction. In: Davies K E, ed. Genome analysis — a practical approach. Oxford: IRL Press 1988; pp 141–152

69. Saiki R K, Gelfand D H, Stoffel S et al. Primer-directed enzymatic amplification of DNA with a thermostable DNA polymerase. Science 1988; 239: 487–491

70. Scharf S J, Horn G T, Erlich H A. Direct cloning and sequence analysis of enzymatically amplified genomic sequences. Science 1986; 233: 1076–1078

71. Innis M A, Myambo K B, Gelfand D H, Brow M A D. DNA sequencing with Thermus aquaticus DNA polymerase and direct sequencing of polymerase chain reaction-amplified DNA. Proc Natl Acad Sci USA 1988; 85: 9436–9440

72. Gyllensten U B, Erlich H A. Generation of single-stranded DNA by the polymerase chain reaction and its application to direct sequencing of the HLA-DQA locus. Proc Natl Acad Sci USA 1988; 85: 7652–7656

73. Morgan G J, Hughes T, Janssen J W G et al. Polymerase chain reaction for detection of residual leukaemia. Lancet 1989; i: 928–929

74. Lee M-S, Chang K-S, Cabanillas F, Freireich E J, Trujillo J M, Stass S A. Detection of minimal residual cells carrying the t(14;18) by DNA sequence amplification. Science 1987; 237: 175–178

75. Cunningham D, Hickish T, Rosin R D, Sauven P, Baron J H, Farrell P J. Polymerase chain reaction for detection of dissemination in gastric lymphoma. Lancet 1989; i: 695–697

76. DiLella A G, Huang W-M, Woo S L C. Screening for phenylketonuria mutations by DNA amplification with the polymerase chain reaction. Lancet 1988; i: 497–499

77. Lench N, Stanier P, Williamson R. Simple non-invasive method to obtain DNA for gene analysis. Lancet 1988; i: 1356–1379

78. Feldman G L, Williamson R, Beaudet A L, O'Brien W E. Prenatal diagnosis of cystic fibrosis by DNA amplification for detection of KM-19 polymorphism. Lancet 1988; ii: 102

79. Kogan S C, Doherty M, Gitschier J. An improved method for prenatal diagnosis of genetic diseases by analysis of amplified DNA sequences. N Engl J Med 317: 1987; 985–990

80. Kulozik A E, Lyons J, Kohne E, Bartram C R, Kleihauer E. Rapid and non-radioactive prenatal diagnosis of β thalassaemia and sickle cell disease: application of the polymerase chain reaction (PCR). Br J Haematol 1988; 70: 455–458

81. Cai S-P, Chang C A, Zhang J-Z, Saiki R K, Erlich H A, Kan Y W. Rapid prenatal diagnosis of β thalassemia using DNA amplification and nonradioactive probes. Blood 1989; 73: 372–374

82. Embury S H, Scharf S J, Saiki R K et al. Rapid prenatal diagnosis of sickle cell anemia by a new method of DNA analysis. N Engl J Med 1987; 316: 656–661

83. Erlich H A, Gelfand D H, Saiki R K. Specific DNA amplification. Nature 1988; 331: 441–442

84. Syvänen A-C, Bengtstrom M, Tenhunen J, Soderlund H. Quantification of polymerase chain reaction products by affinity-based hybrid collection. Nucleic Acids Res 1988; 16: 11327–11338

85. Li H, Gyllensten U B, Cui X, Saiki R K, Erlich H A, Arnheim N. Amplification and analysis of DNA sequences in single human sperm and diploid cells. Nature 1988; 335: 414–417

86. Lo Y-M D, Mehal W Z, Fleming K A. False-positive results and the polymerase chain reaction. Lancet 1988; ii: 679

87. Kwok S, Higuchi R. Avoiding false positives with P C R. Nature 1989; 339: 237–238

88. Yeoh S C, Sargent I L, Redman C W G R, Wordsworth B P, Thein S L. Detection of fetal cells in maternal blood. Prenat Diagn 1991; 11: 117–123

89. Medearis A L, Hensleigh P A, Parks D R, Herzenberg L A. Detection of fetal erythrocytes in maternal blood postpartum with the fluorescence-activated cell sorter. AM J Obstet Gynecol 1984; 148: 290–295

90. Nance S J, Nelson J M, Arndt P A, Hwai-Tai C, Lam H C, Garratty G. Quantitation of fetal–maternal hemorrhage by flow cytometry. Am J Clin Pathol 1989; 91: 288–292

91. Bianchi D W, Flint A F, Pizzimenti M F, Knoll J H M, Latt S A. Isolation of fetal

DNA from nucleated erythrocytes in maternal blood. Proc Natl Acad Sci USA 1990; 87: 3279–3283

92. Iverson G M, Bianchi D W, Cann H M, Herzenberg L A. Detection and isolation of fetal cells from maternal blood using the fluorescence-activated cell sorter (FACS). Prenat Diagn 1981; 1: 61–73

93. Covone A E, Mutton D, Johnson P M, Adinolfi M 1984 Trophoblast cells in peripheral blood from pregnant women. Lancet 1984; ii: 841–843

94. Covone A E, Kozma R, Johnson P M, Latt S A, Adinolfi M. Analysis of peripheral maternal blood samples for the presence of placenta-derived cells using Y-specific probes and McAb H315. Prenat Diagn 1988; 8: 591–607

95. Kozma R, Spring J, Johnson P M, Adinolfi M. Detection of syncytiotrophoblast in maternal peripheral and uterine veins using a monoclonal antibody and flow cytometry. Hum Reprod 1986; 1: 335–336

96. Kozma R, Chapman M, Loke Y W, Johnson P M, Adinolfi M. Detection of trophoblast-like cells in maternal blood using specific monoclonal antibodies. J Reprod Immunol 1987; 11: 55–61

97. Pool C, Aplin J D, Taylor G M, Boyd R D H. Trophoblast cells and maternal blood. Lancet 1987; i: 804–805

98. Bertero M T, Camaschella C, Serra A, Bergui L, Caligaris-Cappio F. Circulating 'trophoblast' cells in pregnancy have maternal genetic markers. Prenat Diagn 1988; 8: 585–590

99. Adinolfi M, Camporese C, Carr T. Gene amplification to detect fetal nucleated cells in pregnant women. Lancet 1989; ii: 328–329

100. Mueller U W, Hawes C S, Wright A E et al. Isolation of fetal trophoblast cells from peripheral blood of pregnant women. Lancet 1990; 336: 197–200

101. Johnson P M, Cheng H M, Molloy C M, Stern C M M, Slade M B. Human trophoblast-specific surface antigens identified using monoclonal antibodies. Am J Reprod Immunol 1981; 1: 246–254

102. Loke Y W, Day S. Monoclonal antibody to human cytotrophoblast. Am J Reprod Immunol 1984; 5: 106–108

103. Lo Y-M D, Patel P, Wainscoat J S, Sampietro M, Gillmer M D G, Fleming K A. Prenatal sex determination by DNA amplification from maternal peripheral blood. Lancet 1989; ii: 1363–1365

104. Lo Y-M D, Patel P, Sampietro M, Gillmer M D G, Fleming K A. Detection of single-copy fetal DNA sequence from maternal blood. Lancet 1990; 335: 1463–1464

105. Camaschella C, Alfarano A, Gottardi E et al. Prenatal diagnosis of fetal haemoglobin Lepore-Boston disease on maternal peripheral blood. Blood 1990; 75: 2101–2106

106. Nakahori Y, Mitani K, Yamada M, Nakagome Y. A human Y-chromosome specific repeated DNA family (DYZ1) consists of a tandem array of pentanucleotides. Nucleic Acids Res 1986; 14: 7569–7580

107. Nakagome Y, Nagafuchi S, Nakahori Y. Prenatal sex determination. Lancet 1990; 335: 291

108. Playfair J H L, Wolfendale M R, Kay H E M. The leucocytes of peripheral blood in the human foetus. Br J Haematol 1963; 9: 336–344

109. Wood W G. Developmental haemopoiesis. In : Hardisty R M, Weatherall D J, eds. Blood and its disorders. 2nd Ed. Oxford: Blackwell Scientific Publications, 1982; pp 75–98

5. Screening tests for pregnancy-induced hypertension

P. Baker   F. Broughton Pipkin

Screening, the deliberate examination of substantial segments of the population in search for disease at its earliest stages, is a logical extension of the role of preventive medicine and one which is becoming increasingly in vogue. Ideally, a screening test should be readily available to the entire population at risk, although this presupposes that one can identify such a population. The concept of a two-tier screening system may be more appropriate, i.e. an initial test followed up by more sophisticated and/or intensive testing on those assessed in the first test as being at increased risk. This review concerns screening tests for pregnancy-induced hypertension (PIH), a condition which has not only remained the most common cause of maternal mortality in England and Wales over recent decades,[1] but which is also responsible for considerable perinatal mortality.[2] A suitable screening test should be cheap, easy to perform and readily interpretable. The hypertensive diseases in pregnancy are common in the Third World, and different screening systems may be appropriate for the Third World as compared to the western world.

For a screening test to be of value, prophylactic measures must be effective. Low-dose aspirin and possibly fish-oil administration appear to reduce the incidence of PIH.[3,4] No treatment is entirely without risk; in particular, there is some concern as to the safety of aspirin ingestion in pregnancy. Some studies[5] suggest that there is an increase in congenital malformations when aspirin is given in early pregnancy, and animal data have shown that aspirin may cause constriction of the fetal ductus arteriosus and may increase the incidence of antepartum and postpartum haemorrhages.[6,7] Such fears may prove to be unfounded, with large studies having found no association between aspirin ingestion and either congenital malformations[8] or persistent pulmonary hypertension.[9] Nevertheless, there is obvious merit in identifying those at high risk of developing the disease, to whom such prophylactic measures should be targeted.

One of the problems in any review concerning PIH is that the unknown aetiology of hypertensive diseases of pregnancy has led to clinical signs such as hypertension and proteinuria not merely diagnosing disease, but defining it. A disease cannot be defined precisely by clinical signs, and this has resulted in a lack of uniformity between authors. This lack of uniformity makes comparisons of the different success rates obtained using diverse techniques by various groups extremely difficult. The advantages of using the definition of PIH as a diastolic blood pressure of 90 mmHg or greater, occurring in a previously normotensive woman after the 20th week of pregnancy, two such consecutive blood pressure recordings having been obtained at least 4 hours apart, and of pre-eclampsia as PIH with the addition of proteinuria >300 mg/24 h urine collection,[10] (accepted by the International Society for the Study of Hypertension in Pregnancy) have been outlined in a previous volume in this series.[11] Unless stated, the definitions used in the studies quoted below approximate to that of Davey & MacGillivray.[10] Similarly, the diagnosis of PIH, and particularly pre-eclampsia, in multiparous subjects is controversial, McCartney[12] finding the characteristic changes of pre-eclampsia on renal biopsy in only 3% of multiparous subjects presenting with acute hypertension in pregnancy. Thus, unless stated otherwise, the subjects in the studies quoted below were primiparous.

A myriad of potential screening tests have been advocated, in keeping with the legion of possible aetiologies that have been proposed, pre-eclampsia having been termed 'the disease of theories' over 70 years ago.[13] This chapter will attempt to review those techniques, — some simple and non-invasive, others sophisticated and invasive, — which have been subjected to prospective trials.

FAMILY HISTORY

Over a century ago, a familial history of the disease was suggested.[14] However, it is only in the last 30 years that research has focused on this aspect, principally due to the persistent and dedicated work of Leon Chesley. His analysis of data collected over a 49-year period concerned the incidences of pre-eclampsia and eclampsia in 147 sisters, 248 daughters, 74 granddaughters and 131 daughters-in-law of women who had eclampsia.[15] The observed incidences fitted closely with a single gene model, with the frequency of the putative gene being 0.25. Other studies have confirmed a genetic and familial predisposition. Arngrimsson et al[16] found a pattern of inheritance through three or four generations in 94 families from the homogenous island population of Iceland, which could fit either a single recessive gene model or a dominant model with incomplete penetrance.

Cheyne et al[17] gave family history questionnaires to 300 women at antenatal booking clinic visits and found that a family history of PIH increased the risk of developing hypertension by over threefold. Although the specificity and sensitivity of this technique were only 74 and 44% respectively, the economical and non-invasive nature of such a screening test may make it a useful adjunct to other methods.

TESTS RELIANT ON BLOOD PRESSURE MEASUREMENTS

Errors in tests which are reliant upon blood pressure recordings are compounded by a necessity to standardize the technique of measurement, and by random and systematic variations in blood pressure. Factors such as posture influence blood pressure, measurements being lowest when the patient is lying in the left lateral position.[18] The position of the arm relative to the heart also affects recordings, each centimetre of vertical height above or below the level of the heart being equivalent to a difference in pressure of 0.7 mmHg.[19] The spontaneous variability of blood pressure in hypertensive pregnant women has long been appreciated.[20] In addition, Murnaghan et al[21] demonstrated that in 16 normotensive patients blood pressure varied with the circadian rhythm, values being highest during the afternoon and early evening. Under stressful conditions, Sleight et al[22] found that a rise in blood pressure could be evoked. This latter factor may well be responsible for many of the elevated blood pressure recordings noted when patients visit their obstetricians. Such factors are compounded by different blood pressure distributions in different populations, for example, higher blood pressure recordings have been found in black people as compared to white people living in the same environment.[33]

One specific difficulty encountered when measuring blood pressure in pregnant women concerns the use of either the 4th or 5th Korotkoff sounds for diastolic pressure. Raftery & Ward[24] demonstrated that in healthy young women, the 5th sound correlated better with diastolic pressure recorded directly from the right brachial artery. However, in pregnancy, use of the 5th sound results in large skewing of data due to the finding of the 5th Korotkoff sound at zero cuff pressure in some pregnant women.[25]

Compliance with current recommendations on blood pressure measurement technique in pregnancy is very poor.[26] Blood pressure recordings will depend upon whether they are taken by the obstetrician, general practitioner or midwife, and whether they are taken at the beginning or end of the visit. For methods based on blood pressure measurements to be effective, increased uniformity of recording measurement is necessary. Home monitoring with automated sphygmomanometers might help to minimize such problems.

Mid-trimester blood pressure

Blood pressure normally falls at the beginning of pregnancy and reaches its lowest level in the second trimester.[25,27] The use of mid-trimester blood pressure recordings as a screening test for PIH is based on a study by Page & Christianson[28] who incorporated 14 833 women of mixed parity during the fifth and sixth months of gestation. They expressed blood pressure as mean arterial pressure (MAP; the diastolic pressure plus one-third of the pulse pressure). There was a steady progression in the incidence of PIH (defined as a MAP >110 mmHg) with each 5 mmHg increment in mid-trimester MAP. A mid-trimester MAP >90 mmHg increased the risk of developing PIH by over fourfold and of developing pre-eclampsia by over threefold.

Several subsequent prospective studies, each of which obtained measurements in over 700 primigravidae, have revealed a wide disparity in predictive values, with false-negative values of 1–18% and false-positive values of 73–87%.[29-31] The advantage of using mid-trimester blood pressure recordings to identify high-risk patients is that such recordings are already measured routinely on all antenatal patients. However, when used as the sole screening criterion, mid-trimester blood pressure recordings select less than half of the women who develop PIH, and less than one-third of those selected subsequently develop PIH.

The roll-over test

Gant et al[32] described what later became known as the roll-over test. They reported that an increase of >20 mmHg in the diastolic blood pressure, when the patient was turned from the left lateral to the supine position, predicted the development of subsequent hypertension in 15 out of 16 women tested at between 28 and 32 weeks' gestation. However, a large proportion of the subjects studied by Gant et al[32] were young Afro-American teenagers of low socioeconomic group, and there are problems in relating these results to other populations. Subsequent reports have indicated that the test is less satisfactory, with Tunbridge & Donnai[33] finding a false-negative rate of 19% and false-positive rate of 80%. Dekker et al[34] found a false-positive rate of 67% and they concluded that the roll-over test was of no value in the prediction of PIH.

There are several flaws in the test. Some patients have unusually low diastolic blood pressures in the left lateral position (<45 mmHg); this can create a false-positive result when the value is compared with the reading in the supine position.[35] An artefactual rise in diastolic blood pressure might be expected when the patient rolls from the left lateral position to the supine position, as the position of the sphygmomanometer cuff relative to the heart will be altered.[34] Furthermore, markedly differing results from the same patient are found when the test is performed on a biweekly basis.[35] Despite the fact that the test is simple to perform and requires only time and personnel rather than elaborate equipment, it has rightly found little place in routine obstetric practice.

Hand-grip test

Isometric exercise is known to cause general sympathetic activation and to increase systemic arterial pressure in healthy adults.[36] Degani et al[37] found that an increase in diastolic pressure >20 mmHg during a hand-grip exercise test at 28–32 weeks' gestation was associated with an increased incidence of PIH. After a constant baseline diastolic blood pressure had been established, each of the 100 subjects compressed an inflated sphygmomanometer cuff for a 3-minute period at maximal and then at 50% of maximal voluntary contraction. A 20 mmHg increase in diastolic blood pressure was considered to be a positive result. The study demonstrated false-negative and false-positive rates of 4 and 19% respectively — rates which were much better than those derived from the roll-over test, performed simultaneously on the same patients (false-negative and false-positive rates of 4 and 87% respectively).

The hand-grip test is not affected by position changes and is safe and easily performed, although it is time-consuming, taking up to 30 minutes to perform. Moreover, in a larger study, using a modified version of the test, Hidaka et al[38] found a false-negative rate of 60%. In addition, although the hand-grip test represents sympathetic nervous system activity, there is little evidence that PIH is mediated by sympathetic activity.[39] Thus, further evaluation is necessary to determine the potential of the technique as a screening test.

FOREARM VENOUS TONE

Abnormalities in venous tone have also been reported in PIH. In a cross-sectional study, Stainer et al[40] found that women with PIH were veno-constricted in the forearm, when compared with normotensive pregnant women. The authors suggested that measurement of venous tone may have potential as a screening test for PIH. However, the number of women studied was small, with only 11 PIH patients (2 of whom were in their second pregnancies). Moreover the degree of overlap was such that only one value of the PIH group lay outside the normal range. A prospective study from the same centre demonstrated similar results, with differences in forearm venous tone occurring at least 6 weeks before the diagnosis of PIH.[41] Patient number was again small (37 subjects, of whom 8 developed PIH) and overlap was again present. Stainer et al[42] reported a correlation between forearm venous tone and haemoglobin concentration; thus forearm venous tone may simply be a marker of plasma volume expansion. Although non-invasive, the technique is time-consuming and requires both temperature control and sophisticated equipment. It would seem to have limited potential as a method of screening the general population.

URINARY ASSAYS

Urinary protein excretion normally increases in pregnancy, and may occasionally rise to 200 mg/24 h urine collection, but it is usually undetectable by conventional laboratory tests.[43] The development of a radioimmunoassay for albumin[44] has made it possible to detect micro-albuminuria in patients who have not yet developed proteinuria as demonstrated by clinical methods. In a study of 199 patients of mixed parity, Nakamura et al[45] found that when a fasting urinary albumin: creatinine ratio of 16 or over was taken to indicate a positive screening test result, the false-negative rate was only 6%, with a false-positive rate of 57%. These data were in marked contrast to those of Lopez-Espinoza et al[46] who, in a smaller study of subjects of mixed parity, found that proteinuric pre-eclampsia was not preceded by a phase of increasing albumin loss which could be detected by sensitive radioimmunoassay techniques. Greater evaluation is necessary before any assessment of this method of screening for PIH can be made.

Taufield et al[47] measured 24-hour urinary calcium excretion, and found lower total and fractional excretion in women with pre-eclampsia as compared to normotensive pregnant women. Rodriguez et al[48] evaluated the value of both microalbuminuria and the calcium : creatinine ratio as predictive tests. They studied 88 normotensive women of mixed parity at 24–34 weeks' gestation, using values of <0.04 ug/ml and >11 ug/ml as positive test results for the calcium : creatinine and albumin values, respectively. The calcium : creatinine ratio outperformed measurement of microalbuminuria, with a false positive rate of 36% and a false-negative rate of 4%. Although these results are encouraging, there was a high proportion of multiparous patients amongst those who developed pre-eclampsia, and as the authors suggested, these results require confirmation before acceptance in other populations.

Blood pressure-depressing systems such as the kallikrein-kinin system may be involved in maintaining a normal blood pressure. Urinary kallikrein excretion has been shown to increase in normotensive pregnancy, whereas in pre-eclampsia reduced levels as compared to non-pregnant subjects have been found.[49] Millar et al[50] demonstrated in a longitudinal study of 305 patients of mixed parity, that measurement of urinary kallikrein to creatinine ratio in a random urine sample collected at the booking visit (16–20 weeks' gestation) could be used to predict patients at risk of developing PIH with a false-negative rate of less than 10% and a false-positive rate of less than 50%.

Difficulties with assay techniques have impeded assessment of the kallikrein-kinin system in PIH.[51] However, Stroud et al[52] have adapted the previous labour-intensive urinary kallikrein assay into a simple automated method — an advance which greatly increases the potential of the technique as a routine screening test.

Ylikorkala & Makila[53] argued that the platelet–vascular changes pathognomonic for pre-eclampsia could be explained by an imbalance between locally produced and acting prostaglandins, prostacyclin and thromboxane A_2, with the imbalance tilted towards the vasoconstrictor, platelet-aggregating actions of thromboxane A_2. Support for this theory is provided by Koullapis et al,[54] who found significantly higher plasma levels of thromboxane B_2 (the stable metabolite of thromboxane A_2) in 19 patients of mixed parity with PIH. Diminished production of the vasodilator prostacyclin may thus be a factor in the aetiology of PIH. In a small study, Fitzgerald et al[55] found reduced levels of 2,3-dinor-6-keto-prostaglandin $F_{1\alpha}$ (a stable urinary metabolite of prostacyclin) in patients who subsequently developed PIH, with the differences apparent in the first trimester. Moreover, in the same patients, they found no difference in the results of the angiotensin II (AII) sensitivity test (see below) between those women who developed PIH and those who remained normotensive. A complex method was used in this study, involving gas chromatography mass spectrometry. Evaluation of potential as a screening test would require study of a larger population with a more easily applied method such as radioimmunoassay.

ROUTINE BLOOD TESTS

Redman et al[56] found that in a study of 332 hypertensive pregnant patients of mixed parity, plasma urate levels were a better indicator of fetal prognosis than blood pressure. In a smaller study, defining elevated blood pressure as an increase of both 30 mmHg systolic and 20 mmHg diastolic blood pressures, they suggested that serial plasma urate measurements gave warning of the disorder before the appearance of other clinical features.[57] Fay et al[58] also demonstrated that in women who subsequently developed PIH, plasma urate measurements rose above those of the control group as early as 4 weeks before delivery, although the difference between the groups was only significant in the week prior to delivery.

Breckenridge[59] had previously noted serum urate to be frequently raised in essential hypertension, finding hyperuricaemia in 58% of patients under treatment for hypertension at the Hammersmith Hospital. Uric acid is filtered through the glomeruli, but is primarily excreted through the tubules and in 71 male patients with borderline and established hypertension, serum uric acid concentrations correlated inversely with renal blood flow per square metre of body surface.[60] Raised serum urate levels are probably better regarded not as a predictive, diagnostic or specific feature of pre-eclampsia, but as a sensitive indicator of impaired renal function and renal blood flow.

The majority of observers have found a reduction in the number of circulating platelets in pre-eclampsia.[61] Redman et al[62] suggested that platelet count might be helpful in monitoring high-risk pregnancies. They found that a reduction in platelet count occurred early in the development of pre-eclampsia, being detectable about 7 weeks prior to delivery. However, the study group chosen were multiparous women with chronic hypertension, in whom a diagnosis of superimposed pre-eclampsia cannot be made with ease. The chosen method of diagnosing pre-eclampsia was that of an elevation in plasma urate which, as discussed above, is probably better regarded as an indicator of impaired renal function. In addition, the variation in counts between patients was such that no importance could be attached to a single low reading. Gibson et al[63] reported that a reduced platelet count is found in only a minority of patients with pre-eclampsia; thus platelet counts cannot be regarded as a good screening test and are probably best considered as a marker of end-stage disease.

CLOTTING ALTERATIONS AND PLATELET ACTIVITY

A discussion of the clotting abnormalities associated with PIH is outside the scope of this chapter, but the topic has been extensively reviewed.[61] However, it appears that enhanced consumption of the various clotting components, secondary to platelet activity, is characteristic of women with pre-eclampsia. Parameters which have been reported to indicate the subsequent development of the disease are antithrombin III and factor VIII consumption. Increased levels of beta-thromboglobulin, a platelet-specific protein released during platelet activation, have also been reported in women with pre-eclampsia.[64] Although these findings have been supported by subsequent studies,[65] prospective studies are needed to assess the potential of the technique as a screening test.

Antithrombin III irreversibly binds factors Xa, VIIa and II, and because of its pivotal role as a modulator, is a sensitive indicator of clotting activity.[66] Weiner & Brandt[67] reported significantly lower levels of antithrombin III activity in women with pre-eclampsia as compared to healthy pregnant women. The level of antithrombin III activity began to decline as

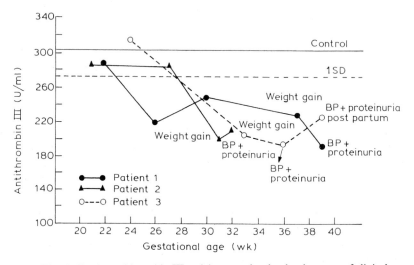

Fig. 5.1 The decline in antithrombin III activity precedes the development of clinical disease in at least some patients. BP = blood pressure. Reprinted from Weiner & Brandt (1982)[67] with permission.

much as 13 weeks prior to the development of clinical manifestations in the three women followed longitudinally who became pre-eclamptic (Fig. 5.1). In a study of 57 women of mixed parity with PIH, Weenink et al[68] also demonstrated a decline in antithrombin III activity in comparison to normotensive pregnancies, with significant differences apparent as early as 28 weeks' gestation. Unfortunately, subsequent studies have been more equivocal, with Oian et al[69] concluding that antithrombin III activity was unaltered in pre-eclampsia, and Pekonen et al[70] only finding significant changes in patients with severe pre-eclampsia (blood pressure >160/110 mmHg and/or proteinuria >5 g/24 h urine collection).

One of the most definitive tests for early coagulation abnormalities in pre-eclampsia is that for demonstrating factor VIII consumption.[71] This depends on the simultaneous measurement of factor VIII clotting activity and factor VIII-related antigen. When the clotting system is activated, the circulating levels of both factors increase rapidly as a secondary response, but because factor VIII clotting activity is destroyed by thrombin, its final level is lower than that of the related antigen and the difference between the two is a reflection of factor VIII consumption. Normal pregnancy is associated with an increase in factor VIII consumption which is further exaggerated if pre-eclampsia develops.[71] In a serial study of women who develop pre-eclampsia, there was a tendency for this change to precede the other changes of pre-eclampsia.[72]

However, such changes in the coagulation system are not sensitive enough to form the basis of an accurate screening test. The coagulation index, developed by Howie et al[73] and derived from fibrin/fibrinogen degradation products, factor VIII activity and platelet counts, proved incapable even of discriminating between patients with mild pre-eclampsia (diastolic blood pressure 90–109 mmHg, proteinuria <300 mg/24 h urine collection) and the normotensive control group when used as a prospective test.[74] Moreover, Pritchard et al[75] described a series of patients with no evidence of any coagulopathy, some of whom developed eclampsia.

DOPPLER ULTRASOUND

In pregnancies complicated by hypertension, the physiological invasion of the spiral arteries is incomplete.[76] However, in a thorough review of utero-placental and fetoplacental circulations in PIH contained in an earlier volume in this series, Hanretty & Whittle[77] concluded that although Doppler waveforms appear to be abnormal in some hypertensive pregnancies, the value of the technique as a screening test is unproven, with major methodological problems existing which may limit any practical application. Moreover, a subsequent study by Steel et al[78] which incorporated over 1000 nulliparous patients screened using Doppler uteroplacental waveforms in early pregnancy (median 18 weeks' gestation), with persistently abnormal waveforms on repeat tests at 24 weeks taken to indicate a positive result, found a false-negative rate of 5% and a false-positive rate of 75%. Steel et al[78] concluded that the test was not helpful for the management of the individual patient.

TESTS RELATED TO ANGIOTENSIN II SENSITIVITY

Alterations in pressor sensitivity to AII in women with PIH are well-documented. In 1968, Talledo et al[79] demonstrated that pre-eclamptic patients showed increased sensitivity to infusions of AII as compared to normotensive pregnant women. Since then several prospective studies have been performed. In 1973, Gant et al[80] reported that primigravid women who later developed PIH in the same pregnancy showed an increased vascular sensitivity to AII as early as the 18th to 22nd weeks of gestation (Fig. 5.2). Their series contained 192 patients, mostly Afro-American teenagers, between 13 and 17 years old. In all, 91% of the subjects who needed more than 8 ng AII/kg per min (on at least one occasion between 28 and 32 weeks' gestation) to elicit an increase in diastolic blood pressure of at least 20 mmHg remained normotensive throughout the pregnancy. Conversely, only 9% of the women who later developed PIH had not shown an increased sensitivity to AII.

There are problems in relating the results of this AII sensitivity test obtained by Gant et al[80] to other populations. Gant et al reported the incidence of PIH in the Dallas population as 37.5%, well above the incidence of approximately 10% found in European populations.[81] The youth and lower socioeconomic status of the Afro-American population, as well as the tendency of negroes to hypertension, may have been pre-

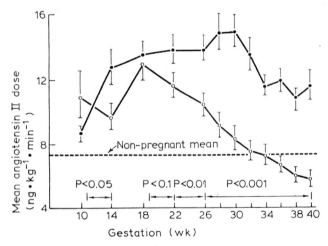

Fig. 5.2   Comparison of mean angiotensin II dose required to raise diastolic blood pressure 20 mmHg in 120 primigravidae who remained normotensive (filled circles) and 72 primigravidae in whom pre-eclampsia occurred (open circles). From Gant et al (1973)[80] with permission.

disposing factors in the etiology of 'PIH' and 'pre-eclampsia', and thus may have influenced the data obtained. Teenagers have been suggested as suffering more frequently from hypertensive disorders in pregnancy.[82]

A search of the literature reveals only five relatively small studies[34,83–86] which have also investigated the prospective value of the AII sensitivity test in the early diagnosis of hypertensive disorders in pregnancy. Oney & Kaulhausen[85] tested an unselected European population, performing an AII infusion on 231 normotensive women between 28 and 32 weeks' gestation. They confirmed the high predictive value of a negative test (0.954), but found a high false-positive rate (approximately 50%). Similar results were obtained by Orozco et al[84] in a small study of 22 South American women of mixed parity; Nakamura et al[86] in a study of 48 Asian women of mixed parity, and by Dekker et al[34] in a study of 90 European women. The mean effective pressor dose of AII in the very different Afro-American, South American, European and Asian populations differed minimally, suggesting that race is not a major factor in determining vascular reactivity to AII.

One dissenting report is that of Morris et al.[83] They examined a small group of young primigravid patients, testing them each week from the 29th to the 32nd week of pregnancy. They found a false-positive rate of 93% and a false-negative rate of 17%, concluding that AII infusions were an unreliable screening test. However, there were methodological differences in this study. Rather than using a sphygmomanometer to measure arterial blood pressure, Morris et al[87] used a Doppler ultrasound device. For unknown reasons, they could not establish a constant baseline diastolic pressure. Therefore they calculated basal diastolic blood pressure from the average of two 30-minute periods in the left lateral recumbent position.

Sensitivity to infused AII is regarded as one of the better predictors of whether PIH will develop later in the pregnancy, and the AII sensitivity test has been used to select patients who should receive preventive treatment, such as low-dose aspirin.[3] Interestingly, Spitz et al[87] demonstrated that the administration of low-dose aspirin to women in the third trimester of pregnancy with increased AII pressor sensitivity caused them to become more refractory to infused AII. These women did not, however, become as refractory to infused AII as normal pregnant women. Fish-oil intake is also associated with a reduction in the AII pressor response in males.[88] Unfortunately, the test is impractical as a screening test for the general population, as it takes several hours to perform, and requires both medical supervision and the placement of an intravenous cannula.

The cause of the altered AII sensitivity in women with PIH is unknown, although Broughton Pipkin[89] suggested that it might be due to alterations in vascular smooth muscle AII receptors. Although receptors for AII, with high affinity and specificity, have been found in a variety of animal vascular tissues[90–92] in humans, vascular tissue is inaccessible and thus difficult to study directly. Platelets have been suggested as an accessible model of smooth muscle cells; not only do the cells share many structural and biochemical characteristics, but similarities between aspects of platelet behaviour and changes in vascular tone have been described.[93,94] Moreover, specific AII binding sites, with many of the characteristics of receptors, have been reported on human platelets,[95,96] and changes in the renin–angiotensin system consequent upon manipulation of dietary sodium intake evoke parallel changes in platelet and arterial muscle AII-binding sites.[97,98]

Measurement of platelet AII binding is a relatively straightforward assay, and can be performed using a single venous blood sample of approximately 20 ml.[99] In normotensive primigravidae, platelet AII binding has been found to fall from 5–8 weeks' gestation.[100] The fall in platelet AII binding in pregnancy thus parallels the diminution in pressor responsiveness to infused AII,[80] as would be expected if platelet AII binding reflects vascular smooth muscle reactivity. Furthermore, significantly higher levels of platelet AII binding have been found in women with established PIH as compared to normotensive primigravidae (Fig. 5.3).[102–104] If platelet AII binding also parallels pressor responsiveness to infused AII in women with PIH, then the differences in levels of binding between normotensive primigravidae and PIH patients should be apparent well before the clinical development of the disease.

In the only prospective evaluation so far of this technique as a screening test for PIH, we have measured platelet AII binding in 34 primigravid pregnant women (between 28 and 32 weeks' gestation), in whom the

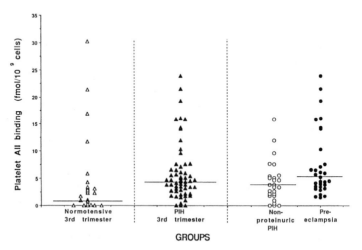

Fig. 5.3   Platelet angiotensin II (AII) binding in 61 patients with pregnancy-induced hypertension (PIH) as compared to 30 women whose pregnancies remained normotensive. The median values of platelet AII binding are indicated by the horizontal bars. Platelet AII binding was significantly higher in the PIH patients as compared to the normotensive subjects ($P<0.0001$). The overall data from the PIH group, and the data obtained when the PIH patients were subdivided on the basis of significant proteinuria, are shown.

pressor response to infused AII was also determined.[101] In order to increase the proportion of patients studied who subsequently developed PIH, the patients were initially recruited on the basis of a casual diastolic blood pressure of 80 mmHg at antenatal clinic (although all the diastolic blood pressures were <70 mmHg prior to the AII infusion). There was a significant correlation found between the values of platelet AII binding and the slope of the curve relating the diastolic pressor response to infused AII, suggesting that colinearity between the two techniques exists and supporting the use of platelet AII binding as a model of vascular smooth muscle pressor responsiveness. Ten of the 34 pregnant women subsequently developed PIH, whereas 24 remained normotensive. Platelet AII binding in the subjects who subsequently developed PIH was significantly higher than in the subjects who remained normotensive. There were, however, no significant differences between the groups in any of the parameters derived from the AII infusion experiments. The use of platelet AII binding alone in predicting the outcome of the pregnancies, as assessed using discriminant analysis, was more successful than when any of the infusion parameters were used, or when either platelet count or serum urate estimation were used, with 77% of patients being correctly classified.

Nakamura et al[86] argued that it was imprudent to predict the outcome of pregnancy on only one performance of the AII sensitivity test, and that it was preferable to perform the test serially in the same patient for accurate evaluation. The high coefficients of variation found using platelet AII binding[99] suggest that the predictive accuracy of this technique might also be improved by serial estimations.

The predictive accuracy of platelet AII binding in assessing the risk of developing PIH was thus at least as great as that previously derived using the AII sensitivity test (with the exception of the original report[80]). Moreover, by including the booking visit systemic blood pressure (information readily available), almost a 90% correct classification was achieved. There is an urgent need for a much larger study to assess the prospective use of platelet AII binding in determining the risk of developing PIH.

Pharmaceutical companies are working on the characterization of platelet AII binding sites. Once this is achieved, the possibility of a direct assay for mass samples becomes reasonable. Serial estimations of platelet AII binding would be preferable, as these might increase the accuracy of the evaluation, and would indicate the optimal gestation to perform the test if a single estimation were deemed to be the most cost-effective. If the results of such a study were to confirm those of this study, then the more invasive, more expensive and more time-consuming AII sensitivity test would surely be redundant.

CONCLUSIONS

As yet there is no practical, acceptable and reliable screening test for PIH

Table 5.1   Potential screening tests for pregnancy-induced hypertension

	Sensitivity (%)	Specificity (%)	+ve predictive value (%)	−ve predictive value (%)	Large study	Confirmatory studies	Simple	Acceptable
Mid-trimester blood pressure estimation[28]	44	87	9	98	✓	✓	✓	✓
Hand-grip test[37]	81	96	81	96	X	✓/X	✓	✓
Urinary albumin: creatinine ratios[45]	64	84	43	94	X	X	✓	✓
Platelet AII binding[103]*	50 {66}*	88 {98}*	60 {70}*	84 {96}*	X	X	✓/X	✓

Values in brackets indicate the results of discriminant analysis when platelet AII binding was combined with the booking visit blood pressure.

that has been thoughoughly tried and tested. The AII sensitivity test, widely regarded as the most reliable predictive test for PIH, is patently unsuitable as a mass screening test. However, there are several techniques which may prove to be appropriate screening tests. The most promising of these are mid-trimester blood pressure estimations, the hand-grip test, urinary microalbumin : creatinine ratios and measurement of platelet AII binding. The results of these four methods are summarized in Table 5.1.

REFERENCES

1. HMSO. Reports on confidential enquiries into maternal death in England and Wales, 1952–1954 to 1982–84. London: HMSO, 1984
2. Chamberlain G, Phillip E, Howlett B, Masters K. British births 1970, vol 2; Obstetric care. London: Heinemann, 1978
3. Wallenburg H C S, Dekker G A, Makovitz J W, Rotmans P. Low dose aspirin prevents pregnancy-induced hypertension and pre-eclampsia in angiotensin sensitive primigravidae. Lancet 1986; i: 1–3
4. Secher N, Olsen S. Fish-oil and pre-eclampsia. Br J Obstet Gynaecol 1990; 97: 1077–1079
5. McNeil J. The possible teratogenic effect of salicylate on the developing fetus: brief summaries of eight suggested cases. Clin Paediatr 1973; 12: 347–350
6. Heymann M A, Rudolph A M Effect of acetylsalicylic acid in the ductus arteriosus and circulation in foetal lambs in utero. Circ Res 1976; 38: 418–422
7. Collins E, Turner G. Maternal effects of regular salicylate ingestion in pregnancy. Lancet 1975; ii: 335–338
8. Slone D, Siskind V, Heineman O P, Manson R R, Kaufman D W, Shapiro S. Aspirin and congenital malformations. Lancet 1976; i: 1373–1375
9. Shapiro S, Siskind V, Manson R R, Heineman O P, Kaufman D W, Slone D. Perinatal mortality and birthweight in relation to aspirin later in pregnancy. Lancet 1976; i: 1375–1376
10. Davey D A, MacGillivray I. The classification and definition of the hypertensive disorders of pregnancy. In: Sharp F, Symonds E M, eds. Hypertension in pregnancy. Ithaca, New York: Perinatology Press, 1986: pp 401–408
11. Davey D A. Hypertensive disorders of pregnancy. In: Studd J, ed. Progress in obstetrics and gynaecology, vol 5. Edinburgh: Churchill Livingstone, 1988: pp 89–107
12. McCartney C P. Pathological anatomy of acute hypertension in pregnancy. Circulation 1964; 30 (suppl II): 37–42
13. Zwiefel P. Eklampsie. In: Doderlein A, ed. Handbuch der Geburtshilfe, vol II. Wiesbaden: Bergmann, 1916: pp 672–723

14. Elliot G T Jr. Case 120: puerperal eclampsia in the eighth month: extraordinary family history: rigid cervix, douche, dilators, forceps. In: Obstetric clinic. New York, Appleton, 1873 : pp 291–293
15. Chesley L C, Cooper D W. Genetics of hypertension in pregnancy: possible single gene control of pre-eclampsia and eclampsia in the descendants of eclamptic women. Br Obstet Gynaecol 1986; 93: 898–908
16. Arngrimsson R, Bjornsson S, Geirsson R T, Bjornsson H, Walker J J, Snaedal G. Genetic and familial predisposition to eclampsia and pre-eclampsia in a defined population. Br J Obstet Gynaecol 1990; 97: 762–769
17. Cheyne H, Bjornsson S, Walker J A family history questionnaire as a predictor of those at risk of developing pregnancy induced hypertension. VIIth World Congress of Hypertension in Pregnancy, Perugia, Italy, 1990. Scientific program p 219
18. Wichman K, Ryden G, Wichman M. The influence of different positions and Korotkoff sounds on the blood pressure measurements in pregnancy. Acta Obstet Gynecol Scand 1984; 118 (Suppl) 25–28
19. Murnaghan G A. Methods of measuring blood pressure. In: Sharp F, Symonds E M, eds. Hypertension in pregnancy. Ithaca, New York: Perinatology Press, 1987: pp 19–28
20. Wiessner A Uber Blutdruckmessungen wahrend der Menstruation und Schwangerschaft. Centralbl Gynaekol 1899; 23: 1335
21. Murnagham G A, Mitchell R H, Ruff S. Circadian variation of blood pressure in pregnancy. In: Bonnar J, MacGillivray I, Symonds E M, eds. Pregnancy hypertension. Lancaster: MTP, 1980: pp 107–112
22. Sleight P, Fox P, Lopez R, Brooks D E. The effect of mental arithmetic on blood pressure variability and baroreflex sensitivity in man. Clin Sci Mol Med 1978; 55: 381–382
23. Editorial. Ethnic factors in disease. Br Med J 1981; 282: 1496–1497
24. Raftery E B, Ward A P. The indirect method of recording blood pressure. Cardiovas Res 1968; 2: 210–268
25. MacGillivray I, Rose G A, Rowe B. Blood pressure survey in pregnancy. Clin Sc 1969; 37: 395–407
26. Perry I J, Wilkinson L S, Shinton R A, Beevers D G. Conflicting views on the measurement of blood pressure in pregnancy. Br J Obstet Gynaecol 1991; 98: 241–243
27. Friedman E A, Neff R K. Pregnancy hypertension. A systematic evaluation of clinical diagnostic criteria. Littleton, Massachusetts: PSG Publishing, 1977
28. Page E W, Christianson R. The impact of mean arterial pressure in the middle trimester upon the outcome of pregnancy. Am J Obstet Gynecol 1976; 125: 740–745
29. Montquin J M, Rainville C, Giroux L et al. A prospective study of blood pressure in pregnancy: prediction of pre-eclampsia. Am J Obstet Gynecol 1985; 151: 191–196
30. Ales K L, Norton M E, Druzin M L. Early prediction of antepartum hypertension. Obstet Gynecol 1989; 73: 928–933
31. Villar M A, Sibai B M. Clinical significance of elevated mean arterial pressure in second trimester and threshold increase in systolic or diastolic blood pressure during third trimester. Am J Obstet Gynecol 1989; 160: 419–423
32. Gant N F, Chand S, Worley R J, Whalley P J, Grosby U D, MacDonald P C. A clinical test useful for predicting the development of acute hypertension in pregnancy. Am J Obstet Gynecol 1974; 120: 1–7
33. Tunbridge R D G, Donnai P. Pregnancy-associated hypertension, a comparison of its prediction by roll-over test and plasma noradrenaline measurement in 100 primigravidae. Br J Obstet Gynaecol 1983; 90: 1027–1032
34. Dekker G A, Makovitz J W, Wallenburg HCS. Prediction of pregnancy-induced hypertensive disorders by angiotensin II sensitivity and supine pressor test. Br J Obstet Gynecol 1990; 97: 817–821
35. Phelan J P. Enhanced prediction of pregnancy-induced hypertension by combining supine pressor test with mean arterial pressure of middle trimester. Am J Obstet Gynecol 1977; 129: 397–400
36. Lind A R, McNicol G W. Circulatory response to sustained hand-grip contractions performed during other exercise. J Physiol 1967; 192: 595–607
37. Degani S, Abinader E, Eibschitz I, Oettinger M, Shapiro I, Sharf M. Isometric

exercise test for predicting gestational hypertension. J Obstet Gynaecol 1985; 65: 652–654

38. Hidaka A, Tomoda S, Kitanaka T, Nakamoto O, Sugawa T. Prediction of pregnancy induced hypertension. VIIth World Congress of Hypertension in Pregnancy, Perugia, Italy, 1990. Scientific program. p 220.

39. Pedersen E B. Autonomic nervous system and vascular reactivity in normal and hypertensive pregnancies. In: Rubin P C ed. Handbook of hypertension, Vol 10: Amsterdam: Elsevier, 1988: pp 152–167

40. Stainer K, Morrison R, Pickles C J, Cowley A J. Abnormalities of peripheral venous tone in women with pregnancy-induced hypertension. Clin Sci 1986; 70: 155–157

41. Stainer K. The peripheral venous system in health and disease. PhD Thesis, University of Nottingham

42. Stainer K, Pickles C J, Kilby M D, Cowley A J. The peripheral vasculature in pregnancy and pregnancy induced hypertension. VIIth World Congress of Hypertension in Pregnancy, Perugia, Italy, 1990. Scientific program. p 315

43. Taylor D J. The epidemiology of hypertension during pregnancy. In: Rubin P C, ed. Handbook of hypertension, vol 10. Amsterdam: Elsevier 1988; pp 223–240

44. Woo J, Floyd M, Cannojn D C, Kahan B. Radioimmunoassay for urinary albumin. Clin Chem 1978; 24: 1464–1467

45. Nakamura T, Ito M, Yoshimura T, Mabe K, Okamura H. Usefulness of the urinary microalbumin/creatinine ratio in predicting pregnancy-induced hypertension. Personal communication, 1992

46. Lopez-Espinoza I, Dhar H, Humphreys S, Redman C W G. Urinary albumin excretion in pregnancy. Br J Obstet Gynaecol 1986; 93: 176–181

47. Taufield P A, Ales K L, Resnick L M, Druzin M L, Gartner J M, Laragh J H. Hypocalcuria in pre-eclampsia. N Eng J Med 1987; 317: 715–718

48. Rodriguez M H, Maskaki D I, Mestman J, Kumar D, Rude R. Calcium/creatinine ratio and microalbuminuria in the prediction of pre-eclampsia. Am J Obstet Gynecol 1988; 159: 1452–1455

49. Karlberg B E, Ryden G, Wichman K. Changes in the renin-angiotensin-aldosterone and kallikrein-kinin systems during normal and hypertensive pregnancy. Acta Obstet Gynecol Scand 1984; 118: (suppl) 17–24

50. Millar J G B, Stroud C S, Campbell S K, Higgins B, Albano J D M, Clark A D. Prediction in early pregnancy of PIH: kallikreins revisited. VIIth World Congress of Hypertension in Pregnancy, Perugia, Italy, 1990. Scientific program p 170

51. Ferris T F. Prostanoids in normal and hypertensive pregnancy. In: Rubin P C, ed. Handbook of hypertension, vol 10: Hypertension in pregnancy. Amsterdam: Elsevier, 1988: pp 102–117

52. Stroud C S, Campbell S K, Albano J D M, Millar J G B. A simple automated method of urinary kallikrein estimation. VIIth World Congress of Hypertension in Pregnancy, Perugia, Italy, 1990. Scientific program p 306

53. Ylikorkala O, Makila U M. Prostacyclin and thromboxane in gynecology and obstetrics. Obstet Gynecol 1985; 152: 318–329

54. Koullapis E N, Nicolaides K H, Collins W P, Rodeck C H, Campbell S. Plasma prostanoids in pregnancy-induced hypertension. Br J Obstet Gynaecol 1982; 89: 617–621

55. Fitzgerald D J, Entman S S, Mulloyk K, FitzGerald G A. Decreased prostacyclin biosynthesis preceding the clinical manifestation of pregnancy-induced hypertension. Circulation 1987; 75: 956–963

56. Redman C W G, Beilin L J, Bonnar J, Wilkinson R H. Plasma urate measurement in predicting fetal death in hypertensive pregnancy. Lancet 1976; i: 1370–1373

57. Redman C W G, Williams G F, Jones D D, Wilkinson R H. Plasma urate and serum deoxycytidylate deaminase measurements for the early diagnosis of pre-eclampsia. Br J Obstet Gynaecol 1977; 84: 904–908

58. Fay R A, Bromham D R, Brooks J A, Gebski V J. Platelets and uric in the prediction of pre-eclampsia. Am J Obstet Gynecol 1985; 152: 1038–1039

59. Breckenridge A. Hypertension and hyperuricaemia. Lancet 1966; i: 15–18

60. Messerli F H, Frohlich E D, Dreslinski G R, Suarez D H, Aristimuno G G. Serum uric acid in essential hypertension; an indicator of renal vascular involvement. Ann Int Med 1980; 93: 817–821

61. Weiner C P. Clotting alterations and pre-eclampsia/eclampsia syndrome. In: Rubin P C, ed. Handbook of hypertension, vol 10. Amsterdam: Elsevier; 1988: pp 241–256

62. Redman C W G, Bonnar J, Beilin L J. Early platelet consumption in pre-eclampsia. Br Med J 1978; 1: 467–469

63. Gibson B, Hunter D, Neame P B, Kelton J G. Thrombocytopenia in pre-eclampsia and eclampsia. Semin Thromb Hemost 1982; 8: 234–247

64. Redman C W G, Allington M J, Bolton F G, Stirrat G M. Plasma beta-thromboglobulin in pre-eclampsia. Lancet 1977; ii: 248

65. Douglas J T, Shah M, Lowe G D O, Belch J J F, Forbes C D, Prentice C R M. Plasma fibrinopeptide A and beta-thromboglobulin in pre-eclampsia and pregnancy hypertension. Thromb Haemost 1982; 47: 54–55

66. Bick R K. Disseminated intravascular coagulation and related syndromes: etiology, pathophysiology, diagnosis and management. Am J Hematol 1978; 5: 265–282

67. Weiner C P, Brandt J. Plasma antithrombin III activity in normal pregnancy. Obstet Gynecol 1982; 56: 601–603

68. Weenink G H, Treffers P E, Kahle L H, Ten Cate J W. Antithrombin III in normal pregnancy. Thromb Res 1982; 26: 281–287

69. Oian P, Omsjo I, Martin Maltau J, Osterud B. Increased sensitivity to thromboplastin synthesis in blood monocytes from pre-eclamptic patients. Br J Obstet Gynaecol 1985; 92: 511–517

70. Pekonen F, Rasi V, Ammala M, Viinikka L, Ylikorkala O. Platelet function and coagulation in normal and preeclamptic pregnancy. Thromb Res 1986; 43: 553–560

71. Denson K W E. The ratio of factor VIII-related antigen and factor VIII biological activity as an index of hypercoagulability and intravascular clotting. Thromb Res 1977; 10: 107–119

72. Redman C W G, Denson K W E, Beilin L J, Bolton F G, Stirrat G M. Factor VIII consumption in pre-eclampsia. Lancet 1977; ii: 1249–1252

73. Howie P W, Purdie D W, Begg C B, Prentice C R M. Use of coagulation tests to predict the clinical progress of pre-eclampsia. Lancet 1976; ii: 323–325

74. Dunlop W, Hill L M, Landon M J, Oxley A, Jones P. Clinical relevance of coagulation and renal changes in pre-eclampsia. Lancet 1978; ii: 346–349

75. Pritchard J A, Cuningham F G, Merson R A. In: Lindheimer M D, Katz A I, Zuspan FP eds. Hypertension in pregnancy. New York: Lea & Febiger, 1976: p 95

76. Brosens I, Dixon H G, Robertson W B. Fetal growth retardation and the arteries of the placental bed. Br J Obstet Gynaecol 1977; 84: 656–664

77. Hanretty K, Whittle M J. The uteroplacental and fetoplacental circulations in clinical practice. In: Studd J, ed. Progress in obstetrics and gynaecology, vol 8. Edinburgh: Churchill Livingstone: 1990: pp 33–48

78. Steel S A, Pearce J M, McParland P, Chamberlain G V P. Early Doppler ultrasound screening in prediction of hypertensive disorders of pregnancy. Lancet 1990; 335: 1548–1551

79. Talledo O E, Chesley L C, Zuspan F P. Renin-angiotensin system in normal and toxemic pregnancies. III. Differential sensitivity to angiotensin II and norepinephrine in toxemia of pregnancy. Am J Obstet Gynecol 1968; 100: 218–221

80. Gant N F, Daley G L, Chand S, Whalley P J, MacDonald P C. A study of angiotensin II pressor response throughout primigravid pregnancy. J Clin Invest 1973; 52: 2682–2689

81. Symonds E M. Hypertension in pregnancy. In: Stallworthy J, Bourne G, eds. Recent advances in obstetrics and gynaecology, no. 13. Edinburgh: Churchill Livingstone, 1979

82. Vollman R F. Rates of toxaemia by age and parity. In: Rippman E T, ed. Die Spatgestose (EPH Gestose). Basel: Schabe, 1970

83. Morris J A, O'Grady J P, Hamilton C, Davidson E C. Vascular reactivity to angiotensin II infusion during gestation. Am J Obstet Gynecol 1978; 130: 379–384

84. Orozco J Z, Pinsker V S, Hernandez E M, Karchmer S. Valor de la prueba de la angiotensina II y del 'roll over test' como metodos predictivos de la enfermedad hipertensiva aguda del embarazo (preeclampsia y eclampsia). Ginecol Obstet Mexico 1979; 46: 235–244

85. Oney T, Kaulhausen H. The value of the angiotensin sensitivity test in the early

diagnosis of hypertensive disorders in pregnancy. Am J Obstet Gynecol 1982; 142: 17–20

86. Nakamura T, Ito M, Matsui K, Yoshimura T, Kawasaki N, Maeyama M. Significance of angiotensin sensitivity test for prediction of pregnancy-induced hypertension. Obstet Gynecol 1986; 67: 388–394

87. Spitz B, Magness R R, Cox S M, Brown C E L, Rosenfeld C R, Gant N F. Low-dose aspirin. 1. Effect on angiotensin II pressor responses and blood prostaglandin concentrations in pregnant women sensitive to angiotensin II. Am J Obstet Gynecol 1988; 159: 1035–1043

88. Leaf A, Weber P C. Cardiovascular effects of n-3 fatty acids. N Eng J Med 1988; 318: 549–557

89. Broughton Pipkin F. The renin-angiotensin system in normal and hypertensive pregnancies. In: Rubin P C, ed. Handbook of hypertension, vol 10: Hypertension in pregnancy. Amsterdam: Elsevier, 1988: pp 118–151

90. Lin S-Y, Goodfriend T L. Angiotensin receptors. Am J Physiol 1970; 218: 1319–1328

91. Aguilera G, Catt K J. Regulation of vascular angiotensin II receptors in the rat during altered sodium intake. Cir Res 1981; 49: 751–758

92. McQueen J, Murray G D, Semple P F. Identification of the angiotensin II receptor in the rat mesenteric artery. Biochem J 1984; 223: 659–671

93. Cameron H A, Ardlie N G. The facilitating effects of adrenaline on platelet aggregation. Prostaglandins Leukot Med 1982; 9: 117–128

94. Cowley A J, Stainer K, Cockbill S, Heptinstall S. Correlation between platelet behaviour and cold induced vasoconstriction in man, and the effects of epoprostenol infusion. Clin Sci 1984; 67: 511–514

95. Moore T J, Williams G H. Angiotensin II receptors on human platelets. Circ Res 1981; 51: 314–320

96. Ding Y-A, Kenyon C J, Semple PF. Receptors for angiotensin II on platelets from man. Clin Sci 1984; 66: 725–731

97. Moore T J, Taylor T, Williams G H. Human platelet angiotensin II receptors: regulation by the circulating angiotensin level. J Clin Endocrinol Metab 1984; 58: 778–782

98. Ding Y-A, Kenyon C J, Semple P F. Regulation of platelet receptors for angiotensin II in man. J Hypertension 1985; 3: 209–212

99. Baker P N, Broughton Pipkin F, Symonds E M. Platelet angiotensin II binding sites and plasma renin concentration, renin substrate and angiotensin II concentration in human pregnancy. Clin Sci 1990; 79: 403–408

100. Baker P N, Broughton Pipkin F, Symonds E M. A prospective study of platelet Angiotensin II binding in pregnancy. Clin Sci 1991; 80 (Suppl 24): 27

101. Baker P N, Broughton Pipkin F, Symonds E M. A comparison of platelet angiotension II binding and the angiotensin II sensitivity test in predicting the development of pregnancy induced hypertension. Clin Sci 1992; 83: 89–95

102. Baker P N, Broughton Pipkin F, Symonds E M. Platelet angiotensin II binding sites in hypertension in pregnancy. Lancet 1989; ii: 1151

103. Baker P N, Broughton Pipkin F, Symonds E M. Platelet AII binding in normotensive and hypertensive pregnancy. Br J Obstet Gynaecol 1991; 98: 436–440

104. Pawlak M A, Macdonald G J. Possible regulatory disorder of angiotensin II receptors in pregnancy-induced hypertension. VIIth World Congress of Hypertension in Pregnancy, Perugia, Italy, 1990. Scientific program; p 247

6. Road traffic accidents in pregnancy — the management and prevention of trauma

M. Griffiths   J. Siddall-Allum   P. W. Reginald
M. McD. Usherwood

Nash[1] has stated that road traffic accidents (RTAs) represent the most common cause of non-obstetric trauma in pregnancy. This view is supported by Rothenberger and colleagues[2] who found vehicular accidents to be the main cause of blunt maternal trauma. The number of maternal deaths from RTAs is apparently small,[3] having fallen — presumably as a result of increased seat belt use — over the last two decades. Morbidity or mortality can occur in the fetus and/or pregnant woman. Major maternal trauma, particularly if involving the maternal pelvis, may subsequently have effects on mode of delivery. Indeed such pelvic trauma prior to pregnancy may also be relevant. Spinal injury resulting in paraplegia, either prior to or during pregnancy, will have a significant bearing on the management of pregnancy and labour and has recently been well-reviewed elsewhere.[4] In such cases spinal injury usually precedes pregnancy and causes management difficulties throughout the antenatal and intra-partum period. Difficulties in such women may arise even in the recognition of the onset of labour if the level of injury is high. Such patients are best managed jointly with spinal injury specialists and possibly are best delivered in maternity units with previous experience of managing such cases.[4]

Until a recent series of case reports by ourselves[5,6] and Slade[7] there seems to have been little attention to the subject of RTAs in pregnancy in the British literature. This markedly contrasts with the number of publications in the North American, Australian and South African journals.

We could find no data on the incidence of significant fetal or maternal injury as a result of RTAs in pregnancy. In the decade before widespread use of seat belts in the USA, Parkinson[8] found four perinatal fetal mortalities due to RTAs among 10 000 deliveries in 1964. If this rate were extrapolated to England and Wales at current birth rates[9] it would imply more than 250 fetal deaths per year.

A review of causes of maternal mortality in Massachusetts covering 1954 to 1985 demonstrated that by the early 1980s the most common cause of maternal mortality was trauma.[10]

ACUTE MANAGEMENT OF PREGNANT VICTIMS OF RTAs

The pregnant woman, following a car accident, may present to her own general practitioner, the Accident & Emergency department, or directly to the maternity unit, seeking assessment and reassurance of fetal wellbeing. Pearce[11a] stated that: 'The management of women surviving road traffic accidents is mainly concerned with resuscitating the mother as this is also the best means of resuscitating the fetus'.

A recent paper by Nash[12] emphasizes the mother's understandable anxiety for her fetus, and highlights the physiological changes during pregnancy which affect interpretation of clinical signs in the woman. Some of these physiological changes may mask effects or delay the diagnosis of major trauma.

The management of trauma in pregnancy is summarized in Figure 6.1.

If the woman has sustained major trauma — and especially if her life is in danger — her condition should be stabilized, since fetal wellbeing is intimately related to maternal wellbeing. However, early contact with obstetricians and also neonatal paediatricians can be helpful. Rothenberger et al[2] found that fetal loss occurred in 80% of women admitted with hypovolaemic shock. These authors concluded that: 'The best chance of fetal survival is to assure maternal survival'.

Difficulties in assessing the pregnant woman include the following:

1. The enlarged uterus makes assessment of abdominal organs such as the liver and spleen difficult.
2. Changes in cardiovascular physiology such as a decrease in peripheral blood pressure in the second trimester, increased circulatory volume and increased heart rate, together can mask blood loss of perhaps 25–30%[11b].
3. Changes in the respiratory physiology such as increased tidal volume lead to a mild respiratory alkalosis. An arterial partial pressure of carbon dioxide of 40 mmHg at term is likely to indicate maternal and fetal acidosis.[12]

Hoff and colleagues[13] have shown the use of the Injury Severity Score to be the most useful predictor of fetal demise (and therefore an indicator of a need to consider delivery where compatible with good maternal outcome). The same authors also found that maternal blood pressure and heart rate were poor predictors of fetal demise, whilst arterial pH and partial pressure of oxygen had some value

In cases where maternal injury is minimal, then prompt fetal assessment should be made, since cases have been reported where fetal trauma proved to be more significant than that sustained by the mother.[5,6,14]

Quick assessment by abdominal palpation and auscultation of the fetal heart may reassure the mother, but does not confer any prognostic value. It is important to take maternal blood for a Kleihauer test, since this may

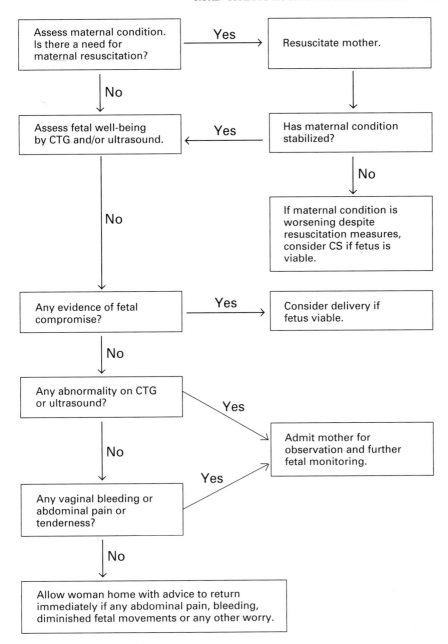

Fig. 6.1 Flow chart to show management of trauma in pregnancy, with respect to fetal well-being.

detect a concealed retroplacental bleed. Fetomaternal haemorrhage is more common with an anteriorly located placenta.[16]

Women who are Rhesus-negative should be given anti-D immunoglobulin. An ultrasound scan may be useful in determining gestation, presentation, viability and placental topography. Cardiotocography (CTG) provides a visual record of fetal heart rate and uterine activity. In the presence of abdominal pain, vaginal bleeding or heart rate abnormality on auscultation, the woman should be admitted to the maternity unit for assessment with ultrasound and CTG, since early delivery may well be indicated.

We would suggest that anyone who sees a pregnant victim of an RTA, and who is able to assure her that all is well, should also advise her to seek prompt advice if pain or bleeding occurs within the next 48 hours, since abruption may present within this time.[17] It is not necessary *routinely* to admit all women for observation at initial presentation. Higgins & Garite[17] reported a single case of late abruption occurring after more than 24 hours; their experience led them to recommend CTG monitoring for 48 hours after admission with severe trauma. Goodwin & Breen[18] felt that prolonged observation of more than a couple of hours was not necessary in women 'who lack obstetric findings on initial presentation'.

Pearce[11a] recommends that the fetus should be monitored by CTG for 4 hours. We believe that for some women without injuries and where initial fetal assessment is satisfactory, then such lengthy monitoring might be unnecessary, whilst even 4 hours would not prevent loss due to late abruption.[17] We would recommend initial assessment of a fetus which has reached viability by CTG. In the absence of any maternal injuries and with the reassurance of a satisfactory CTG, the woman could be allowed home with advice to return if any bleeding, abdominal pain or anxiety regarding fetal movement developed.

Where there are significant maternal skeletal injuries these must be dealt with: management is only slightly altered with the fetus in mind. X-rays should be performed when indicated,[11a] whenever possible with shielding to the abdomen.[16] Particularly in pregnancy, prolonged immobilization or anaesthetic procedures carry an increased risk of thromboembolic disease: prophylaxis with heparin should be considered when close control of coagulation is required. Particularly during the third trimester aortocaval compression should be avoided — again particularly during procedures under anaesthetic — by appropriate use of lateral tilt.[19]

If abdominal visceral trauma is suspected, it should be borne in mind (as outlined above) that abdominal signs may be masked. In such cases early laparotomy or peritoneal lavage may be appropriate.[20] Due to the combination of the masking of clinical signs on abdominal examination by the enlarging pregnant uterus and the physiological changes in the circulation, severe intra-abdominal injury may be present with less obvious signs than might be expected in the non-pregnant woman. This effect should probably be mitigated by an earlier recourse to invasive procedures or laparotomy.

Particularly during the third trimester, if a need for laparotomy arises there may well be a consideration for a synchronous caesarean section. Caesarean section should only be performed for independent obstetric indications, or where the large gravid uterus makes surgical access impossible.

Sadly in some cases of maternal mortality, postmortem caesarean section may be considered. In the majority of cases this has been associated with a bad fetal outcome, but not invariably so. Lopez-Zeno and colleagues[21] reported on a case where there was a delay of more than 20 min after maternal demise before delivery — resulting in the birth of 'a clinically normal child'. Anecdotal cases even suggest that 'perimortem section' may be associated with maternal recovery.[16,22,23] In such cases it is likely that the return of blood from the pregnant uterus and decreased pressure on abdominal vessels due to the fetus and placenta lead to an increased return via the inferior vena cava to the right side of the heart.

SEAT BELTS IN PREGNANCY

The wearing of seat belts by drivers and front seat passengers has been compulsory in the UK since January 1983. This legislation has clearly prevented many deaths and serious injuries. Subsequent legislation has addressed the use of restraints by children and rear seat passengers. Under current legislation drivers or front seat passengers of private motor cars may only omit to wear a seat belt if they possess a certificate exempting them from this requirement on medical grounds. It is frequently the case that pregnant women may find the use of seat belts uncomfortable,[24] and as a result pregnant women often fail to wear seat belts.[6,25,26]

Although it may seem reasonable to assume that both mother and fetus will be safest if, whilst travelling by car, the woman is properly restrained by a well-fitting seat belt,[14,27,28] this view is not universally accepted, nor are seat belts always properly fitted.

We have recently reported three cases[5,6] which to some extent demonstrate the hazards to the fetus of ill-fitting seat belts, as well as the hazards of failing to wear a restraint.

The first case was of a woman involved, at 36 weeks of pregnancy, as a front seat passenger in an RTA. She had been wearing a conventional seat belt. The subsequent pattern of her injuries suggests that the lap portion of her seat belt had been positioned over her lower abdomen. She suffered a number of chest and abdominal injuries. In the Accident & Emergency department no fetal heart was heard and subsequent ultrasound confirmed fetal demise. After resuscitation labour was induced. A Kleihauer test performed previously had shown the presence of fetal cells in the maternal circulation. After spontaneous delivery of a fresh stillborn infant, the placenta was delivered in two halves. The placenta had been traumatically bisected by the too highly placed lap strap.

The second case occurred at 31 weeks of pregnancy. This woman was similarly involved in an RTA, again wearing a conventional seat belt. Once more the pattern of her injuries indicated that the lap portion of her seat belt had been lying over the lower abdomen. She was examined by her general practitioner, who could hear no fetal heart. She was transferred to a maternity unit and ultrasound scan once more confirmed fetal death. Kleihauer test also showed a large fetomaternal haemorrhage. Maternal injuries were minor. Labour was induced. Subsequent examination of the placenta showed retroplacental thrombus, with adjacent areas of intraplacental haemorrhage.

The third woman was not wearing a seat belt. At 35 weeks' gestation she was involved in an RTA as a driver and was flung against the steering wheel. Although she presented to the Accident & Emergency department no maternal injuries were evident. Initial observations and investigations, including a CTG and ultrasound scan, were normal. As the patient complained of abdominal discomfort, she was admitted for observations. Ninety minutes after admission a further CTG demonstrated a prolonged fetal bradycardia. At emergency caesarean section there was no maternal visceral injury or abruption. The fetus was liveborn but acidotic and anaemic. Despite resuscitation — including transfusion — the condition of the baby deteriorated. An ultrasound scan showed no evidence of intracranial haemorrhage, but suggested an intra-abdominal bleed. At laparotomy a ruptured spleen was demonstrated and splenectomy performed. Despite strenuous efforts the baby died 24 hours later with disseminated intravascular coagulopathy.

In the first two cases potentially more serious maternal injuries were prevented by the use of seat belts; nevertheless in all three cases major fetal and/or placental injury resulted in in utero or early neonatal death. As in the third case, severe or lethal fetal injuries can occur with only minor or no maternal injury.[29] Questioning a number of pregnant and recently pregnant women revealed that the lap portion of the seat belt is almost always worn dangerously high.

It is often assumed that the deceleration forces due to an emergency stop do not exceed 1 **g**. However a value of 1.2 **g** may be more realistic. This would result in a pressure via the belt of the order of 2 lb/in^2 (0.145 kg/cm^2). A collision with an immovable object, such as a solid wall, would probably be associated with deceleration equal to 15–40 **g** (at speeds up to 70 mph or 112 km/h) and result in belt pressures up to about 60 lb/in^2 (4.4 kg/cm^2).[31]

When the pregnant woman is involved in an RTA the fetus may be endangered by one or more of three possible mechanisms — *indirect trauma*, whereby severe injuries to the mother result in maternal shock, severely compromising placental bed blood flow;[30] *direct trauma*, where blunt or sharp injury to the maternal abdomen also injures the fetus or placenta; or by *deceleration injury*.[32] It should be borne in mind that within the confines of the uterus the fetus is a relatively unrestrained 'passenger'. If the 'fetal vehicle' — the mother — is rapidly decelerated, as in an RTA, then the fetus too will be decelerated by the limits of the uterine cavity and rapid deceleration of delicate fetal structures might lead to visceral trauma, as in the third case.

Recently Murdoch Eaton and colleagues[33] have shown that direct fetal trauma via the maternal abdomen can lead to intraventricular haemorrhages. She reported two cases, one with resolution of the haemorrhage and one where the haemorrhage contributed to the death of the infant. Neither fetus was delivered until more than 2 weeks after the trauma, and no cranial abnormality was suspected until after delivery. Perhaps a fetus which survives an RTA might be assessed by an ultrasonographer whilst still in utero for evidence of intraventricular haemorrhage.

Indirect trauma can best be prevented by protecting the mother from major injury, by use of seat belts or other restraints, and by accident prevention. Direct trauma from blunt injury is also prevented by restraints, which protect the maternal abdomen — and so the fetus — from damage from the steering-wheel or any other source of injury. However in this context an ill-fitting restraint is capable of causing blunt trauma to the fetus and placenta (as in the first two cases discussed above.) As long as the fetus remains an unrestrained 'passenger' within the uterus, deceleration injuries cannot be totally prevented.

In the UK front seat restraints are almost invariably of the three-point fixing type, with horizontal lap strap and diagonal shoulder strap. Shoulder harnesses are rarely seen. In other parts of the world (and less so recently) both diagonal-only and lap-only belts have been used; the former is also presently seen for use as a rear seat restraint, as well as in aircraft. Diagonal-only restraints have been associated with frequent failure, when the passenger is not effectively restrained; they provide inadequate protection and may cause severe intra-abdominal trauma, due to sharp flexion over the belt.[34] The recommendation that pregnant women should wear only the diagonal component of a three-point fixing belt and sit on the lap strap — made by Fakhoury & Gibson,[35] who restated the earlier controversial advice of McCallum,[24] — is therefore to be deprecated, and was described by Herbert[36] as positively dangerous. The use of lap-only belts fails to restrain the upper body, giving incomplete protection of any RTA victim, with particular risk of head and facial injuries to the mother.[34] There is also evidence that this type of restraint is associated with an *increased* risk of fetal trauma.[28] Lap-only belts, or the use of only the lap portion of a three-point restraint, are associated with forced flexion of the mother over the lap belt, resulting in uterine compression and distortion. This forced flexion is prevented by the diagonal component of the three-point restraint.[11a] The use of lap-only restraints by pregnant women should therefore be avoided.

The conventional three-point fixing restraint offers excellent protection in the event of collision to anyone travelling by car. Whether the wearer be a pregnant woman or not, the belt should be properly fitted to prevent seat belt injury to abdominal viscera. This type of belt is designed to restrain a passenger via the skeleton. The diagonal strap should pass over the shoulder and chest, without impinging on the abdomen; the lap strap should lie across the upper thighs, so restraining the femurs and/or pelvis; this placement should avoid maternal visceral injury.

Crosby[37] observed that maternal mortality was less for drivers than front or rear seat passengers — this was however due to a lesser risk of ejection for *unrestrained* drivers compared to *unrestrained* passengers. No differences would therefore be anticipated between driver and front or rear seat passengers if all are properly restrained.

A case reported by Fakhoury & Gibson[35] involved a pregnant woman with seat belt injuries to the lower abdomen (indicating to us that the seat belt was incorrectly fitted) and causing fetal death due to multiple injuries. The authors had not considered that the pattern of maternal injuries indicated that the lap strap had been worn too high. They concluded that the fetal death resulted from the dangers of the use of seat belts with lap straps by pregnant women. Slade[7] recently reported a case of posterior uterine rupture in a woman wearing an incorrectly fitting seat belt; we believe though that the author in the illustrations to his case report has still recommended seat belt fitting which impinges on the pregnant abdomen, and is thus unsafe.

In the pregnant passenger or motorist, the positioning of the seat belt should not differ from what ought to be used for the non-pregnant wearer — the diagonal strap should pass between the breasts, the lap strap should again lie on the thighs. The basic rule should be to place the straps above and below the 'bump', not over it. We have contacted the Royal Society for the Prevention of Accidents (RoSPA) who agreed with this advice.[38] This view is supported by Herbert,[36] who recommended placing the lap strap 'as low as possible below the bulge' and Pearce.[11a] Incorrect placement is hazardous to the fetus, as demonstrated by our own reports and those of Attico and colleagues[26] and Matthews.[25]

In a large series of cases reported by Pepperell and colleagues[39] severe maternal injury was only found in women not wearing seat belts. In their report many cases of maternal and fetal trauma were labelled as 'seat belt injury'. It seems certain that most, if not all, of these cases were actually due to too high positioning of the lap strap. The authors of this paper concluded that: 'The wearing of seat belts would appear to protect the pregnant woman from severe extragenital injury likely to cause her death, but may well increase the risk of placental abruption or uterine rupture'. This conclusion was strongly criticized by Lane[40] and Herbert & Henderson.[41] We would simply advise that the mother and her fetus are both best protected by a properly fitted restraint.

The use of conventional seat belts in pregnancy was recently addressed by an article in a midwifery journal.[42] This article, which may have influenced beliefs among midwives and antenatal class teachers, emphasized the dangers of seat belts, considering that they can cause fetal injury and miscarriage. The author appears not to have considered that such risks should not apply to properly fitted seat belts or that the dangers are far greater for unrestrained mothers.

RoSPA felt that our experience suggested that there was a need for education of pregnant women in the correct use of seat belts in pregnancy. They suggested that this education might be carried out in antenatal classes.[38] We were already aware of anecdotal reports of potentially dangerous advice given to women by doctors and midwives.

In view of this suggestion by RoSPA and our worries concerning inappropriate advice sometimes being given we decided to survey the teaching given to women in antenatal classes regarding seat belt use.[15] The survey involved 30 maternity units representing a range of teaching hospital and district general hospital units drawn from all the health regions of England and Wales. We found that only a minority (46%) of hospital-based antenatal classes routinely gave advice regarding seat belt use in pregnancy; most of the others felt able to give advice if specifically asked. The advice given was extremely varied, ranging from appropriate advice regarding correct fitting of seat belts, through various potentially hazardous modifications, to advice that seat belts need not be worn in pregnancy.

Where modifications to seat belt fitting were recommended, most simply suggested that the belt should 'fit comfortably'. Three respondents however suggested different modifications — one to 'fit the bump', one to pad the belt with a folded towel or piece of foam (in order to spread the impact), while the third suggested the use of the diagonal strap alone. As outlined above, we would consider the latter to be extremely dangerous advice; the former approximates to our own advice and that of RoSPA. The second advice — the use of padding, as also recommended by Matthews[25] — is *potentially* dangerous as the padding might spread the force of the impact on to the abdominal contents. Alternatively, the padding might well slip in the event of a collision, rendering the seat belt less effective.

No antenatal class teacher believed that in the event of an RTA either the mother or her fetus would be safest if a seat belt was avoided. Despite this a significant minority (42%) sometimes advised a pregnant woman to seek a certificate from her general practitioner exempting her from wearing a seat belt. More sinister still was one unit where advice had been sought from the local police, who apparently had advised that pregnant women were exempted from seat belt regulations and that they did not require such a certificate (this respondent therefore 'never' advised women to obtain an exemption certificate).

We are concerned that as yet little attention is given to the subject of seat belt use by pregnant women in antenatal classes. Where advice is given or available it is not necessarily appropriate. This is in no way a criticism of teachers, who have largely adopted a common sense approach; rather it reflects a deficiency within health professionals generally, — a deficiency which ought to be simple to correct.

Correct seat belt use could be simply taught by demonstration or by viewing a video. Particularly if joint maternal and fetal safety were emphasized, once taught, women are likely to heed the advice in both the current and any subsequent pregnancy.

Chang and colleagues[43] considered the attitudes and practices among American obstetricians. Whilst the majority (71.6%) considered that maternal passenger safety should be discussed by the obstetrician with the pregnant woman, a quarter were themselves unsure what advice to give (of those who were sure it is unclear how many gave correct advice), and fewer than a third actually did discuss the matter routinely.

Chang and colleagues also noted a dearth of teaching materials available. This deficiency still remains today.

MATERNAL PELVIC INJURIES — MODE OF DELIVERY

Maternal pelvic injuries may initially result in genital tract trauma, which must be sought and appropriately treated. Subsequently acquired pelvic abnormalities, asymmetry or instability may interfere with the progress of labour and caesarean section may be indicated. Little or no work has assessed this question. Simple lateral X-ray pelvimetry is unlikely to yield sufficient information. Full pelvimetry, preferably using computed tomography scanning, may have some role in such cases. We would recommend that the woman's previous obstetric history be taken into account, together with engagement of the presenting part, clinical assessment of the pelvis, assessment of the medical condition of the mother and her views. Individual cases will require individual management.

The advice of an orthopaedic surgeon might usefully be obtained concerning the extent of pelvic deformity and/or the instability of recent fractures. Golan et al[44] reviewed the literature concerning recent pelvic fractures. They concluded that in the absence of gross deformity vaginal delivery may be permitted. Caesarean section may be required in 5–10% of cases where there is deformity. In a similar review Crosby[37] stated that 'delivery through a recently fractured pelvis is not attended by serious complications and labor should be allowed be allowed to continue in the absence of gross pelvic deformity'. He did also acknowledge that bladder or urethral injuries might occur in such deliveries.

CONCLUSIONS

Major maternal trauma in pregnancy should be treated as outside pregnancy, but secondary consideration should be given to the fetus. Pregnancy may mask physical signs and physiological changes in pregnancy may have some bearing on management. In the absence of significant maternal trauma, major fetal injury may still occur, therefore after initial assessment of the mother efforts should be directed at confirming fetal wellbeing.

The pregnant woman and her fetus are both best protected in the event of an RTA if she is properly restrained by a correctly fitting three-point fixing seat belt. Such a restraint offers excellent protection to the mother and protects the fetus against direct and indirect trauma. Unfortunately even adequate maternal restraint may not protect against fetal deceleration injury.

Incorrectly fitted seat belts offer less protection to the mother and may present a potential hazard to the fetus as a cause of direct trauma. This potential hazard could easily be avoided if women were taught how to wear restraints properly. Teaching on this subject in many antenatal classes run by maternity units appears to be deficient either by its total absence or in other cases in its correctness. This deficiency should be addressed by obstetricians, midwives, health visitors and others concerned with the care of pregnant women.

The design of seat belts which are more easily correctly fitted should perhaps be considered. Within the last few months a seat belt accessory for pregnant women has been marketed in the UK (Comfitum; Electrolux Klippan). This device is designed to pull the lap strap down below the pregnant abdomen. Its use may help some women but the design is not ideal; it can only be used when trousers are worn. Proper seat belt use might appropriately be included in the test for a driving licence.

Whether driving or a passenger, all pregnant women should wear properly fitting seat belts at all times when travelling by car.

ACKNOWLEDGEMENTS

We are grateful for the advice of Robert Cummins and other members of the RoSPA National Road Safety Committee.

REFERENCES

1. Nash P. Cited in Alert to A&E over accident toll on foetus. Hosp Doctor 1990; October 11, p.18
2. Rothenberger D, Quattlebaum F W, Perry J F, Zabel J, Fischer R P. Blunt maternal trauma : a review of 103 cases. J Trauma 1978; 18: 173–179
3. Turnbull A, Tindall V R, Beard R W et al. Report on confidential enquiries into maternal deaths in England & Wales 1982–1984. London: HMSO, 1989
4. Hughes S J, Short D J, Usherwood M McD, Tebbutt H. Management of the pregnant woman with spinal cord injuries. Br J Obstet Gynaecol 1991; 98: 513–518
5. Griffiths M, Hillman G, Usherwood M McD. Seat belt injury in pregnancy resulting in fetal death: two case reports. Br J Obstet Gynecol 1991; 98: 320–321

6. Siddall-Allum J, Kaler S, Reginald P W, Hughes J. Splenic rupture in utero following a road traffic accident. Br J Obstet Gynaecol 1991; 98: 318–319

7. Slade R J . Posterior rupture of a gravid uterus following a road traffic accident. J Obstet Gynecol 1991; 11: 45–46

8. Parkinson E B. Perinatal loss due to external trauma to the uterus. Am J Obstet Gynecol 1964; 90: 30–33

9. Macfarlane A, Mugford M . Birth counts. Statistics of pregnancy and childbirth. London: HMSO, 1984

10. Sachs B P, Brown D A J, Driscoll S G et al. Maternal mortality in Massachusetts. Trends and prevention. N Engl J Med 1987; 316: 667–672

11a. Pearce M . Seat belts in pregnancy. Br Med J 1992; 304: 586–587

11b. Auerbach P S. Trauma in the pregnant patient. Top Emerg Med 1979; 1: 133–145

12. Nash P. ABC of trauma: trauma in pregnancy. Br Med J 1990; 301: 974–976

13. Hoff W S, D'Amelio L F, Tinkoff G H et al. Maternal predictors of fetal demise in trauma during pregnancy. Surg Gynecol Obstet 1991; 172: 175–180

14. Stuart G C E, Harding P G R, Davies E M. Blunt abdominal trauma in pregnancy. Can Med Assoc J 1980; 122: 901–905

15. Griffiths M, Usherwood M McD, Reginald P W. Ante natal teaching of the use of seat belts in pregnancy. Br Med J 1992; 304: 614

16. Pearlman M D, Tintinalli J E, Lorenz R P. Blunt trauma during pregnancy. N Engl J Med 1990; 323: 1609–1613

17. Higgins S D, Garite T J. Late abruptio placenta in trauma patients: implications for monitoring. Obstet Gynecol 1984; 63: 10s–12s

18. Goodwin T M, Breen M T. Pregnancy outcome and fetomaternal hemorrhage after noncatastrophic trauma. Am J Obstet Gynecol 1990; 162: 665–671

19. Kerr M G, Scott D B, Samuel E. Studies of inferior vena cava in late pregnancy. Br Med J 1964; i: 532–533

20. Rothenberger D, Quattlebaum F W, Zabel J, Fischer R P. Diagnostic peritoneal lavage for blunt trauma in pregnant women. Am J Obstet Gynecol 1977; 129: 479–481

21. Lopez-Zeno J A, Carlo W A, O'Grady J P, Fanaroff AA. Infant survival following delayed cesarean section delivery. Obstet Gynecol 1990; 76: 991–992

22. Brennan L, Halfacre J. Trauma in pregnancy. Br Med J 1990; 301: 1332

23. Nash P, Driscoll P. Trauma in pregnancy. Br Med J 1990 301: 1332

24. McCallum G. Use of seat belts during pregnancy. Med J Aust 1982; 2: 115

25. Matthews C D. Incorrectly used seat belt associated with uterine rupture following vehicular collision. Am J Obstet Gynecol 1975; 121: 1115–1116

26. Attico N B, Smith R J, FitzPatrick M B, Keneally M. Automobile safety restraints for pregnant women and children. J Reprod Med 1986; 31: 187–192

27. Crosby W M, Costiloe J P. Safety of lap-belt restraint for pregnant victims of automobile collisions. N Engl J Med 1971; 284: 632–636

28. Crosby W M, King A I, Stout L C. Fetal survival following impact: improvement with shoulder harness restraint. Am J Obstet Gynecol 1972; 112: 1101–1106

29. Stafford P A, Biddinger P W, Zumwalt R E. Lethal intrauterine fetal trauma. Am J Obstet Gynecol 1988; 159: 485–489

30. Sherer D M, Schenker J G. Accidental injury during pregnancy. Obstet Gynecol Surv 1989; 44: 330–337

31. Reed G. Personal communication, 1992

32. Connor E, Curran J. In utero traumatic intra-abdominal deceleration injury to the fetus. A case report. Am J Obstet Gynecol 125: 567–569

33. Murdoch Eaton D G, Ahmed Y, Dubowitz L M S. Maternal trauma and cerebral lesions in preterm infants. Case reports. Br J Obstet Gynaecol 1991; 98: 1292–1294

34. Schoenfeld A, Ziv E, Stein L, Zaidel D, Ovadia J. Seat belts in pregnancy and the obstetrician. Obstet Gynecol Surv 1987; 42: 275–282

35. Fakhoury G W, Gibson J R M. Seat belt hazards in pregnancy: case report. Br J Obstet Gynaecol 1986; 93: 395–396

36. Herbert D C. Use of seat belts during pregnancy. Med J Aust 1982; 2: 115

37. Crosby W M. Trauma during pregnancy: maternal and fetal injury. Obstet Gynecol Surv1974; 29: 683–699

38. Cummins R. Personal communication. 1990

39. Pepperell R J, Rubinstein E, MacIsaac I A. Motor-car accidents during pregnancy. Med J Aust 1977; 1: 203–205
40. Lane J C. Motor-car accidents during pregnancy. Med J Aust 1977; 1: 669–670
41. Herbert D C, Henderson J M. Motor-car accidents during pregnancy. Med J Aust 1977; 1: 670–671
42. Markos A R. Use of conventional seat-belts in pregnancy. Midwife Health Visitor Commun Nurse 1990; 26: 256–258
43. Chang A, Christal S, O'Sullivan T. Automobile passenger education for pregnant women and infants. J Reprod Med 1985; 30: 849–853
44. Golan A, Sandbank O, Teare A J. Trauma in late pregnancy. A report of 15 cases. S Afr Med J 1980; 57: 161–165

7. Non-prescription drugs and pregnancy

W. F. Rayburn   E. A. Conover

Despite a growing awareness of the need to avoid drugs, pregnant women take many medications. The typical pregnant woman takes one to three drugs besides vitamin supplements or iron.[1,2] Drug ingestion is common throughout pregnancy, exposing the fetus during such critical periods as organogenesis and just prior to labor and delivery. Non-prescription drugs, particularly non-narcotic analgesics, are taken more often than prescribed medications during pregnancy.[1-3] The obstetrician may not know the patient is taking such drugs, and the patient may not recognize their potential for harm.

Any study of the effects of a non-prescription drug on the developing fetus raises several questions. Agents available over the counter for at least the past 15 years may have been studied by the Collaborative Perinatal Project[4] or the Boston Collaborative Drug Surveillance Program.[5,6] Although valuable, data from these studies are not always conclusive and do not help in evaluating newer non-prescription drugs or those infrequently taken during pregnancy. Other drug studies usually involve small series or case reports which may be biased or merely reflect the patients' background risk for birth defects regardless of exposure.

For many drugs, the only data come from animal studies which involve the parenteral administration of doses high enough to cause maternal morbidity. In addition, these studies may not accurately reflect human risk because of interspecies differences. When the only information on a drug is based on case reports or animal studies, that drug is often avoided by the inquiring pregnant patient, unless the benefits are clearly shown to outweigh the risks.

While information about prescription drug use may be scant or difficult to interpret, assessing the risks with non-prescription medications is even more difficult. The *Physician's Desk Reference for Non-Prescription Drugs*[7] often reveals little or no information about warnings during pregnancy. Many drugs contain combinations of both active and inactive ingredients, confusing the discussion of any single ingredient. A drug's label may not show doses, although the lowest effective dose is often used. Recognizing these limitations, recommendations will be offered for use of specific groups of non-prescription drugs during pregnancy.

MILD ANALGESICS

Mild analgesics are the drugs most commonly taken during pregnancy.[1,3] This category includes acetaminophen (paracetamol), aspirin, and ibuprofen. Acetaminophen, rather than aspirin, is considered to be the analgesic and antipyretic of choice during pregnancy. No increase has been found in the frequency of congenital anomalies in offspring of women who took acetaminophen during the first trimester or those who took this drug any time during gestation.[4,6,7] Nephrotoxicity and hepatotoxicity occur rarely as complications of overdosage in adults, and these conditions have also been observed among infants born to women who took large therapeutic or toxic doses late in pregnancy.

Aspirin is an oral analgesic and antipyretic that is a non-steroidal anti-inflammatory agent. Very large doses have been shown to be teratogenic in many animals. Human case-controlled studies have reported associations between congenital malformations and aspirin use early in gestation[8] (Fierler, 1985), but a consistent outcome attributable to the drug has not been uncovered.[4,7] In addition, two large studies did not find any evidence of aspirin-induced teratogenicity.[9,10] Therefore, any increase in risk in humans, if present, is relatively small.

Most concern about aspirin involves its chronic use during the third trimester. Since it is a prostaglandin synthetase inhibitor, aspirin decreases platelet adhesiveness and aggregation; premature babies whose mothers have taken aspirin within 1 week of delivery have an increased incidence of intracranial bleeding.[11] Chronic aspirin exposure in utero may also cause premature closure of the fetal ductus arteriosus. Because of these potential side-effects, the Food and Drug Administration recommends that women not use aspirin during the last 3 months of pregnancy unless prescribed by their physician.[12]

Ibuprofen is another non-steroidal anti-inflammatory analgesic. Only recently has it been available as a non-prescription drug, and thus evidence regarding its reproductive effects is limited. Ibuprofen is not teratogenic in rats or rabbits at doses several times larger than those used in humans. No increased frequency of malformations has been observed among infants whose mothers took ibuprofen during the first trimester.[7] Intrauterine closure of the ductus arteriosus from ibuprofen has been demonstrated in rodents, but effects on humans late in pregnancy are unknown.[13]

ANTACIDS AND BOWEL PREPARATIONS

Antacids and oral bowel preparations are the second most commonly used group of non-prescription drugs during pregnancy. These agents should be taken only after diet manipulation and conservative treatment have been unsuccessful for treating dyspepsia, constipation, or diarrhea. Patients should be informed that in some cases these products may actually exacerbate diarrhea or constipation.

Most antacids contain calcium carbonate, aluminum, sodium bicarbonate, or magnesium. A buffered preparation of calcium carbonate is often recommended. Moderate use would appear to present minimal risk to the fetus and may also enhance maternal nutrition. Some antacids also contain sodium bicarbonate. Frequent use of this alkaline sodium salt can produce metabolic alkalosis and fluid overload in both mother and offspring. There have been no studies in either laboratory animals or human pregnancy regarding the reproductive toxicity of magnesium carbonate.

Aluminum and its reproductive toxicity have received little study, perhaps because aluminum was once thought to be poorly absorbed. However, 12–31% of the oral aluminum intake may be absorbed. Animal studies indicate that maternally administered aluminum crosses the placenta and accumulates in fetal tissues, causing an increase in fetal death as well as abnormal skeletal growth and impaired learning and memory in surviving offspring.[14,15] No data as yet suggest that comparable toxic effects occur frequently in human pregnancies. However, the unlimited use of aluminum-containing antacids is not recommended.

Kaolin, a clay composed of hydrated aluminum silicate, is administered orally in the treatment of diarrhea. The agent is not teratogenic in rats, but no epidemiological studies have examined its use in human pregnancy. Consumption of large amounts of kaolin, as in cases of geophagia, may be associated with anemia.[16] In addition, there are some indications that the use of kaolin-containing agents may serve as a significant source of aluminum loading during pregnancy. Short-term therapy is likely safe, but there appears to be little clinical evidence to support the long-term use of kaolin-containing medications during pregnancy.

Bismuth subsalicylate (e.g. Pepto Bismol) is frequently used for relief of indigestion, nausea and vomiting, and diarrhea. The use of bismuth salts during pregnancy is somewhat controversial. Bismuth is concentrated in the placenta and readily transferred to the fetus, where it may bind to numerous tissues including the bones.[17] No increased frequency of congenital anomalies has been noted,[4] but no effort has been made to look for subtle effects such as deposition on bone. The salicylate component of bismuth subsalicylate has also raised concerns, because it may decrease platelet adhesiveness and aggregation as well as increase the risk of premature closure of the fetal ductus arteriosus. Therefore, we recommend that medications containing bismuth subsalicylate be used in small quantities or avoided completely during pregnancy.

Docusate, an emulsifying agent used as a stool softener, has not been found to be associated with any malformations.[4,6,7] As with many laxatives, docusate used in excess may produce hypomagnesemia. In one case, maternal overuse of this agent throughout pregnancy was associated with symptomatic hypomagnesemia in the neonate.[18]

Phenolphthalein, a laxative/cathartic, has not been found to be associated with an increased frequency of congenital anomalies when used during the first 4 lunar months of pregnancy.[4] Overdose with this laxative can lead to fluid and electrolyte deficits resulting from excessive catharsis.[18] Moderate use, however, has not been reported to cause adverse reproductive effects.

COLD MEDICATIONS

Most cold and cough medications contain a combination of decongestants, antitussives, expectorants, and mild analgesics. Nasal congestion is a primary complaint. Decongestants alone are often delivered as either oral capsules or nasal sprays. These products dry the nasal mucosa passageways by stimulating alpha-adrenergic receptors. Most studies involving decongestants have not found a significant risk for malformations, but because of theoretical concerns about the risk for vascular-mediated birth defects, they should be reserved for cases of significant maternal discomfort.[4] Perhaps of greater concern is whether these alpha-stimulating drugs induce maternal hypertension or reduce uterine blood flow when taken at doses which produce therapeutic effects.

Many clinicians consider pseudoephedrine to be the drug of choice for pregnant women who require a decongestant. Studies have shown that only a small percentage of the agent crosses the placenta to the fetus and that pseudoephedrine may have a relatively mild vasoconstrictive effect. The frequency of malformations was no higher than expected among the offspring of women who took pseudoephedrine at any time during pregnancy.[4,6,7] One study involving 12 women who took a single dose of pseudoephedrine between 26 and 40 weeks of gestation found no significant alterations in uterine or fetal circulation.[19] In addition, it has been shown that ephedrine, an isomer of pseudoephedrine, does not alter intravillous blood flow.[20] Exposure to ephedrine during the first trimester has not been associated with increases in any kind of birth defects.[4,6,7]

Epidemiological studies of congenital anomalies among infants born to women who took phenylephrine during pregnancy have produced inconsistent results. The Collaborative Perinatal Project included 1249 pregnancies exposed to phenylephrine during the first 4 lunar months and found a weak but statistically significant association with the occurrence of congenital anomalies.[4] These included ear and eye defects, syndactyly, hip dislocation, musculoskeletal deformities, and umbilical herniation. In contrast, the Boston Collaborative Drug Surveillance Project[7] found the frequency of malformations to be no greater than expected among 225 infants born to women treated with phenylephrine during the first trimester. Two case control studies involving 390 and 298 children found an increased risk for congenital heart disease in infants exposed to phenylephrine early in pregnancy.[8,21] Of equal or greater concern is the fact that phenylephrine and other alpha-adrenergic agonists may induce maternal hypertension and reduce uterine blood flow when used at doses comparable to those which produce therapeutic effects.

As with phenylephrine, epidemiological studies regarding the risk of malformations among infants exposed to phenylpropanolamine in utero have produced inconsistent results. The Collaborative Perinatal Project monitored 726 pregnancies exposed to phenylpropanolamine during the first trimester and found a possible association between the use of this agent and hypospadias, ear and eye malformations, polydactyly, and pectus excavatum.[4] In contrast, the Boston Collaborative Drug Surveillance Program found the frequency of malformations was no greater than expected among more than 350 infants born to women who took phenyl-propanolamine during the first trimester.[4,7] Like phenylephrine, phenylpro-panolamine may result in decreased uterine blood flow and maternal hypertension.[22] Oxymetazoline is an alpha-adrenergic agonist used in long-acting nasal decongestant sprays. The frequency of congenital anomalies is not greater than expected among the infants exposed to oxymetazoline during the first trimester of pregnancy.[6,7] No decrease in blood flow to the uterine arcuate artery, fetal descending aorta, and umbilical artery occurred after a one-time dose was used in normotensive pregnant women.[23] Caution is merited, though, because nasal sprays are absorbed systemically and thus may present an exposure to the fetus; in addition, some women may develop rebound congestion and subsequently overdose themselves with this drug.

Dextromethorphan is a commonly used antitussive. Among the offspring of women who used dextromethorphan during the first trimester of pregnancy, the frequency of malformations was no greater than expected.[4,6,7]

Guaifenesin and terpin hydrate (a cyclic alcohol) are used as expectorants. The frequency of malformations with either compound was no greater than expected among the children of women who took guaifenesin during the first trimester of pregnancy.[4,6,7]

ANTIHISTAMINES

Antihistamines are useful to treat hayfever. Aside from slight drying of nasal secretions and induction of drowsiness, antihistamines are not effective in relieving cold symptoms. Although most have a low risk for teratogenicity, an association between exposure during the last 2 weeks of pregnancy to antihistamines and retrolental fibroplasia in premature infants has been reported.[24] Examples of antihistamines in non-prescription products include brompheniramine, chlorpheniramine, diphenhydramine, and pyrilamine.

The frequency of congenital anomalies was not increased among the infants of women who took brompheniramine during the first trimester.[6,7] The Collaborative Perinatal Project found a slightly increased frequency of congenital anomalies among the children of 65 women who took brompheniramine during the first 4 lunar months of pregnancy, but the increase was due to minor defects that occurred in varying rates at participating institutions.[4] One retrospective study found that first-trimester exposure to diphenhydramine was more common among children born with oral clefts than those without clefts, but the finding was not substantiated in the larger collaborative studies. Currently, research is being conducted into the question of whether pyrilamine and a related agent, methapyrilamine, are carcinogens; they have been associated with an increased risk of malformations.[4]

CIGARETTE-SMOKING CESSATION PRODUCTS

Overwhelming evidence shows that maternal smoking has harmful effects on the fetus. A widely accepted mechanism of these adverse effects has not been established, but a chronic reduction of placental blood flow by nicotine and fetal hypoxia from carbon monoxide may be contributory. It seems obvious that pregnant women should be encouraged to quit smoking or at the very least limit their use of tobacco as much as possible.

Lobeline, a non-prescription medication to curb smoking, is a plant alkaloid that has effects similar to nicotine. Lobeline may inhibit the synthesis of sex steroids when applied to rat granulosa cells and testicular cells in culture.[25] The Collaborative Perinatal Project, studying a small group of women who used lobelia plant extract as an antitussive during the first 4 months of pregnancy, found no increased incidence of fetal malformations.[4] Other than these two reports, there is no evidence regarding the reproductive toxicity of lobeline in either laboratory animals or humans. Therefore, it is unclear whether using lobeline as an aid to smoking cessation presents a lower risk than use of cigarettes. Instead, it would seem reasonable to try non-medication strategies such as behavioral modification techniques.

DERMATOLOGIC PREPARATIONS

Several dermatologic preparations are available over the counter as acne treatments, dandruff shampoos, first-aid ointments, and surface anesthetics. Because of their topical application, their potential for reproductive toxicity has received little attention. However, some agents are absorbed in relatively large amounts and thus may present exposure to the fetus.

Benzoyl peroxide, the active ingredient in many topical acne medications, has an antibacterial effect. Approximately 5% of benzoyl peroxide is absorbed through the skin. No studies have examined its reproductive toxicity in either animals or humans. However, the relatively low level of systemic absorption should provide a partial protective factor.

Resorcinol is an aromatic alcohol used topically in the treatment of acne, seborrhea, eczema, and psoriasis. Resorcinol may be absorbed after topical application, but has not been found to be teratogenic in rats, rabbits, or humans at any time during the pregnancy.[4,26]

Selenium sulfide is used in topical preparations for the treatment of dandruff and fungal infections of the scalp and skin. Information available on selenium-containing compounds used in industry reveals that in mice it crosses the placenta readily, causing a decrease in birth weight and reducing neonatal survival.[27] In humans, a cluster of miscarriages has been reported in a small group of women exposed occupationally to selenium.[28] While these data may not directly apply to women exposed to selenium through dandruff shampoo, caution should be employed in using frequent or large amounts of this agent.

Bacitracin, an antimicrobial, is often incorporated into topical antiseptics. No relationship between first-trimester exposure and adverse pregnancy outcome has been shown.[4] Polymyxin B, another topical antimicrobial, is not teratogenic in rats or rabbits and is without apparent adverse effects in humans.[4]

Benzocaine is a surface anesthetic of the amide class. The frequency of congenital anomalies has not been shown to be significantly greater than expected among children exposed in utero to benzocaine during the first 4 months of pregnancy.[4]

SCABICIDES

Non-prescription treatments for lice frequently contain a combination of pyrethrin and piperonyl butoxide. To our knowledge, there have been no studies regarding the use of pyrethrin during human pregnancy. Investigations in mice, rats, and rabbits have not suggested teratogenicity, although large doses have produced an increased number of resorptions.[29] Piperonyl butoxide is added to pyrethrin insecticides to enhance activity. Large doses of piperonyl butoxide ($\geq$500 mg/kg) have not been shown to be teratogenic in rats and mice, but may be teratogenic in rabbits.[30] As with the pyrethrins, there are no studies regarding the possible human reproductive toxicity of this agent.

Scabicides should be used with caution during pregnancy. Before treatment, it is important to confirm infestation. If a patient needs to use the agent, we suggest that she use gloves to minimize systemic absorption. The patient should check to be sure that the first treatment was unsuccessful before considering a second application. A second use should be made no sooner than 24 hours after the first; usually 7–10 days are required to kill newly hatched lice. Each family member should also be examined carefully and, if infected, should be treated promptly to avoid spread or reinfection. Contaminated clothing or other articles should be dry-cleaned, boiled, or otherwise treated until decontaminated.

MOTION SICKNESS

Dimenhydrinate and meclizine are two antihistamines in non-prescription products for preventing motion sickness. The Collaborative Perinatal Project studied 319 mothers with first-trimester exposure to dimenhydrinate; the total incidence of malformations was not increased, although a possible association with cardiovascular defects and inguinal hernia was suggested.[4] The statistical significance of these findings is unknown, and independent confirmation is required. Dimenhydrinate can result in increased uterine activity and has been implicated anecdotally as a cause of premature labor.[31] This effect is most prevalent in the latter part of pregnancy.

Although meclizine hydrochloride causes clefting in rodents, the frequency of congenital anomalies in general is no greater than expected among children born to women who used meclizine in the first trimester.[32-34] A weak association has been reported between maternal use of meclizine in the first trimester and malformations of the ear or eye, but this has not been observed in other studies.[4]

DIET PILLS

A variety of non-prescription diet pills are sometimes taken in early gestation before pregnancy is diagnosed. Phenylpropanolamine alone or in combination with caffeine is the principal ingredient. It is a stimulant that is structurally similar to epinephrine. Decreased uterine blood flow and maternal hypertension are theoretically possible.

Phentermine is another sympathomimetic amine which serves as an appetite suppressant. There are no studies regarding its reproductive toxicity in the human. Animals exposed to a similar agent, chlorphentermine, do not show an increased risk for malformations but do demonstrate lipidosis in fetal and maternal organs. Whether or not this creates long-term adverse effects in the exposed fetus is unknown.[35]

Certain diet pills contain guar gum. No increase in abnormal pregnancy outcome has been shown with large doses of guar in the diet of pregnant rats,[36] but there are no studies in human pregnancy.

Many weight reduction aids contain caffeine. While caffeine in small amounts appears to present minimal risk during pregnancy, large quantities for long periods may result in an increased risk for pregnancy loss, low birth weight, and perhaps malformations.[37]

CONCLUSIONS

Non-prescription drugs are taken more commonly than prescription medications during pregnancy. Requests for non-prescription drugs often increase rather than decrease as gestation advances because of an increase in maternal symptoms such as backache, nasal congestion, headache, and weakness. Initial and periodic prenatal examinations should include a questioning and documentation of any specific non-prescription drugs, since many patients may not perceive these medications as being important to report.

Limited information exists on the safety of non-prescription drugs during pregnancy, so caution should be employed. It is not safe to assume that these products are without reproductive toxicity, particularly in women with other medical conditions. We would recommend choosing products with the fewest ingredients and lowest dose to treat the individual symptoms adequately. Patients should be instructed to follow the directions and use the medication only while symptoms are present.

REFERENCES

1. Rayburn W F, Wible-Kant J, Bledsoe P. Changing trends in drug use during pregnancy. J Reprod Med 1982; 27: 569–575
2. Buitendijk S, Bracken M B. Medication in early pregnancy: prevalence of use and relationship to maternal characteristics. Am J Obstet Gynecol 1991; 165(1): 33–40
3. Rubin P C. Prescribing in pregnancy. Br Med J 1986; 293: 1415
4. Heinonen O P, Slone D, Shapiro S. Birth defects and drugs in pregnancy. Littleton, Ma, Publishing Sciences Group, 1977
5. Jick H, Holmes L B, Hunter J R. First-trimester drug use and congenital disorders. JAMA 1981; 246: 343–346
6. Aselton P A, Jick H, Milunsky A. First-trimester drug use and congenital disorders. Obstet Gynecol 1985; 65: 451–455
7. Physician's desk reference for non-prescription drugs. Oradell, NJ: Medical Economics, 1992
8. Zierler S, Rothman K J. Congenital heart disease in relation to maternal use of benedectin and other drugs in early pregnancy. N Engl J Med 1985; 313(6): 347–352
9. Slone D, Siskind V, Heinonen O P. Aspirin and congenital malformations. Lancet 1976; i: 1373–1375
10. Werler M M, Mitchell A, Shapiro S. The relation of aspirin use during the first trimester of pregnancy to congenital cardiac defects. N Engl J Med 1989; 321: 1639–1642
11. Runtack C M, Guggenhein M, Rumack B, Peterson R, Johnson M, Braithwaite N. Neonatal intracranial hemorrhage and maternal use of aspirin. Obstet Gynecol 1981; 58: 52S–56S
12. Food and Drug Administration Labeling for oral and rectal over-the-counter aspirin and aspirin-containing drug products: final rule. Fed Register 1990; 55: 27776–27784
13. Momma K, Takeuchi H. Constriction of the fetal ductus arteriosus by non-steroidal anti-inflammatory drugs. Prostaglandins 1983; 26: 631–643
14. Benett R W. Experimental studies on the effects of aluminum on pregnancy and fetal development. Anat Anz 1975; 138 (suppl): 356–378
15. Yokel R A. Toxicity of gestational and aluminum exposure to the maternal rabbit in offspring. Toxicol Appl Pharmacol 1985; 79: 121–133
16. Patterson E C, Staszak D. Effects of geophagia (kaolin ingestion) on the maternal blood and in embryonic development in the pregnant rat. J Nutr 1977; 107: 2020–2025
17. Thompson H E. The transfer of bismuth into the fetal circulation after maternal administration of sobisminol. Am Syph 1941; 25: 725–730
18. Schindler A M. Isolated neonatal hypomagnesaemia associated with maternal overuse of stool softener. Lancet 1984; ii: 822
19. Smith C, Rayburn W, Anderson J, Duckworth A. Effect of a single dose of oral

pseudoephedrine on uterine and fetal Doppler blood flow. Obstet Gynecol 1990; 76: 803–806

20. Hollmen A I. Intervillous blood flow during cesarean section with prophylactic ephedrine and epidural anesthesia. Acta Anaesthesiol Scand 1984; 28: 296–400

21. Rothman K J, Fyler D C, Goldblatt A, Kreidberg M B. Exogenous hormones and other drug exposures of children with congenital heart disease. Am J Epidemiol 1979; 109: 433–439

22. Horowitz J D, Howest L, Christophidis N et al. Hypertensive responses induced by phenylpropanolamine in anorectic and decongestant preparations. Lancet 1980; i: 60–61

23. Rayburn W F, Anderson J, Smith C, Appel L, Davis S. Uterine and fetal Doppler flow changes from a single dose of long-acting intranasal decongestant. Obstet Gynecol 1990; 76: 180–182

24. Zierler S, Purohit D. Prenatal antihistamine exposure and retrolental fibroplasia. Am J Epidemiol 1986; 123: 192–196

25. Kasson B G, Hsuch A S. Nicotinic cholinergic antagonists inhibit androgen biosynthesis by cultured rat testicular cells. Endocrinology 1985; 117: 1874–1880

26. Spengler J, Osterburg I, Korte R. Teratogenic evaluation of p-toluenediamene sulphate, resorcinol and p-amniophenol in rats and rabbits. Teratology 1986; 33: 31A

27. Schroeder H A, Mitchener M. Toxic effects of trace elements on the reproduction of mice and rats. Arch Environ Health 1971; 23: 102–106

28. Robertson D S F. Selenium — a possible teratogen? Lancet 1970; i: 518–519

29. Khera K S. Teratogenicity study on pyrethrum and rotenone (natural origin) in pregnant rats. J Toxicol Environ Health 1982; 10: 111–119

30. Schwetz B A, Murray F, Staples R. Teratology studies on the metabolic inhibitors. SKF-525A and piperonyl butoxide in mice and rabbits. Toxicol Appl Pharmacol 1976; 37: 150–151

31. Watt L O. Oxytocic effects of dimenhydrihate in obstetrics. Can Med Assoc J 1961; 84: 533–534

32. Milkovich L, Van den Berg B J. An evaluation of the teratogenicity of certain anti-nauseant drugs. Am J Obstet Gynecol 1976; 125: 244–248

33. Melin G W. Drugs in the first trimester of pregnancy and the fetal life of *Homo sapiens*. Am J Obstet Gynecol 1964; 90: 1169–1180

34. Nelson M M, Forfar J O. Associations between drugs administered during pregnancy and congenital abnormalities of the fetus. Br Med J 1971; 1: 523–527

35. Thoma-Laurie D. Neonatal toxicity in rats following in-utero exposure to chlorphentermine or phentermine. Toxicology 1982; 24: 85–94

36. Collins T F, Welsh J, Black T, Graham S, O'Donnell M. Study on the teratogenic potential of guar gum. Food Chem Toxicol 1987; 25: 807–814

37. Narod S A, deSanjose S, Victoria C. Coffee during pregnancy: a reproductive hazard? Am J Obstet Gynecol 1991; 164: 1109–1114

8. Antimicrobials in pregnancy

C. J. Kelleher   L. D. Cardozo

Antimicrobials (antibiotics, antifungals, antiseptics and antivirals) are the most commonly prescribed drugs during pregnancy. Infections can lead to significant morbidity and an adverse outcome for the mother, the baby, or both. Many congenital and neonatal infections can be avoided by the timely use of antimicrobial agents. The use of these drugs is not limited to the treatment of established infection. They may be employed as prophylactic agents and with the advent of ever-increasing intervention in obstetric practice, the role of antimicrobials in the prevention of infection has become an important aspect of obstetric management.

ANTIBIOTICS

The general principle that drugs should not be administered to pregnant women unless the benefits outweigh the risks applies equally well to antibiotics as to other forms of medication. The armamentarium of antibiotics is constantly changing due to both commercial pressure and bacterial resistance, and unless vigilance is maintained women may well be exposed to drugs during pregnancy, the effects of which are poorly understood.

The majority of drugs, antibiotics included, will carry the warning: 'To be used with caution in women of child-bearing age'. In some cases, possibly as a result of experimental work on animals, pregnancy will be listed as a contraindication to their use. It is very difficult to obtain ethical committee approval for the trial of any drugs during pregnancy, thus prescribing for pregnant women may be difficult. Many of the newer preparations are unavailable during pregnancy, so the prescriber must resort to second-line and possibly inferior treatment. In addition a doctor may be confronted by a patient who finds that she is pregnant after completing or shortly after commencing a course of antibiotics, and thus it is important to know the effects of these drugs on the developing fetus.

SAFETY OF ANTIBIOTICS IN PREGNANCY

Most of the information available regarding the effects of antibiotics in early pregnancy has been obtained by accident, when neither the woman nor her physician have suspected that she was pregnant at the time of administration. Alternatively antibiotics may be prescribed when the benefit of a particular treatment has been thought to outweigh the possible risks. Most physicians continue to prescribe during pregnancy those antibiotics with which they are familiar, and which have already been used extensively with little or no documented evidence of adverse side-effects. Adverse reactions to drugs are usually notified to the Committee on Safety of Medicines through the yellow card scheme.

Many antibiotics have side-effects and can cause anaphylaxis in pregnant as well as non-pregnant individuals. These side-effects are well-established, and reported in the various drug data sheets produced by the pharmaceutical companies and the *British National Formulary*. Of particular concern in pregnancy are the teratogenic and toxic effects of these drugs on the unborn fetus or neonate.

There is no evidence that any of the antimicrobial agents approved for general use in pregnancy are teratogenic in humans, with the possible exception of tetracyclines and rifampicin. Some sulphonamides are teratogenic in animals[1] and as a result of such findings the long-acting sulphonamide sulphadimethoxypyrimidine was withdrawn.[2] The increased risk of kernicterus associated with the use of sulphonamides contraindicates these drugs in the later weeks of pregnancy.

Tetracyclines, co-trimoxazole, and 5-fluorocytosine have all been shown to be teratogenic in laboratory animals.[3,4] No adverse effects of co-trimoxazole have been reported in pregnant women and it has been widely used during pregnancy.[5]

Very high doses of metronidazole have been shown to be carcinogenic in rodents,[6a] although this has not been substantiated in women.

Tetracyclines form complexes with calcium in the bones and teeth of the developing fetus during the middle to the end of pregnancy, resulting in yellow discoloration of the teeth and enamel hypoplasia[6b]. They have also been associated with reports of bone growth retardation and congenital cataracts. In addition to effects on the fetus, these drugs in larger doses are linked with maternal hepatotoxicity through a direct action on the liver as a result of the altered physiology of this organ in the pregnant state.

The aminoglycosides, e.g. gentamicin, have been extensively studied throughout pregnancy in view of the risk of ototoxicity and nephrotoxicity. Conway & Birt[7] reported minor degrees of eighth nerve dysfunction in 8 out of 17 children who had been exposed to streptomycin during intrauterine life. Other investigators have shown this to be a rare occurrence.[8] Kanamycin, which does not cross the placenta in significant amounts, has been shown to produce little evidence of toxic effects.[9a,b] Gentamicin is a valuable drug for the treatment of severe or potentially life-threatening infections. The safety of this drug during pregnancy has not been fully established and it is known to cross the placenta in significant amounts.

Chloramphenicol has not been shown to produce adverse effects on the developing fetus in the first or second trimesters despite its toxic side-effects in the mother.[8] This drug does however produce serious side-effects if used in the third trimester. In extreme cases it can result in the circulatory collapse of the neonate — 'Grey baby syndrome'.[10]

The beta-lactam antibiotics, e.g amoxycillin, are well-established in obstetric practice and have not been associated with side-effects beyond those experienced by non-pregnant women. Erythromycin is a useful alternative to penicillin in those with a history of penicillin allergy. No teratogenic or toxic effects on the fetus have been experienced with erythromycin, although isolated cases of hepatotoxicity have been reported in the mother.[11] The newer antibiotics, e.g. Augmentin, which contain a beta-lactamase inhibitor, appear to be safe to use in pregnancy, but are more expensive.

Nitrofurantoin has been shown to be a safe agent and has been used for more than 30 years in the treatment of urinary tract infection with few documented toxic effects. This drug is however contraindicated in

Table 8.1 FDA classification of drugs

Category	Description
A	No fetal risk: proven safe for use during pregnancy
B	Fetal risk not demonstrated in animal or human studies
C	Fetal risk unknown: no adequate human studies
D	Some evidence of fetal risk: may be necessary to use drug in pregnancy

Table 8.2 Antibiotics by FDA classification

Antibiotic	A	B	C	D
Penicillins (e.g. amoxycillin)		X		
Penicillin combined with beta-lactamase inhibitor (e.g. augmentin)		X		
Cephalosporins (e.g. cefuroxime)		X		
Aminoglycosides (e.g. gentamicin)			X	
Aminoglycosides (e.g. streptomycin)				X

Table 8.3 FDA classification of other antibiotics

Antibiotic	A	B	C	D
Chloramphenicol			X	
Metronidazole		X		
Sulphonamides		X		
Tetracyclines				X
Trimethoprim			X	
Nitrofurantoin		X		
Erythromycin		X		

patients with renal impairment because of the risk of toxic serum levels developing.

In an attempt to highlight safer prescribing of antibiotics during pregnancy the Food and Drug Administration (FDA) of the USA designed a classification scheme based on the known side-effects of commonly prescribed antibiotics. The major groups of this classification are summarized in Table 8.1.[12] A summary of the more commonly used antibiotics and their FDA classification is given in Tables 8.2 and 8.3.

ANTIBIOTICS AS PROPHYLACTIC AGENTS

Over the last 50 years the use of antibiotics has changed from their established role in the treatment of infection to one of preventing infection. The discovery that short courses and even single doses of antibiotic prophylaxis can decrease the infection rate resulting from a procedure has led to the widespread introduction of antibiotic prophylaxis into obstetric practice. This has been most widely adopted in the prevention of postoperative infection following caesarean section.

PROPHYLAXIS AND CAESAREAN SECTION

The worldwide increase in caesarean section rates has led to an increase in surgical morbidity associated with delivery. The infection rate following caesarean section has been reported at 11–85%.[13,14] This compares unfavourably with that following normal delivery — less than 10%.[15,16] This has led to a search for both important predisposing risk factors and effective means of prophylaxis. Postoperative genital tract infection is a serious complication causing significant morbidity, both immediate and, in some cases, long-term. In severe cases it can even threaten the mother's life. Several recent reports have revealed an increase in the virulence of group A streptococcus linked to a re-emergence of exotoxin A. This has resulted in a number of fatalities after caesarean section, all of which could possibly have been prevented by the adoption of a policy of routine antibiotic prophylaxis for this procedure.[17] Antibiotic prophylaxis has however failed to find widespread favour in the UK despite its extensive use in the USA.[18]

Attempts at prophylaxis were first documented in 1943. Richards[19] reported that the use of sulpha compounds decreased infectious morbidity. Heseltine & Thelen[20] used local applications of sulphas under the bladder flap, but concluded that, far from reducing morbidity, this practice had the side-effect of markedly increasing adhesion formation. Keetel & Plass[21] studied the use of an intramuscular injection of penicillin as prophylaxis after vaginal delivery, and showed a small decrease in the post-delivery infection rate. Although they concluded that this form of therapy would be far better suited to use in caesarean section patients, this further study was never performed.

The results of most studies assessing the efficacy of prophylactic antibiotics have been in favour of the administration of some form of prophylaxis, although not in all cases.

The major factors to be taken into account are the background morbidity of infectious complications at different institutions, the benefit of using antibiotics in cases considered to be of low risk, and the consequences for both the neonate and mother associated with using antibiotics on such a wide scale. The risk of organism resistance must be considered with blanket prescription of antimicrobials.

It is also important to weigh the cost of antibiotic prophylaxis against the alleviation of morbidity. Mugford et al[22] showed that antibiotic prophylaxis was cost-effective by decreasing the duration of inpatient stay following caesarean section. Evidence appears to be in favour of antibiotic prophylaxis for caesarean section, but the best regimen has yet to be decided.

Prophylactic antibiotics appear to act in two principal ways, namely by destroying some bacteria and slowing the growth of others. They also alter the characteristics of the serosanguinous fluid that collects in the pelvic cavity postoperatively, rendering it less suitable to support the growth of microorganisms. Other possible mechanisms of action include interference with the production of bacterial proteases and interference with the attachment of bacteria to mucosal surfaces. In addition, antibiotics may, in a way that is not completely understood, enhance the host's phagocytic capacity.[23]

Burke[23] has demonstrated that the timing of antibiotic delivery to injured tissue is of critical importance to its efficacy as a prophylactic measure. The greatest benefit is obtained when the dose is administered just before or coincident with the time of maximal bacterial contamination and tissue trauma.

Paediatricians have voiced concern that antibiotics employed prior to delivery increase the risk of immediate or delayed infection in the neonate with resistant organisms. There may also be difficulty in the microbiological identification of causative organisms in cases of neonatal sepsis. Indeed it is true that the most commonly used prophylactic agents, namely the penicillins and cephalosporins, readily cross from the mother to fetus and amniotic fluid, but studies have failed to show that the neonates are at increased risk of complications of this nature.[24] Alternatively antibiotic prophylaxis can still be given usefully after clamping of the cord. Gordon et al[24] showed that the administration of ampicillin after clamping of the cord was as effective as giving it before the operation.

DEFINING INFECTIOUS MORBIDITY

The incidence of infectious complications is significantly higher with caesarean section than following vaginal delivery.[13–16] The very large spread of reported incidence of caesarean section infectious morbidity — 11–85% — suggests that there is a vast difference in the infection rate at different institutions, and also a difference in the inclusion criteria in different studies.[25] The Joint Committee on Maternal Welfare has defined febrile morbidity, the commonest indication for postoperative antibiotic prescription, as a temperature of 38° C or greater on any 2 of the first 10 postoperative days, excluding the first 24 hours, and measured at least four times daily.[26]

Wound infection is defined as the presence of induration, serosanguineous discharge, or dehiscence with purulent discharge with or without a positive microbiological culture.

Genital tract infection is a clinical diagnosis initially, with pain and tenderness of the uterus, and the existence of purulent discharge from the cervix confirmed by positive microbiological culture on a high vaginal swab.

Urinary tract infection is a microbiological diagnosis made by the identification (greater than $10^5/l$) of organisms in a clean-catch midstream urine specimen.

It is true that one of the major risk factors must be the background infection rate at a particular institution. A report from Zimbabwe concluded that all cases of caesarean section carried out in that country warranted prophylactic antibiotics.[27] Whilst the same conclusion has been reached by several researchers closer to home, others have attempted to identify specific risk factors for postoperative infective morbidity to enable us to be more selective in the introduction of prophylaxis.

A recent study at King's College Hospital analysed morbidity following caesarean sections not covered by prophylactic antibiotics. This study showed that 80 of 221 patients had evidence of infection postoperatively and were commenced on antibiotic therapy at that time. The study also showed that the duration of inpatient admission was significantly prolonged by infectious morbidity.[28]

IDENTIFYING PATIENTS WHO ARE AT RISK

Several groups of patients at high risk of developing postoperative infection have been identified by a number of studies. All cases of emergency caesarean section, in particular those urgent cases without proper preoperative cleaning, can be considered to be at risk. Green et al[29] analysed 15 variables, and showed that anaemia, labour and a general anaesthetic were all major risk factors. The use of internal fetal monitoring,[30] duration of caesarean section lasting more than 1 hour, rupture of membranes for greater than 6 hours[31] and the collection postoperatively of a haematoma significantly increase the risk. Obesity, low socioeconomic status, age below 24 years, induction of labour and previous abdominal surgery are all

Table 8.4   Risk factors for postoperative infection

Emergency Caesarean section
Ruptured membranes > 6 hours
Intrapartum infection
Obesity
Prolonged surgery > 1 hour
Anaemia
Haematoma formation
Low socioeconomic class
Age < 24 years
Induction of labour
Internal fetal monitoring
Previous abdominal surgery

contributory factors.[32,33] A summary of the major risk factors for post-operative infection is listed in Table 8.4.

Early studies included all patients undergoing caesarean section and made no attempt to identify those groups at high risk. Despite extensive research, no universal agreement exists as to what constitutes the high-risk case. Gibbs & Weinstein[34] were the first to report in a controlled manner the risks of infection in their patient population. They found that, regardless of whether or not patients were undergoing primary or repeat caesarean section, the risk of infection was high when prophylactic antibiotics were not used. Johnson et al[35] on the other hand found that patients undergoing elective repeat caesarean section were at low risk and did not benefit from antibiotic prophylaxis. Obviously some confusion prevails, and although those at particularly high risk can be identified with relative ease, a large proportion of the patients who would benefit from prophylactic antibiotics may not fit clearly into this high-risk category.

Recent research suggests that women undergoing elective low-risk caesarean section may well also benefit from antibiotic prophylaxis. Mallaret et al[36] have attempted to clarify this viewpoint by studying the benefit of prophylactic antibiotics in 266 women undergoing caesarean section without high risk of postoperative infectious morbidity. They showed that antibiotic prophylaxis using a single dose of cefotetan after cord clamping was cost-effective in reducing hospital stay due to infection, and significantly reduced infection rates compared to their control placebo group.[36,37]

There is a good argument for giving prophylactic antibiotics to all patients undergoing caesarean section. The benefit of such a policy would depend on the background infection rate at different institutions. The evidence is certainly strongly in favour of prophylactic antibiotic coverage of all emergency caesareans, and all those with other significant risk factors.

SELECTING AN AGENT

Many different antibiotics used either alone or in combination have been employed for prophylaxis with proven efficacy. The difficulty in comparing drugs is that the majority of studies have varied with respect to patient populations, time, duration, route of administration, and morbidity criteria, as well as major bias potential due to lack of prospective blinding of the subjects and controls.

The aminoglycosides, because of the risk of ototoxicity and nephrotoxicity, and because they require a second drug to provide adequate coverage, should not be considered for prophylaxis. Similarly, because of the potential for maternal hepatotoxicity and toxic fetal effects, the tetracyclines are not suitable for this purpose.

Of the remaining classes of antibiotics, the penicillins and cephalosporins seem the obvious choice. They have been studied in the fields of obstetrics and gynaecology and have been shown to be equally effective as prophylactic agents.[16] There seems to be little evidence that adding metronidazole will increase their prophylactic effect.[18]

Ideally a drug should be selected that is relatively inexpensive, and which would not be the first-line drug employed for the treatment of serious life - threatening sepsis. Extrapolating from the most recent studies, it appears that the duration of adequate drug levels in the tissues need not be prolonged.[25,38-40] Therefore most drugs with a reasonable half-life (1–2 hours) should be effective when given in single doses or as a short course of maximum three doses.

Since so many different drugs with varying spectra of activity have been shown to be effective, it seems unnecessary for the drug to be active against all of the organisms present in the cervicovaginal flora. Although these organisms are frequently isolated from post-caesarean section infections, simply decreasing their concentration (rather than eradicating them completely) appears to be effective in reducing infectious morbidity.

By decreasing the incidence of postoperative infective morbidity, the use of postoperative antibiotics is also decreased. This has two additional effects, namely the avoidance of prolonged courses of treatment, and secondly offsetting the financial cost of prophylaxis. Gerber et al[41] showed that single-dose perioperative prophylaxis with cefotiam and metronidazole decreased postoperative prescribing of antibiotics from 26.3 to 13.3%. They also concluded that single-dose prophylaxis was effective in decreasing morbidity compared to a non-treatment group.

PROPHYLAXIS OR TREATMENT?

Early studies of antibiotic prophylaxis used a prolonged regimen consisting of an initial dose prior to the incision followed by 3–5 days of antibiotic therapy.[13,42] Several investigators have shown that such a regimen is therapeutic, and have recommended a shorter three-dose course. This practice of multiple-dose prophylaxis has continued.[43]

In 1983 Hawrylyshyn et al[44] reported a significant decrease in postoperative infections after a single 2 g dose of cefoxitin given as the umbilical cord was clamped. Several other studies have confirmed this important result.[38,45–47] Despite the fact that short prophylactic regimens have been adopted, the optimum number of doses remains in dispute. A practical and cost-effective approach would seem to be the introduction and close clinical audit of single-dose prophylaxis.

Intraoperative antibiotic irrigation of the uterus, wound or peritoneal cavity has been shown by investigation to be an effective form of prophylaxis. This technique exerts its primary effect by providing a high concentration of antibiotic directly at the site of injured tissue, but systemic absorption of antibiotic occurs, and this must account for at least some of the prophylactic effect. This route of administration has however been shown to have little advantage over the normal parenteral administration of antibiotics during the operation. Use of systemic antibiotics in conjunction with intraoperative irrigation does not enhance the efficacy of prophylaxis.[4] Therefore there is no justification for combining both methods.[48]

THE APPEARANCE OF RESISTANCE

Selective pressure by the frequent use of antibiotics has already altered the efficacy of some frequently used antibiotics. In many hospitals, for instance, the majority of coliforms are now resistant to ampicillin. Moellering et al[49] using a computer analysis were able to show that an increase in the prevalence of infections due to gentamicin-resistant organisms coincided with the increased use of the drug at the Massachusetts General Hospital.

Inevitably some patients will develop infection despite antibiotic prophylaxis. It is well-documented that prophylaxis induces changes in the normal bacterial flora. The likelihood of infection with resistant organisms must be borne in mind when investigating and treating a patient who has become infected postoperatively despite antibiotic prophylaxis. Antibiotics used for the treatment of serious infections have not been used as prophylactic agents. These measures have ensured that organism resistance has not emerged as a major problem.[50]

VAGINAL DELIVERY

Recently various authors have reinvestigated the practice of vaginal douching during delivery. Stray-Pederson et al[51] showed that douching during delivery with 2 mg/ml chlorhexidine reduced the transmission of maternal infection to the neonate. During the course of this study they also noted that maternal infectious morbidity was reduced not only for vaginal delivery but also for caesarean section.

Heittmann & Benrubie[52] looked at the efficacy of prophylactic antibiotics when used for instrumental forceps delivery. Despite the fact that they were able to show a small decrease in the post-delivery infection rate, they felt that with an infection rate as low as 3.5% antibiotic prophylaxis was unwarranted.

PREMATURE RUPTURE OF THE MEMBRANES

Cervical colonization probably plays a role in the aetiology of premature rupture of the membranes (PROM — rupture of the membranes before the onset of labour). Even if chorioamnionitis were to be the cause of PROM, the infection of the membranes or the amniotic fluid is usually subclinical for a long period of time. PROM also results from other causes and no firm agreement exists regarding the benefit of prophylactic antibiotics.

Alger et al[53] isolated *Chlamydia trachomatis* three times more often from cases of PROM than from a control group, and in the same study *Streptococcus agalactiae* (Group B Streptococcus, GBS) were isolated from 16% of the patients with PROM compared to 4% of the control group. When *Neisseria gonorrhoeae* is isolated, the incidence of PROM is reported to be as high as 75%.[54] The presence of the Mycoplasmas is a possible causative factor in PROM, premature labour, and postpartum infective morbidity.[55,56] Some of the common infections thought to be associated with PROM are listed in Table 8.5.

Several large studies[53,57,58] have shown that prophylaxis with ampicillin or erythromycin can prevent the onset of chorioamnionitis following PROM. Morales et al[58] found that ampicillin prophylaxis reduced the incidence of clinical chorioamnionitis from 26 to 4%, and of neonatal sepsis from 10 to 5%. Whilst *C. trachomatis* and *Mycoplasma* sp. are found in many cases of PROM, their pathogenic effect is much less clear.[59]

The duration of prophylaxis is another problem. Whilst caesarean section and other surgical procedures may benefit from one to three doses of antibiotic prophylaxis, PROM initiates a defect in the barrier to infection of the host, leaving the amniotic cavity exposed for a long period of time. It is also well documented that some women are chronic carriers of Group B streptococci, and that this colonization can reappear even after effective antibiotic treatment. Presumably if antibiotic prophylaxis were thought to be necessary, then the course of treatment would need to be extended until delivery.

In 1989 Ohlsson performed an extensive study reviewing the results of 27 randomized trials of prophylactic antibiotics in PROM.[60] His conclusion

Table 8.5 Infectious causes of PROM

Authors	Organism
Alger et al (1988)[53]	*Chlamydia trachomatis* *Streptococcus agalactiae*
Naessens et al (1989)[54]	*Neisseria gonnorhoeae*
Lang et al (1989)[55] Williams et al 1987[56]	*Mycoplasma* sp.

was that antibiotic prophylaxis has been shown to be of no proven benefit in this condition.

A more common approach to management of PROM is the routine microbiological screening of such women, and intervention with specific antibiotic treatment after the isolation of relevant pathogens.[61] This attitude of expectant treatment may inevitably lead to a delay in the treatment of certain cases, but as there is so far no clear evidence that prophylaxis is of proven benefit, it seems to be the logical course of action. Amniocentesis to detect the presence of infection decreases the risk of subclinical infection remaining unrecognized.

PRETERM LABOUR

About 20% of preterm labours (labour before 37 completed weeks of gestation) are due to obstetric complications such as antepartum haemorrhage, pre-eclampsia, or multiple pregnancy, and around 40% due to premature membrane rupture. A proportion are also due to acute pyrexial illnesses, e.g. urinary tract infection. Of the remaining cases a large portion may be due to cervicovaginal or intrauterine infection.[62–66] Despite the evidence suggestive of an infective aetiology in premature labour, there has been little investigation of the use of antibiotic therapy in idiopathic preterm labour. Morales et al[58] found a statistically significant delay from the time of admission in premature labour to the time of delivery after ampicillin or erythromycin prophylaxis, but Newton et al[67] using a similar regime found no such effect.

The best course of action therefore would seem to be correct microbiological examination, and targeting those cases at risk with specific antimicrobial therapy.

Recently a randomized controlled trial from South Africa[67a] has shown that an antibiotic regimen of ampicillin and metronidazole can prolong pregnancy in women in active preterm labour with intact membranes.

ANTIBIOTICS AND CERVICAL CERCLAGE

The treatment of cervical incompetence with cervical cerclage is well-established. The operation is usually performed as an elective procedure at 13–17 weeks, although interval sutures are also used at some centres. Occasionally sutures are inserted at later gestations as a salvage procedure. The technique is associated with an increased risk of premature labour, although the use of tocolytics and prostaglandin synthase inhibitors may avert this complication. Surprisingly, despite the heavy colonization of the cervix and vagina at this gestation, clinical infections are very rare. Procedures carried out at later gestations are far more likely to be complicated by infectious sequelae. In a study carried out by Charles & Edwards,[68] the infection rate of late operations was shown to be nearly three times that of the early procedures.

It has been demonstrated that the cervicovaginal flora can change significantly following cervical cerclage. Chryssikopoulos et al[69] studied 319 patients and found that the percentage of women with normal flora decreased from 65 to 32% after the operation. The bacteria which increased the most postoperatively were *Escherichia coli*, *Clostridium welchii* (*C. perfringens*), *Streptococcus agalactiae* (GBS) and *Staphylococcus aureus*.

Several authors have recommended the prescription of prophylactic antibiotics to those cases carried out after 18 weeks' gestation.[68,70] However Kessler et al[71] showed that ampicillin prophylaxis in these cases was of little value in decreasing the infection rate.

It would be impossible and probably detrimental to try and eradicate the vaginal flora following cervical cerclage. Prophylactic antibiotics would have to be given for a prolonged period of time to achieve this goal in view of the fact that most pregnancies carry on to term following cervical cerclage. Inevitably antibiotic resistance would develop, compounding the initial problem. It seems reasonable to take microbiology swabs at the time of surgery, and maintain microbiological vigilance throughout the course of the confinement. If this policy were adopted then specific infections could be treated as they arise with suitably targeted antibiotic treatment, obviating the need for prolonged courses of antibiotics of doubtful benefit.

URINARY TRACT INFECTIONS IN PREGNANCY

Infection can affect the urinary tract in pregnancy in three different ways — asymptomatic bacteriuria, acute cystitis, and acute pyelonephritis (Table 8.6). Some patients may enter pregnancy with long-standing urinary tract problems and these can be exacerbated by infection, leading to a deterioration in renal function in pregnancy. Many patients will also be catheterized during their labour, especially those with an epidural block or prior to caesarean section and instrumental delivery.

Asymptomatic bacteriuria affects 2–10% of pregnant women — a similar incidence to that seen in the non-pregnant state when it is often a transient self-limiting phenomenon.[72] Due to the physiological changes of normal pregnancy, 25% of pregnant women with untreated bacteriuria will develop symptomatic urinary tract infections.

In view of the high incidence of asymptomatic bacteriuria and the

Table 8.6   Incidence of urinary tract infections in pregnancy

Asymptomatic bacteriuria — 2–10% of pregnant women
25% will develop symptomatic bacteriuria
Acute pyelonephritis can follow
Acute cystitis — 1% of pregnant women
Acute pyelonephritis — 1–2% of pregnant women
7% develop bacteraemia

possible prevention of pyelonephritis, most centres now routinely screen all pregnant women in the antenatal clinic. Although the treatment of asymptomatic bacteriuria outside pregnancy remains controversial, the increased risk of upper urinary tract involvement in pregnancy with its attendant risks for both mother and fetus indicates that all women with bacteriuria in pregnancy should be treated. If such a policy were adopted then 80% of cases of antenatal pyelonephritis could be prevented.[73]

The choice of antibiotic is limited by the safety of prescribing in pregnancy. The beta-lactam antibiotics (penicillins and cephalosporins) are probably the safest to use whilst sulphonamides, septrin and amino-glycosides, all of which are efficacious in non-pregnant women, are contraindicated due to their possible harmful effects on the fetus.[74] Single-dose treatment has the advantages of cost, compliance, and minimizing adverse effects, but there is a higher risk of long-term recurrence. Jakobi et al[75] showed that single-dose therapy with amoxycillin cured only 75% of women and in addition that failure of this form of treatment might be due to renal rather than bladder bacteriuria. At present therefore a standard course of antibiotic therapy for 7–14 days should be prescribed.[73]

Acute cystitis occurs in approximately 1% of women and is a common cause of preterm labour. It is more common in the second trimester, and is not usually preceded by asymptomatic bacteriuria. Prior to commencing treatment, urine microscopy and culture of a clean-catch midstream urine specimen should be performed.

Acute pyelonephritis is one of the commonest indications for antenatal hospital admission during pregnancy and affects 1–2% of pregnant women. The condition is usually a sequel to asymptomatic bacteriuria and can thus be prevented by routine screening.[76]

Bacteraemia occurs in about 7% of cases and septic shock in 1–2% of cases.[77] Therefore treatment should be started with parenteral antibiotics and rehydration in hospital following the acquisition of blood and urine for culture. The initial choice of antibiotic should include a broad-spectrum penicillin or cephalosporin depending on local sensitivities, and then be tailored by appropriate microbiological cultures and sensitivities, as well as the patient's condition. Treatment should be continued parenterally until she shows sign of significant improvement — usually about 5 days — and then switched to oral therapy for a further 10 days. The recurrence rate following successful treatment of this type is of the order of 10%, a figure which does not seem to be affected greatly by long-term antibiotic prophylaxis.[78]

Recurrent bacteriuria which is difficult to eradicate is often associated with an abnormality of the urinary tract. This condition warrants pro-phylaxis throughout pregnancy and the puerperium, with extra precautions during labour. Investigation of the urinary tract should normally be under-taken at least 3 months after pregnancy to allow for the pregnancy-related anatomical and physiological changes to resolve.

Many patients have a transurethral catheter passed during labour or delivery. A recent study at King's College Hospital showed that as many as 29% of women are catheterized in association with parturition.[79] This study looked at 556 labouring women and failed to show any increase in urinary tract infection or urinary symptoms amongst the women who were catheterized during labour. This conflicts with data from other studies which have shown that catheter-associated infections are acquired by an average of about 7% per day during the first 10 days of catheterization.[80, 81] The discrepancy is probably due to the very short duration of catheterization in the King's study group. Another recent study of post-caesarean section patients analysing data from 1985 and 1987 reported a high incidence of bacteriuria and urinary tract infection in this group.[82] In their study bacteriuria ranged from 25 to 34% and clinical urinary tract infection from 2 to 6%.

Application of polymicrobial ointment to the urethral meatus provides little extra benefit when compared with good aseptic technique of catheterization.[80, 83] The recommendation is to take a catheter specimen of urine for culture on removal of the catheter and treat infection when it arises.

As colonization of the periurethral mucosa is derived from the faecal flora, decontamination of the digestive tract from potentially pathogenic microorganisms has been tried. Vollard et al[81] achieved a significant reduction in the prevalence of bacteriuria using a combination of norfloxacin and amphotericin B. Systemic antimicrobial therapy decreases the frequency of infection in long-term catheterized patients, but this favourable effect is usually limited to a few days due to the emergence of resistant strains. As the duration of catheterization is usually brief in obstetric patients this form of intervention does not seem to be appropriate. The use of norfloxacin has also been restricted by the manufacturers to non-pregnant women.

SPECIFIC INFECTIONS

Most organisms are so frequently isolated from the cervicovaginal flora that specific effects on the neonate cannot be easily predicted. Several microorganisms which are frequently detected are know to lead to significant fetal and maternal morbidity. A summary of some of the more common uses of antimicrobials to treat or prevent infection in pregnancy is given in Table 8.7.

GROUP B STREPTOCOCCUS

GBS are commonly found in the cervicovaginal flora. Neonates can become colonized by vertical transmission and as many as 5–20% of these develop life-threatening septicaemia.[90,91] This is often difficult to treat due to the effect of bacterial toxins on the neonatal lungs and kidneys.

The main problem in preventing this condition is identification of the

Table 8.7   Common uses of antimicrobials in pregnancy

Condition	Medication	Authors
Caesarean section prophylaxis	Penicillin or cephalosporin	Mallarat et al (1990)[36] Schwarz & Grolle (1981)[16]
	?Metronidazole	Duff (1987)[18]
Premature membrane rupture	Antibiotics of little prophylactic benefit	Ohlsson (1989)[60]
Urinary tract infection	Penicillin or cephalosporin	McNeely (1988)[73]
Group B streptococci	Penicillin prophylaxis	Tuppurdinen & Hallman (1989)[84]
	Chlorhexidine gel	Kollee et al (1989)[85]
Chlamydia trachomatis	Erythromycin Clindamycin/amoxycillin	Schachter et al (1986)[86] Crombleholme et al (1990)[87]
Malaria	Chloroquine	Some *Plasmodium falciparum*-resistant
Neisseria gonorrhoeae	Penicillin or spectinomycin/ cephalosporin	Alternative choices for resistance or penicillin allergy. *Chlamydia trachomatis* often also present
Acute chorioamnionitis	Broad-spectrum parenteral antibiotics	Treatment to start promptly. No general consensus as to the best antibiotic choice. Gilstrap (1990)[88]
Toxoplasmosis	Spiramycin or pyrimethamine/ sulphonamide combination	For acute infection of fetus Walpole et al (1991)[89]

carrier. Once isolated, these patients can be given prophylaxis with penicillin which is effective in eradicating the bacteria for a short period of time only. Colonization almost inevitably recurs when the treatment is stopped. In addition GBS colonization is intermittent rather than constant in those identified as carriers, and thus a number of patients would be missed if antenatal screening was to be made policy.[92] Intrapartum prophylaxis with penicillin effectively prevents vertical transmission.[84] Another approach is the vaginal application of chlorhexidine gel to those known to be carriers. Kollee et al[85] showed that this treatment is very effective in preventing vertical transmission during vaginal delivery. None of the neonates born to mothers known to be carriers at the time of delivery were found to be colonized with GBS. At the Aker Hospital[93] 2430 unselected consecutive parturients were shown to have a reduction of 77% in colonization of the neonates with GBS following the routine douching of labouring women with a 2% solution of chlorhexidine. Recently, Burman et al 1992[93a] have shown that antepartum chlorhexidine disinfection of the vagina reduced early morbidity among infants born to carriers of GBS. These results are comparable to those seen after penicillin prophylaxis.

CHLAMYDIA TRACHOMATIS

Chlamydia trachomatis is a well-established cause of pelvic inflammatory disease in the mother (endometritis or salpingitis) and conjunctivitis and pneumonitis in newborn infants. Uncertainty still prevails as to the relationship between chlamydia infection and PROM, preterm birth and puerperal infection. The prevalence of genital chlamydial infection varies depending on the population under study, being highest amongst non-Caucasian groups of less than 24 years of age. The vast majority of neonatal chlamydial infections occur during delivery;[94,95] however infection has been associated with breast-feeding,[96] and cases have been documented prior to birth.[97] Vertical transmission during vaginal delivery occurs in 50–70% of infants born to infected mothers.[98]

Various studies have examined the possible roles of maternal chlamydial infection in adverse pregnancy outcome. Suggested complications include PROM, preterm labour, low birth weight (less than 2500 g), intrauterine growth retardation, stillbirth, as well as intrapartum and postpartum maternal and neonatal infectious morbidity.[99,100] Several investigators have shown that the treatment of chlamydial infection during pregnancy decreases the incidence of the above adverse outcomes.[101,102]

To prevent neonatal morbidity, identification and treatment of maternal chlamydial infection during pregnancy is required. Schachter et al[86] offered treatment with oral erythromycin 400 mg four times a day for 7 days to 184 pregnant women at 36 weeks' gestation. Thirty-two women refused treatment and served as the control group for the study. Chlamydial infection or colonization occurred in only 7% of the treatment group as compared to 50% of the controls. Several studies have documented poor compliance with erythromycin therapy due to adverse gastrointestinal side-effects during pregnancy. In such cases a reduced dose of erythromycin or use of agents such as clindamycin and amoxicillin may be better tolerated.[87] Both clindamycin and amoxicillin appear to be effective in the treatment of chlamydia during pregnancy.[103] In all cases the partner should be treated to prevent reinfection.

VIRAL INFECTIONS

The vertical transmission of herpes genitalis with resultant disseminated infection and encephalitis in the neonate led to the adoption of a policy of elective caesarean section within 4 hours of membrane rupture for all those with active herpetic lesions at the time of labour.[104] Recent evidence however suggests that in cases of secondary herpetic infection, transfer of maternal antibodies to the fetus probably takes place, and this passive immunity offers protection against herpetic infection during vaginal delivery. Prober et al[105] reported a series of 34 neonates which showed no sign of herpetic infection following vaginal delivery of women with asymptomatic recurrent herpes at the time of labour. The value of weekly viral cultures must be questioned in the light of this knowledge and the fact that the likelihood of a woman with recurrent herpes shedding the virus asymptomatically at the time of delivery is of the order of 1.4%.

In cases of primary active genital herpes at the time of delivery, caesarean section should be the mode of delivery, within 4 hours of membrane rupture.

Acyclovir has been used successfully both in the treatment of herpetic disease of neonates, and also in the elimination of virus shedding and shortening of the eruption time in patients infected around term.[106,107] This form of treatment has been shown to be effective in cases of secondary herpes, and when given on average for 8 days prior to delivery has been demonstrated to eliminate virus secretion at the time of delivery.

TOXOPLASMOSIS

Congenital toxoplasmosis is characterized by the classical triad of hydrocephalus, chorioretinitis and intracerebral calcifications. Most cases of neonatal infection however will remain subclinical. There is a substantial risk of delayed infection up to a year of age, and repeated investigation until this time is important in order categorically to rule out infection.[108] The incidence of congenital infection is highest when maternal infection is acquired in the third trimester, whilst severity is worst when acquired in the first trimester. About 50% of mothers who acquire the infection during pregnancy will give birth to affected infants if not treated.[109] The incidence of congenital toxoplasmosis varies from 0.5 to 6.5 cases per thousand live births. Serologic screening is required before or very early in pregnancy to identify seronegative women at risk of becoming infected during pregnancy.[89,109]

Every mother who develops acute infection during pregnancy should be treated. Treatment is with spiramycin that achieves high levels in the placenta. If the fetus is affected then pyrimethamine and sulphonamides are administered from the fourth month. Chemotherapy reduces the incidence of congenital toxoplasmosis and the severity of the disease in the newborn. Intrauterine infection can be detected by fetal blood sampling, by amniocentesis and ultrasound examination.[110]

There have been isolated reports of pancytopenia following pyrimethamine and sulphamethoxydiazine therapy during pregnancy.[111] Women have however made an uneventful recovery following treatment with steroids, antibiotics, folinic acid and blood transfusion. Other cases have documented allergy to spiramycin during pregnancy when used in the treatment of toxoplasmosis.[112]

CANDIDA ALBICANS

Vulvovaginal candidiasis is a common cause of women presenting to either their general practitioner or to a hospital-based clinic. It has been estimated that 75% of women worldwide will suffer from the condition at some time during their lives.[113] *Candida albicans* acts as an opportunistic pathogen: attack rates are much more common in the pregnant woman.[114] Increased circulating levels of oestrogen and progesterone raise the glycogen content of vaginal epithelial cells, which favours the proliferation, adherence and germination of the yeast. These hormones may also directly stimulate the growth of *C. albicans*. In the final trimester the decrease in cell-mediated immunity of the mother will also lead to an increase in symptomatic episodes. Not only is the number of episodes increased but treatment with topical agents is much less successful during the third trimester, often leading to frequent recurrence of the condition.

Two major groups of drugs are used for the treatment of candidiasis during pregnancy — the polyenes, and the imidazoles. The polyenes were developed in the early 1950s, the best known being nystatin. They are both fungicidal and fungistatic but have no action against bacteria or viruses. From the patient's point of view they are not the final answer. The candidiasis tends to recur, and the pessaries tend to leak and stain the underclothes.

The imidazoles were introduced in the 1970s, the best known being clotrimazole (Canesten). They have a wide range of antifungal activity, some antibacterial activity but no antiviral activity. They can be taken in shorter courses, and some formulations have special adherent bases to prevent unwanted leakage from the vagina. Many of the imidazoles however carry the warning to avoid or use with caution during pregnancy. Fulconazole (Diflucan), which has been used with such efficacy in recurrent candidal infections, is at present contraindicated during pregnancy.[115]

Cases of candidal septicaemia have been recorded during pregnancy, when there has usually been an additional predisposing cause. In these cases 5-fluorocytosine and amphotericin B have proved successful forms of therapy.[116]

Although candidal colonization is common during pregnancy, candida is seldom the cause of chorioamnionitis. Occasional cases have been reported, usually associated with the presence of an intrauterine contraceptive device or cervical cerclage.[117] In these rare cases systemic treatment or delivery are the only options.

CONCLUSIONS

Antimicrobials have many applications in obstetrics. The selection of an appropriate agent is to a great extent dictated by the principle of safe prescribing during pregnancy. Many agents have however been shown to be both safe and effective when used in pregnancy and this has allowed us to extend their application in obstetric management. The increasing practice of interventional obstetrics has increased our need for successful microbiological vigilance and prophylactic intervention. The recognition of neonatal infectious morbidity has led to improved methods of detection and treatment of those at risk.

REFERENCES

1. Leading article. Teratogenic effects of sulphonamides. Br Med J 1965; 1: 142
2. Green K G. Bimez and teratogenic action. Br Med J 1963; 1: 56
3. Carter M P, Wilson F. Antibiotics and congenital malformation. Lancet 1968; i: 1267–1268
4. Carter M P, Wilson F. Clinical pitfalls in retrospective and prospective drug teratogenicity studies. Dev Med Child Neurol 1963; 5: 371–380
5. Williams J D, Brumfitt W, Condie A P et al. The treatment of bacteriuria in pregnant women with sulphamethoxazole and trimethoprim. A microbiological, clinical, and toxicological study. Postgrad Med J 45 (suppl): 71–75
6a. Rustia M, Shubick P. Induction of lung tumours and malignant lymphomas in mice by metronidazole. J Natl Cancer Inst 1972; 48: 721–726
6b. Leading article. Tetracyclines in pregnancy. Br Med J 1965; 1: 743–744
7. Conway N, Birt B D. Streptomycin in pregnancy. Effect on the fetal ear. Br Med J 1965; 2: 260–263
8. Adamsons K, Joelsson J. The effects of pharmacological agents upon fetus and newborn. Am J Obstet Gynecol 1966; 96: 437–440
9a. Good R, Johnson G. The placental transfer of kanamycin during late pregnancy. Obstet Gynecol 1971; 38: 60–72
9b. Eikenwald H F. Some observations on dosage and toxicity of kanamycin in premature and full term infants. Ann NY Acad Sci 1966; 132: 984–989
10. Gilstrap L C, Cunningham F G. Drugs and medications in pregnancy. Supplement 13. Williams obstetrics. Norwalk, CT: Appleton-Lange, 1987
11. Tolman K G, Sannella J J, Freston J W. Chemical structure of erythromycin and hepatotoxicity. Ann Intern Med 1974; 81: 58–61
12. Federal Drug Administration (FDA). Pregnancy categories for prescription drugs. FDA Drug Bull 1979: September
13. Moro M, Andrews M. Prophylactic antibiotics in caesarean section. Obstet Gynecol 1974; 44: 688–692
14. Weissberg S M, Edwards N L, O'Leary J A. Prophylactic antibiotics in caesarean section. Obstet Gynecol 1971; 38: 290–293
15. Gibbs R S. Clinical risk factors for puerperal infection. Am J Obstet Gynecol 1980; 55: 178–184
16. Swartz W H, Grolle K. The use of prophylactic antibiotics in caesarean section. J Reprod Med 1981; 26: 595–609
17. Languy M, Malledent Y, N'Guyen Q et al. Fatal maternal streptococcus A infection after caesarean section. Ann Fr Anesth Reanim 1990; 9: 477–449
18. Duff P. Prophylactic antibiotics for caesarean delivery: a simple cost effective strategy for prevention of postoperative morbidity. Am J Obstet Gynecol 1987; 157: 794–798
19. Richards W R. An evolution of the use of sulfonamide drugs in certain gynaecological operations. Am J Obstet Gynecol 1943; 46: 541
20. Heseltine H C, Thelen C. Sulfonamides as a prophylatic agent in conjunction with caesarean section. Am J Obstet Gynecol 1946; 52: 813
21. Keetel W C, Plass E D. Prophylactic administration of penicillin to obstetric patients. JAMA 1959; 142: 324
22. Mugford M, Kingston J, Chalmers I. Reducing the incidence of infection after caesarean section: implications of prophylaxis with antibiotics for hospital resources. Br Med J 1989; 299: 1003–1006
23. Burke J F. Preventive antibiotic management in surgery. Ann Rev Med 1973; 24: 289–294
24. Gordon H R, Phelps D, Blanchard K Prophylactic caesarean section antibiotics.

Maternal and neonatal morbidity before and after cord clamping. Obstet Gynecol 1979; 53: 151–156

25. Gjonnaess H. Antimicrobial prophylaxis in gynaecological and obstetric surgery. Scan J Infect Dis 1990; 70 (suppl): 52–67

26. Isaac B Unexplained fever. Boston, Ma: CRC Press, 1991

27. King C. Infection following caesarean section: a study of the literature and cases with emphasis on prevention. Cent Afr J Med 1989; 35: 556–570

28. Kelleher C J, Cardozo L D. A study of the morbidity associated with caesarean section at a London teaching hospital. Unpublished data

29. Green S L, Sarrubi F A, Bishop E H. Prophylactic antibiotics in high risk caesarean sections. Obstet Gynecol 1978; 51: 569

30. Wong R, Gee C L, Ledger W J. Prophylactic use of cefalozin in monitored obstetric patients undergoing caesarean section. Obstet Gynecol 51: 407

31. Kreutner A K, DelBene V E, Delamar D et al. Perioperative antibiotic prophylaxis in caesarean section. Obstet Gynecol 1978; 52: 279

32. Suonio S, Saarikoski S, Vohlonen I, Kauhanen O. Risk factors for fever, endometritis and wound infection after abdominal delivery. Int J Gynecol Obstet 1989; 29: 135–142

33. Moberg P J, Schedvins K. Use of cefuroxime in preventing post caesarean infection in high risk patients. Gynaecol Obstet Invest 1989; 28: 19–22

34. Gibbs R S, Weinstein A J. Bacteriologic effects of prophylactic antibiotics in caesarean section. Am J Obstet Gynecol 1976; 126: 226

35. Johnson S R, Ohm Smith M, Galask R P. Prophylactic antibiotics in obstetrics and gynaecology. In: Zuspan FP, Christian CD, eds. Controversy in obstetrics and gynaecology, vol 3. Philadelphia: WB Saunders, 1983

36. Mallaret M R, Blatter J P, Racinet C et al. Economic benefit of using antibiotics prophylactically in caesarean sections with little risk of infection. J Gynecol Obstet Biol Reprod Paris 1990; 19: 1061–1064

37. Racinet C, Mallaret M R, Ravier M et al. Antibiotic prophylaxis in caesarean sections without high risk of infection. Therapeutic trial of cefotetan versus placebo. Presse Med 1990; 19: 1755–1758

38. Galask R P, Weiner C. Comparison of single dose cefmetazole and cefotetan prophylaxis in women undergoing primary caesarean section. J Antimicrob Chemother 1989; 23 (suppl D): 105–108

39. Chan A C, Leung A K. Single dose prophylactic antibiotics in caesarean sections. Aust N Z J Obstet Gynaecol 1989; 29: 107–109

40. Howie P W, Davey P G. Prophylactic antibiotics in caesarean section. Important role but not always necessary. Br Med J 1990; 300: 2–3

41. Gerber B, Retzke F, Wilken H. Effectiveness of perioperative preventative use of antibiotics with ampicillin/gentamycin or cefotiam in abdominal caesarean section. Zentralbl Gynakol 1989; 111: 658–663

42. Morrison J C, Coxwell W L, Kennedy B S et al. The use of prophylactic antibiotics in patients undergoing caesarean section. Surg Gynecol Obstet 1973; 136: 425

43. Crombleholme W R, Green J R, Ohm-Smith M et al. Prophylaxis in caesarean section with cefmetazole and cefoxitin. J Antimicrob Chemother 1989; 23 (suppl): 97–104

44. Hawrylyshyn P A, Bernstein P, Papsin F R. Short term antibiotic prophylaxis in high risk patients following caesarean section. An J Obstet Gynecol 1983; 156: 285

45. Ganesh V, Apuzzio J J, Dispenziere B et al. Single dose trimethoprim-sulfamethoxazole prophylaxis for caesarean section. Am J Obstet Gynecol 1986; 154: 1113

46. Saltzman D H, Eron L J, Kay H H et al. Single dose antibiotic prophylaxis in high risk patients undergoing caesarean section. Obstet Gynecol 1985; 65: 655

47. Gonik B. Single versus three dose cefotaxime prophylaxis for caesarean section. Obstet Gynecol 1985; 65: 189

48. Elliot J P, Flaherty J F. Comparison of lavage or intravenous antibiotics at caesarean section. Obstet Gynecol 1986; 67: 29–32

49. Moellering R C, Wennersten C, Kunz L J et al. Emergence of gentamycin resistant bacteria: experience with tobramycin therapy of infections due to gentamycin resistant organisms. J Infect Dis 1976; 134 (suppl) : 540

50. Gibbs S, St Clair P J, Castillo M S, Castenada Y S. Bacteriologic effects of antibiotic prophylaxis in high risk caesarean section. Obstet Gynecol 1981; 57: 277–282

51. Stray-Pederson B, Hafstad A, Grøgaard J et al. The prevalence of cervical microorganisms during labour and the effect of intrapartum vaginal douching on neonatal colonization. Int J Maternal Fetal Med 1992; in press (see Gjonnaess [25])
52. Heitmann J A, Benrubi G I. Efficacy of prophylactic antibiotics for prevention of endometritis after forceps delivery. South Med J 1989; 82: 960–962
53. Alger L S, Lovchik J C, Hebel J R et al. The association of *Chlamydia trachomatis*, *Neisseria gonorrhoeae*, and Group B streptococcus with preterm rupture of the membranes and pregnancy outcome. Am J Obstet Gynecol 1988; 159: 397–404
54. Naessens A, Foulon W, Breynaert J et al. Postpartum bacteraemia and placental colonization with genital mycoplasmas and pregnancy outcome. Am J Obstet Gynecol 1989; 160: 647–650
55. Lang U, Schmid K, Braems G et al. Cervical mycoplasmas and pregnancy outcome. Vol. 1st World Congress for infectious diseases in Obstetrics and Gynaecology, Hawaii, p 61
56. Williams C M, Okada D M, Marshall J R et al. Clinical and microbiological risk evaluation for post caesarean section endometritis by multivariate discriminant analysis. Role of intraoperative mycoplasma, aerobes, and anaerobes. Am J Obstet Gynecol 1987; 156: 967–974
57. Amon E, Lewis S V, Sibau B M et al. Ampicillin in preterm premature rupture of membranes. A prospective randomised study. Am J Obstet Gynecol 1988; 159: 539
58. Morales W J, Angel J L, O'Brien W F et al. Use of ampicillin and corticosteroids in premature rupture of membranes. A randomised study. Obstet Gynecol 1989; 73: 721–726
59. Mardh P A, Helin I, Bobeck S et al. Colonisation pregnant and puerperal women and neonates with *Chlamydia trachomatis*. Br J Vener Dis 1980; 56: 96–100
60. Ohlsson A. Treatments of premature rupture of the membranes. A meta-analysis. Am J Obstet Gynecol 1989; 160: 890–906
61. Lettau R, Oberhauser F. Bacteriological examinations in cases of premature rupture of the membranes. Vol .1st World congress for infectious diseases in Obstetrics and Gynaecology, Hawaii, p 58
62. Morales W J, Angel J L, O'Brien W F et al. A randomised study of antibiotic therapy in idiopathic preterm labour. Obstet Gynecol 72: 829–833
63. Skoll M A, Moretti M L, Sibai B M. The incidence of positive amniotic fluid cultures in patients in preterm labour with intact membranes. Am J Obstet Gynecol 1989; 161: 813–816
64. Romero R, Sirtori M, Oyarzun E et al. Infection and labour. Prevalence, microbiology, and clinical significance of intraamniotic infection in women with preterm labour and intact membranes. Am J Obstet Gynecol 1989; 161: 817–824
65. Martin D H, Loutsky L, Eschenbach D A et al. Prematurity and perinatal mortality in pregnancies complicated by maternal Chlamydia trachomatis infections. JAMA 1982; 247: 1585–88
66. Minkoff H, Gruenbaum A N, Schwarz R H et al. Risk factors for prematurity and premature membrane rupture. A prospective study of vaginal flora in pregnancy. Am J Obstet Gynecol 1984; 150: 965–972
67. Newton E R, Dinsmoor M J, Gibbs R S. A randomised blinded placebo controlled trial of antibiotics in idiopathic preterm labour. Obstet Gynecol 1989; 74: 562–566
67a. Norman K, Pattinson R, De Sousa J, De Jong P. PRAM: a preterm labour randomised controlled trial investigating antibiotic intervention on a multicentre basis. Proceedings of 26th British Congress of Obstetrics and Gynaecology, Manchester, 7–10th July 1992, Abstracts (Part I) 3
68. Charles D, Edwards W R. Infectious complications of cervical cerclage. Am J Obstet Gynecol 1981; 141: 1065–1071
69. Chryssikopoulos A, Botis D, Vitoratos N et al. Cervical incompetence: a 24 year review. Int J Gynaecol Obstet 1988; 26: 245–253
70. Faro S. Antibiotic prophylaxis. Obstet Gynecol Infect 1989; 16: 279–289
71. Kessler I, Shoham Z, Lancet M et al. Complications associated with genital colonization in pregnancies with and without cerclage. Int J Gynaecol Obstet 1988; 27: 359–363
72. Williams J D. Bacteriuria in pregnancy. In: Asscher A W, Brumfitt W, eds. Microbial disease in nephrology. Chichester: Wiley, 1986: pp 159–181

73. McNeely S G Jr. Treatment of urinary tract infection in pregnancy. Clin Obstet Gynecol 1988; 31: 480–487
74. Chow A W, Jewesson P J. Pharmacokinetics and the safety of antimicrobial agents during pregnancy. Rev Infect Dis 1985; 7: 287–313
75. Jakobi P, Neiger R, Mertzbach D, Paldi E. Single dose antimicrobial therapy for the treatment of asymptomatic bacteriuria in pregnancy. Am J Obstet Gynecol 1987; 156: 1148–1152
76. Gilstrap L C, Leveno K J, Cunningham F G et al. Renal infection and pregnancy outcome. Am J Obstet Gynecol 1981; 141: 709
77. Duff Pyelonephritis in pregnancy. Clin Obstet Gynecol 1984; 27: 17–31
78. Lenke R R, Van Dorsten J P, Schrifin B S. Pyelonephritis in pregnancy. A prospective randomised trial to prevent recurrent disease evaluating suppressive therapy with nitrofurantoin and close surveillance. Am J Obstet Gynecol 1983; 146: 953–955
79. Barnick C G W, Cardozo L. The lower urinary tract in pregnancy, labour and the puerperium. Prog Obstet Gynaecol 1991; 9: 195–206
80. Kunin C M. Detection, prevention and management of urinary tract infections. 4th ed. Philadelphia, PA: Lea & Febiger, 1987
81. Vollard E J, Clasener H A L, Zambon J V et al. Prevention of catheter associated Gram negative bacilluria with norfloxacin by selective decontamination of the bowel and high urinary concentration. J Antimicrob Chemother 1989; 23: 915–922
82. Leigh D A, Emmanuel F X, Sedgwick J, Dean R. Post operative urinary tract infection and wound infection in women undergoing caesarean section. A comparison of two study periods in 1985 and 1987. J Hosp Infect 1990; 15: 107–116
83. Stickler D J, Chawla J C. The role of antiseptics in the management of patients with long term indwelling bladder catheters. J Hosp Infect 1987; 10: 219–228
84. Tuppurainen N, Hallman M. Prevention of neonatal Group B streptococcal disease. Intrapartum detection and chemoprophylaxis of heavily colonised parturients. Obstet Gynecol 1989; 73: 583–587
85. Kollee L A A, Speyer I, Vankuijek M A P et al. Prevention of Group B streptococci transmission during delivery by vaginal application of chlorhexidine gel. Eur J Obstet Gynaecol Reprod Biol 1989; 31: 47–51
86. Schanchter J, Sweet R L, Grossman M, Landers D, Robbie M, Bishop E. Experience with the routine use of erythromycin for chlamydial infections during pregnancy. N Engl J Med 1986; 314: 276–279
87. Crombleholme W R, Schachter J, Grossman M, Landers D V, Sweet R L. Amoxycillin therapy for Chlamydia trachomatis during pregnancy. Obstet Gynecol 1990; 75: 752–756
88. Gilstrap L C. Acute chorioamnionitis. In: Gilstrap L C, Faro S, eds. Infections in pregnancy. New York: Wiley/Liss, 1990: 38–44
89. Walpole I R, Hodgen N, Bower C. Congenital toxoplasmosis: a large survey in Western Australia. Med J Aust 1991; 154: 720–4724
90. Boyer K M, Gotoff S P. Prevention of early onset neonatal Group B streptococcal disease with selective intrapartum chemoprophylaxis. N Engl J Med 1986; 314: 1665–1669
91. Lim D V, Kanarek K S, Peterson M E. Magnitude of colonisation and sepsis by Group B streptococci in newborn infants. Current Microbiol 1982; 7: 99–101
92. Lewin E B, Amsten M S. Natural history of Group B streptococcus colonisation and its therapy during pregnancy. Am J Obstet Gynecol 1981; 139: 512–515
93. Halvard G. Antimicrobial prophylaxis in gynaecological and obstetric surgery. Scand J Infect Dis 1990; 70 (suppl): 52–67
93a. Burman L G, Christensen P, Christensen K et al. Prevention of excess morbidity associated with group B streptococci by vaginal chlorhexidine disinfection during labour. Lancet 1992; 340 (8811): 65–69
94. Judson F N. Assessing the number of genital chlamydial infections in the United States. J Reprod Med 1985; 30: 269–272
95. Heggie A, Lumicao G G, Stuart L A, Gyves M T. Chlamydia trachomatis infection in mothers and infants. A prospective study. Am J Dis Child 1981; 135: 507–511
96. Frommel G T, Rothenberg R, Wang S P, Mcintosh K. Chlamydia infection of mothers and infants. Paediatrics 1979; 95: 28–32
97. Thorp J M, Katz V L, Fowler L J, Kurtzman J T, Bowes W A. Fetal death from

chlamydial infection across intact amniotic membranes. Am J Obstet Gynecol 1989; 161: 1245–1246

98. Schachter J, Grossman M, Sweet R L et al. Prospective study of perinatal transmission of *Chlamydia trachomatis*. JAMA 1986; 255: 3374–3377

99. Gravett M G, Nelson H P, DeRouen T, Critchlow C, Eschenbach D A, Holmes K K. Independent association of bacterial vaginosis and *Chlamydia trachomatis* infection with adverse pregnancy outcome. JAMA 256: 1899–1903

100. The Johns Hopkins Study Group for cervicitis and adverse pregnancy outcome. Association of *Chlamydia trachomatis* and *Mycoplasma hominis* with intrauterine growth retardation and preterm delivery. Am J Epidemiology 1989; 129: 1247–1251

101. Ryan G M, Abdella T N, McNelley S G, Baselski V S, Drummond D E. *Chlamydia trachomatis* infection during pregnancy and effect of treatment on outcome. Am J Obstet Gynecol 1990; 162: 34–39

102. Cohen I, Veille J C, Calkins B M. Improved pregnancy outcome following successful treatment of chlamydial infection. JAMA 1990; 263: 3160–3168

103. McNeely S G, Ryan G M, Baselski V. Treatment of chlamydia infection of the cervix during pregnancy. Sex Transm Dis 1989; 16: 60–62

104. Gibbs R S. Genital herpes in pregnancy. Obstet Gynecol Rep 1988; 1: 102–108

105. Prober C G, Sullender W M, Yasukawa L L et al. Low risk of herpes simplex virus infection in neonates exposed to the virus at the time of vaginal delivery to mothers with recurrent genital herpes simplex virus infections. N Engl J Med 1987; 316: 240–244

106. Salo O P, Lassus A, Hovi T, Fiddian A P. Double blind placebo controlled trial of oral acyclovir in recurrent genital herpes. Eur J Sex Transm Dis 1983; 1: 95–98

107. Nilson A E, Aasen T. Efficacy of oral acyclovir in the treatment of initial and recurrent genital herpes. Lancet 1982; ii: 571–573

108. Tietze P E, Jones J E. Parasites during pregnancy. Prim Care 1991; 18: 75–99

109. Foulon W, Naessens A, Mahler T, de Waele M, de Catte L, de Meuter F. Prenatal diagnosis of congenital toxoplasmosis. Obstet Gynecol 1990; 76: 769–772

110. Hohlfeld P, Forestier F, Marion S, Thulliez P, Marcon P, Daffos F. *Toxoplasma gondii* infection during pregnancy: T lymphocyte subpopulations in mothers and fetuses. Pediatr Infect Dis J 1990; 9: 878–881

111. Pajor A. Pancytopenia in a patient given pyrimethamine and sulphamethoxidiazine during pregnancy. Arch Gynecol Obstet 1990; 247: 215–217

112. Ostlere L S, Langtry J A, Staughton R C. Allergy to spiramycin during prophylactic treatment of fetal toxoplasmosis. Br Med J 1991; 302: 970

113. Sobel J D. Epidemiology and pathenogenesis of recurrent vulvovaginal candidiasis. Am J Obstet Gynecol 1985; 158: 924–934

114. Morton R S, Rashid S. Candidal vaginitis, natural history predisposing factors and prevention. Proc R Soc Med 1977; 70 (suppl 4): 3–6

115. Richardson R G. (ed) Fluconazole and its role in vaginal candidiasis. London: Royal Society of Medicine Services, 1989

116. Potasman I, Leibovitz Z, Sharf M. Candida sepsis in pregnancy and the postpartum period. Rev Infect Dis 1991; 13: 146–149

117. Donders G G, Moerman P, Caudron J, Van Assche F A. Intra-uterine Candida infection: a report of four infected fetusses from two mothers. Eur J Obstet Gynecol Reprod Biol 1991; 38: 233–238

9. The role of infection in the pathogenesis of preterm labour

R. F. Lamont   N. Fisk

The rate of preterm delivery varies from country to country and from institution to institution, but probably lies between 5 and 10% of all births. Despite this, preterm birth accounts for a disproportionate percentage of perinatal deaths, although morbidity and mortality fall with increasing gestational age and increasing birth weight. Rush et al[2] have reported that 85% of neonatal deaths not due to lethal congenital malformation occur in infants with gestational ages between 32 and 37 weeks. While the survival rate for very low birth weight infants (less than 1500 g) has improved greatly over the last three decades, the incidence of major handicap remains unchanged at 6–7% of all preterm births.[3] The decline in perinatal mortality is largely attributable to improved neonatal intensive care which has been achieved at great expense. The estimated cost of neonatal intensive care in the USA in 1980 exceeded $460 000 000. If all neonates had been born at term, the estimated cost would have been just $50 000 000. The social and emotional cost of perinatal mortality and morbidity associated with preterm birth is immeasurable.[4]

The aetiology of preterm labour (PTL) is poorly understood, but certain associated factors are known. Sociobiological variables such as small stature, low maternal weight, age and poor socioeconomic status are frequently found in women who deliver preterm. The incidence of spontaneous preterm delivery also increases significantly according to the number of previous abortions, whether spontaneous or induced, especially if they occurred during the second trimester. The highest risk of all occurs in women with two or more previous preterm births who have a 70% chance of repeating the process.[5]

Complications of the current pregnancy such as antepartum haemorrhage, pre-eclamptic toxaemia, anatomical abnormalities of the uterus, fetal abnormalities, and multiple pregnancy may also result in PTL and delivery. In approximately 50–60% of cases, one or more of the above associations may be found.

PREDICTION AND PREVENTION OF PRETERM LABOUR

Several scoring systems based on these associated factors have been proposed in an attempt to predict spontaneous PTL.[6] Unfortunately, these rely heavily on past obstetric history and are inappropriate for nulliparous women. Even if factors relating to the current pregnancy are included, then it may be possible to predict 75% of preterm births, but this is at the expense of placing 35% of all women in the at-risk category.[7,8] The hazards of applying unnecessary intervention to numerous false-positive scores must be balanced against the possible advantages accruing to each true positive among those treated. To date, some 20 risk assessment systems have been advocated to predict PTL, but this large number attests to the fact that none is ideal.

Even if a scoring system could be produced whereby those women who will deliver preterm could be accurately predicted, prophylactic measures to prevent PTL have been unsuccessful. In properly controlled trials, rest and cervical cerclage have not proven beneficial in this regard. Although there have been isolated reports of success with long-term oral[9] and parenteral[10] administration of beta-agonists or with a combination approach,[11] the utility of beta-agonists for PTL prophylaxis is unproven.[12]

EVIDENCE IMPLICATING INFECTION AS A CAUSE OF PRETERM LABOUR

To date, the evidence which implicates infection as a cause of preterm birth falls into two broad categories. Firstly, there is the increased risk of infection associated with preterm birth manifest clinically, bacteriologically and histologically in both neonates and mothers. Secondly, there is the association of various organisms with prematurity and preterm premature rupture of the membranes (PPROM).

Chorioamnionitis

Placentitis, funicitis (inflammation of the umbilical cord) and amnionitis are found most frequently in association with preterm birth.[13] In the past, chorioamnionitis was thought to be induced by non-infectious agents or factors such as changes in pH, anoxia or meconium.[14] This confusion probably arose because many organisms such as mycoplasmas which cause chorioamnionitis would not have been recovered in the past without more sophisticated methods. In addition, the fragility of some bacteria, like gonococci and chlamydiae, and the administration of antibiotics to the mother may have influenced the success of cultures. Finally, many positive cultures were classified as irrelevant in the past because the organisms grown were considered non-pathogenic. It is now established, however, that many organisms of low virulence may be pathogenic to the fetus and newborn[15] and may enhance the pathogenicity of other bacteria.[16]

Inflammation is a generalized, host response mechanism to a variety of stimuli including infection, trauma and immune phenomena. It is now accepted that most inflammatory lesions of the chorion and amnion and umbilical cord are due to infection.[17] Despite the apparent non-specificity of inflammation, its presence is important as it may be a key event in the initiation of PTL. Bacteria have been recovered from 72% of placentae of women with clinical and histological evidence of chorionamnionitis.[18] The identification of chorioamnionitis has important clinical implications for the preterm infant. Russell[19] compared two groups with and without chorioamnionitis and found that:

1. The absence of chorioamnionitis excluded significant neonatal sepsis within the first 48 hours of life.
2. Sepsis which was manifest from the third day onwards was not related to the presence of chorioamnionitis and was therefore probably not acquired in utero.
3. Fifty-seven of 247 neonates with chorioamnionitis developed probable sepsis compared with no cases of sepsis in those with no chorioamnionitis .
4. Forty-seven of 247 neonates with chorioamnionitis died in the perinatal period compared with only 4 in those without chorioamnionitis.
5. Infants with chorioamnionitis born near term of afebrile mothers with membranes ruptured for less than 24 hours had no infectious problems. In contrast, preterm infants born at less than 33 weeks of febrile mothers whose membranes had been ruptured for more than 48 hours had a perinatal mortality of 50% with all survivors showing evidence of sepsis. This suggests that the interrelationship between ruptured membranes, the onset of labour and infection are different in term and PTL.

Naeye & Peters[20] found a higher incidence of chorioamnionitis in the placentae of women delivering between 20 and 28 weeks (23%) compared to women delivering between 33 and 37 weeks (11%). Guzick & Winn[21] found that 25% of preterm deliveries could be attributed to histopathological evidence of chorioamnionitis either alone or with PPROM. They concluded that occult intrapartum infection of the genital tract is an important cause of preterm delivery. Hillier et al[22] found that patients delivering preterm were five times more likely to have histological chorioamnionitis than those delivering at term.

Clinical and laboratory indices of infection

The clinical signs of chorioamnionitis are unreliable. Pyrexia and purulent vaginal discharge occur as late manifestations; fetal and maternal tachycardia may be secondary to sympathomimetic tocolytics; uterine tenderness and contractions can be non-specific, and leukocytosis is affected by pregnancy, labour and the use of steroids.[23] With the removal of many of these influences postpartum, the diagnosis of endometritis becomes a more accurate reflection of chorioamnionitis. Daikoku et al[24] noted a doubling in the incidence of postpartum endometritis in women delivering preterm compared to term, irrespective of whether the membranes were ruptured (19 versus 8%) or intact (13 versus 6% respectively).

Elevations in C-reactive protein (CRP) have been reported in association with clinical and histological features of infection in women with PTL and PPROM. CRP is an acute-phase reactant of hepatic origin and is released in response to general mediators of tissue inflammation such as interleukin-1 (IL-1), so it is not surprising that this association is far greater in the presence of histological chorioamnionitis compared to that diagnosed clinically.[25] Raised CRP has a sensitivity of 67–88% and specificity of 68–100% for chorioamnionitis in PPROM[26,27] and is considered to be superior to other currently available laboratory and clinical antenatal indicators of infection.[28–30] Between 27 and 55% of patients with PPROM, and 33–61% of those in PTL with intact membranes have elevated CRP.[31] The range of these frequencies reflects the controversy surrounding the appropriate upper limit of normal, which ranges from 7 to 40 mg/l.[30,32] Two groups have reported that women in PTL with elevated CRP were significantly more likely to be refractory to tocolytic therapy, implicating underlying infection as the cause of the PTL in those cases.[32,33] Those women who are refractory to the use of tocolytics have an increased risk of infection[34] and survival is known to be less in those babies born after 32 weeks where tocolytics were used in the presence of contractions and ruptured membranes.[1]

Amniotic fluid specimens for laboratory analysis have been obtained by transabdominal amniocentesis or aspiration of liquor amnii using an intrauterine pressure catheter. Leukocytes in the amniotic fluid have been reported to be associated with subsequent infection,[35] although most workers have found considerable overlap between infected and non-infected groups, precluding its use as a diagnostic test.[36–38] Nevertheless, the absence of leukocytes in the amniotic fluid correlates well with absence of infection.[37,39] More accurately, the detection of leukocyte esterases in amniotic fluid predicts amniotic fluid colonization[40] and clinical amnionitis.[41] Positive cultures in amniotic fluid obtained by amniocentesis occur in 3–48% of patients in PTL,[15,42] with a mean of 16% in a pooled series. Those with positive cultures were more likely to develop chorioamnionitis (58%), to be refractory to tocolytics (65%) and to rupture their membrane spontaneously (40%) compared to those with negative amniotic fluid cultures.[43] Women in labour with PPROM are less likely to undergo amniocentesis successfully compared to those with PPROM not in labour. These figures are therefore likely to be an underestimate, but a significantly increased incidence of positive cultures in women in PTL with contractions and ruptured membranes has been found compared to those with PPROM (39 versus 25%).[31]

Intact membranes are not necessarily a barrier to infection.[38,44] Indeed, intra-amniotic infection with intact membranes has been postulated as an explanation for the early onset of neonatal Group B streptococcal (GBS) infection, since fatal sepsis in the newborn may be observed too soon after membrane rupture to be acquired by passage through the birth canal.

Amniotic fluid glucose concentration has been suggested as a rapid, sensitive, inexpensive test for the detection of intra-amniotic infection in women with PTL and intact membranes.[45]

Preterm premature rupture of the membranes

Although infection is implicated in the aetiology of both PTL and PPROM, histological and microbiological evidence of infection is found more commonly in the presence of ruptured membranes.[19,31,46,47] Between 6 and 12% of pregnancies are complicated by spontaneous rupture of the membranes before labour begins and this is referred to as premature rupture of the membranes. When this situation arises before 37 completed weeks of pregnancy the condition is defined as preterm premature rupture of the membranes (PPROM), which occurs in 2–3% of pregnancies and approximately one-third of preterm deliveries.[48] Management requires balancing the risks of infection associated with prolongation of pregnancy against the risks of immaturity if delivery ensues spontaneously or through obstetric intervention.

The factors responsible for PPROM are unknown, but the clinical impression that patients with PPROM arrive on the labour ward in groups led to the suggestion that PPROM may be related to a drop in barometric pressure.[49] This has been refuted by Witter[50] and Marks et al[51] who found no correlation between PPROM, barometric pressure and the lunar phases.

There is a definite relationship between PPROM and infection, though whether this is cause or effect is unclear. Under different circumstances each may be the cause of the other. Cederquist et al[52] noted two peaks in the incidence of infection following rupture of the membranes, one before 12 hours and another after 72 hours. Using RANKIT analysis in 37 women with PPROM complicated by amniotic fluid infection syndrome, Romem et al[53] noted the existence of three separate clusters in duration of ruptured membranes: short (mean 6 hours), medium (40 hours) and long (210 hours) incubation periods. These authors suggested that in this first group, infection was the cause of membrane rupture.

The fetal risks of PPROM are due to prematurity, infection and the physical anomalies caused by the chronic absence of liquor. The earlier in gestation that membranes rupture, the longer it takes for labour to ensue.[54] When membranes rupture at term, 80–90% of women will be in labour after 24 hours but when the membranes rupture prematurely at 28 weeks, 25% of women are still not in labour after 1 week. Pulmonary hypoplasia and skeletal deformities as a result of oligohydramnios and fetal compression are well-recognized.[55]

The incidence of neonatal infection following PPROM has been reported to be between 0.5 and 25%. The difference in quoted rates can be explained by the criteria used to define infection, i.e. by positive blood cultures or clinical impression.[56,57]

Rush[58] found bacterial colonization in 41% of neonates after PPROM compared to 28% after premature rupture of the membranes at term and 23% of term infants after elective amniotomy. The incidence of amniotic fluid colonization has been estimated to be as high as 10% of term pregnancies in labour[59] though these organisms are likely to be of low virulence. After reaching the amniotic fluid bacteria may be aspirated by the fetus causing pneumonia, enter the auditory canal and cause otitis or meningitis, or the newborn may be clinically uninfected.

Bacteria which are able to cause disease in either the mother or the neonate have been shown to comprise part of the endogenous flora of the vagina and cervix of pregnant women. These women are often asymptomatic, even when subsequent infection of the newborn occurs. Whether or not infection precedes or results from PPROM, it must not be forgotten that the major complication of PPROM is PTL and delivery with all the innate and associated iatrogenic complications.[48]

Neonatal and maternal morbidity from infection

At worst, infection can cause intrauterine death of the fetus or overwhelming neonatal infection and death. While perinatal mortality is easily quantifiable, infant morbidity as a consequence of infection is much more difficult to estimate. In those infants who survive, infection may cause damage in two ways. Firstly, there may be direct infective damage to immature organs before their anatomical, physiological or biochemical adaptations to extrauterine life are complete.

Alternatively, the long-term sequelae may result from the methods used to treat the infection, such as intermittent positive pressure ventilation, parenteral infusions or antibiotics like gentamicin and chloramphenicol.

Pryse-Davies & Hurley[60] obtained histological and microbiological data over a 10-year period from 835 neonatal necropsies. Bacteria were isolated from approximately 40, 20 and 10% of bronchial secretions, heart blood and cerebrospinal fluid of these infants respectively. Histological evidence of infection was found in 27.3% and an infective cause of death given in 3% of all babies. The incidence of disseminated infection (deemed present when an organism was cultured from heart blood as well as from one other site) was 14.3%. The most frequently encountered bacteria were *Pseudomonas* sp., *Escherichia coli*, staphylococci, streptococci and *Klebsiella aerogenes*, comprising 86% of the isolations in disseminated infection. Pryse-Davies & Hurley concluded that infection was an important cause of perinatal death.[60]

Infectious morbidity in preterm neonates is about 10 times greater than that for term neonates and amniotic fluid infection syndrome (congenital pneumonia and chorioamnionitis) was the most frequent cause of death in the United States Collaborative Perinatal Project.[61] Preterm neonates are known to have significantly higher rates of sepsis, including pneumonia, gastroenteritis and skin infections.[62] This might be due to the increased susceptibility of the preterm neonate to infection but could be attributed to intrauterine infection leading to preterm birth. It has been proposed that the onset of PTL women with intrauterine infection may be part of the normal maternal host defence mechanisms against infection.[31]

Maternal infectious morbidity follows a similar pattern, being more common after preterm than term delivery. Intrapartum fever is more common in association with PTL, while endometritis is two or three times more common following preterm birth.[24] There is also evidence that women with a history of pelvic inflammatory disease or previous intra-uterine contraceptive device usage are at relatively increased risk (odds ratio 2.4 and 2.3 respectively) of preterm birth than women without these risk factors.[63]

Coitus

Textbooks of obstetrics normally cite the findings of Pugh & Fernandez[64] as evidence that sexual intercourse during pregnancy causes no harm. Their study claimed to find no harmful effects but showed that PPROM, PTL and antepartum haemorrhage were associated with shorter intervals since the last coitus compared with pregnancies without such complications. More recently, Goorgakopoulos et al[65] found no increase in coital or orgasmic frequency between women who laboured preterm and those who delivered spontaneously at term.

A larger study of coitus during pregnancy, conducted by Zachau-Christiansen & Ross[66] found a relationship between low birth weight and coitus, but the authors concluded that coitus was not of aetiological importance in preterm delivery. In 1981, Naeye et al[67] found that coitus during pregnancy was strongly associated with birth weight of less than 2500 g and an excess of perinatal deaths. A significant proportion of the increase in perinatal mortality associated with coitus is due to the amniotic fluid bacterial infection.

This was partly due to an increase in the severity of infection. The strong association between coitus and infection is independent of other factors known to predispose to infection, i.e. low socioeconomic status, non-white race, cervical incompetence and a prolonged labour.[68]

In pursuit of a causal relationship Naeye & Ross[69] carried out a prospective study of 501 pregnancies among mainly Zulu women in a clinic near Durban, South Africa. Three groups were studied with roughly equal numbers. One group refrained from coitus during the pregnancy; a second group engaged in coitus but used condoms and the third group had coitus without the use of condoms. Chorioamnionitis limited to the extraplacental membranes was frequent only when coitus without a condom had taken place within 2 days of delivery. Preterm delivery and birthweight under 2500 g were most frequent when there had been recent coitus and an amniotic fluid infection was present. Spontaneous rupture of the membranes was most frequent when there had been recent coitus with orgasm and the membranes were inflamed. This study would appear to confirm that coitus during pregnancy is associated with an increased frequency of acute chorioamnionitis and amniotic fluid infections but the study was performed in what may be considered to be a high-risk population.

Coitus may predispose to chorioamnionitis through the actions of seminal fluid which facilitate the passage of bacteria through the cervical mucous plug to infect the fetal membranes. Proteolytic enzymes in the seminal fluid have been shown to increase the permeability of cervical mucus.[70] Bacteria can also attach themselves to mobile spermatozoa which may facilitate their penetration through the cervical mucous plug.[71] Uterine contractions are a feature of orgasm[72] and the resulting sharp increase in intrauterine pressure may further predispose to membrane rupture.[73,74]

The fact that the frequency of amniotic infections and their complications were nearly as low in those using condoms in the Durban study as those who abstained from coitus suggests a direct or indirect action of seminal fluid rather than a mechanical effect of coitus alone.

Urinary tract infection

About 3% of pregnancies are complicated by asymptomatic bacteriuria and about 30% of these will progress to become symptomatic if left untreated. Acute pyelonephritis is associated with preterm labour,[75,76] but the relationship between asymptomatic bacteriuria, preterm delivery and low birth weight is less clear and remains controversial.

A meta-analysis by Romero et al found that women with asymptomatic bacteriuria had a higher rate of preterm births and low birth weight than non-bacteriuric women, and eradication of asymptomatic bacteriuria with antibiotics reduces the rate of preterm birth and low birth weight.[31] It has been proposed that this reduction in the incidence of preterm birth and low birth weight is not due to prevention of pyelonephritis. Rather, an alternative hypothesis suggests that bacteriuria is an indicator of abnormal genital colonization and antibiotics, used to treat urinary tract infection, eradicate genital tract pathogens, which reduces the chance of ascending infection and chorioamnionitis.

Intrauterine infection

The plethora of terms used to describe intrauterine infection is confusing and highlight the differing definitions and nomenclature used in North

America and Europe. In the USA, 'amniotic fluid infection' describes histological inflammation of the chorionic membranes, whereas 'intra-amniotic infection' is defined as the presence of microorganisms in amniotic fluid retrieved by amniocentesis, irrespective of the presence or absence of clinical signs of infection (fever, uterine tenderness, foul-smelling vaginal discharge, fetal or maternal tachycardia). 'Chorioamnionitis' in the USA is defined as the clinical syndrome described above, associated with microbial invasion of the amniotic fluid.[31] In the UK, chorioamnionitis is used interchangeably with all these terms but should indicate whether this is based on clinical or histological criteria.

The clinical manifestations of any infection are related to a multitude of factors including the size of inoculum, virulism of the microorganism, host defence mechanisms, the specific time of clinical observation, and the clinical definition of infection. Microorganisms may gain access to the amniotic cavity and the fetus through a number of pathways. The most important is the ascending route from the upper vagina and cervix. Histological chorioamnionitis is most common and severe at the site of membrane rupture and bacteria identified in cases of congenital neonatal infections are similar to those found in the genital tract. Histological chorioamnionitis is found more commonly in first-born twins and is not found in isolation in second twins. As the membranes of the first twin are generally apposed to the cervix, this is taken as evidence in favour of ascending infection.[31] Rupture of the membranes is not a prerequisite for intra-amniotic infection, as bacteria are capable of crossing intact membranes.[77] Many studies have shown positive amniotic fluid cultures within a short time of membrane rupture, and no correlation between duration of rupture and the incidence of positive culture.[37] Cederquist et al[52] found an early peak in neonatal cord immunoglobulin levels following ruptured membranes, suggesting that some infants were infected before membrane rupture.

ENDOGENOUS VAGINAL FLORA IN PREGNANCY

Quantitative studies comparing pregnant women with non-pregnant pre-menopausal women have shown that the vaginal flora is more abundant[78] and more homogeneous[79] in pregnancy. In both pregnant and non-pregnant women, counts of anaerobic bacteria are greater than aerobic. *Lactobacillus* sp. are numerically dominant in pregnancy, and lactobacilli are more common and anaerobes less common when compared to the non-pregnant state. From quantitative data, *Escherichia coli* and *Bacteroides fragilis* appear to be numerically under-represented in the vaginal flora in pregnancy. While some genital infections are due to exogenous pathogens like *Neisseria gonorrhoeae*, the majority are endogenous. This suggests that either some endogenous organisms possess greater virulence than previously recognized or their virulence changes during pregnancy.

Change of vaginal flora throughout pregnancy

Goplerud et al[80] reported on the endocervical flora of pregnant women during the first, second and third trimesters of pregnancy, the third postpartum day and the sixth postpartum week. The prevalence of significant organisms varied between groups but some general trends emerged. Several groups of microorganisms, such as anaerobic cocci and Gram-negative rods, declined during pregnancy with the most substantial decrease being in the anaerobic flora. Moberg et al[81] noted that anaerobic organisms decreased from early pregnancy to labour, whereas aerobic organisms remained relatively constant. Aerobic lactobacilli and yeasts on the other hand increased as the pregnancy progressed.[80]

In summary, the endogenous microbial flora of the vagina and cervix in pregnancy is homogeneous and mainly composed of organisms of low virulence. However, a mixture of aerobic and anaerobic species, which are often found in association with post-abortal sepsis and puerperal endometritis, can be detected.[82] The total flora in pregnancy is more abundant than in the non-pregnant state although the number of anaerobes is actually reduced. Aerobic organisms remain relatively constant while the number of lactobacilli increases and the number of anaerobes decreases progressively throughout pregnancy. These physiological alterations that occur during normal pregnancy may serve to protect the fetus. The vaginal flora appears to become progressively more benign during pregnancy, so that at birth it predominantly comprises of organisms that do not pose a significant hazard to the fetus passing through the heavily colonized birth canal.

VAGINAL ORGANISMS ASSOCIATED WITH PRETERM LABOUR AND DELIVERY

Several organisms have been associated with preterm birth and low birth weight. The strength of this association varies with the organism studied but only rarely have the various organisms been studied simultaneously.[46,83]

Group B haemolytic streptococcus

The reported mortality from GBS is 55%,[84] with low birth weight infants at particular risk. In a prospective study of 6700 parturients, Regan et al[85] demonstrated a significantly increased incidence of PPROM and preterm delivery among women colonized with GBS. After 34 weeks' gestation, of 94 mothers colonized with GBS, 25% experienced PPROM compared to only 8.8% of the total population ($P<0.005$).

Gonococcus

Neisseria gonorrhoeae has been found in association with amniotic fluid infection syndrome.[86] Women colonized with gonococcus have been found to have a 55% incidence of PPROM[87] and a 67% incidence of preterm birth.[88]

Anaerobes

There are some data which support *Bacteroides* sp. and other anaerobes as being implicated in the aetiology of PTL. Miller et al[15] and Bobbit et al[89] have recorded an incidence of *Bacteroides* sp. colonization of liquor in 25% of women in PTL with intact membranes. Evaldson et al[90] found *Bacteroides fragilis* in the cervix, amniotic fluid or placentae of 23% of women with PPROM. Wahbeh et al[91] performed transabdominal amniocentesis in 33 women in spontaneous PTL before 35 weeks with intact membranes. Bacteria were isolated from 7 women (21.2%) and anaerobic bacteria were isolated from all 7 women. Lamont et al[46] found anaerobic organisms in about 50% of women admitted in PTL with abnormal genital colonization.

Listeria

Data concerning the risk of preterm delivery in offspring of mothers with listeriosis are difficult to obtain because of the non-specific clinical nature of the disease and the difficulty in growing the organism. Those infants infected in utero appear to be delivered early.[92] Relier[93] found that 49 of 76 infants with listeriosis delivered spontaneously between 27 and 36 weeks' gestation.

The genital mycoplasmas

Mycoplasmas and ureaplasmas are a distinct group of microorganisms differing in important biological characteristics from bacteria, viruses, fungi, protozoa and chlamydiae.[94] While genital mycoplasmas are well-recorded as being associated with diseases of the genital tract in women, such as Bartholin's abscess, vaginitis and cervicitis, pelvic inflammatory disease, post-abortal sepsis and postpartum fever,[95] increasing interest is being paid to the role of genital mycoplasmas in disorders of reproduction such as infertility, habitual abortion and stillbirth.[96]

Shurin et al[97] claimed a significantly increased incidence of ureaplasma colonization in infants whose placentae showed chorioamnionitis. They further suggested that since *Ureaplasma urealyticum* was previously considered to be of little virulence, and therefore not specifically cultured, this might explain why chorioamnionitis was reported as occurring in uninfected pregnancies. Kass et al[98] in a prospective study, tested the hypothesis that ureaplasmas might be associated with an excess risk of preterm delivery and found that significantly more low birth weight infants showed a fourfold increase in neonatal antibody titres to *Ureaplasma urealyticum*. They also found that this excess risk of PTL could be reduced by administration of erythromycin.

Embree et al[99] studied 446 high-risk pregnancies. Ureaplasmas but not mycoplasmas were recovered significantly more often from the study group than from the control group. Isolation of both *Mycoplasma hominis* and ureaplasmas was associated with chorioamnionitis. Conversely, ureaplasmas but not *Mycoplasma hominis* were associated with preterm birth, low birth weight and intrauterine growth retardation.

Blanco et al[100] compared 52 women with clinical intra-amniotic infection to matched controls. *Mycoplasma hominis* was isolated in 35% of study patients compared with 8% of controls (p<0.01). Kundsin et al[101] found significantly more ureaplasmas colonized the inner aspect of the chorion of infants who were born preterm, weighed less than 2500 g or received neonatal intensive care. Lamont et al[83] found that 89% of women admitted in PTL between 26 and 34 weeks' gestation were colonized by *Mycoplasma hominis*, *Ureaplasma urealyticum* or *Chlamydia trachomatis*. The evidence is accumulating to link mycoplasmas and ureaplasmas with sporadic or recurrent miscarriage as well as PTL.[83,102]

Other organisms

Organisms commonly associated with vaginitis, such as trichomonas, are more common in the vaginal flora during pregnancy. Taylor[103] stated that 'failure to treat a severe case of *Trichomonas vaginalis* during the last two trimesters of pregnancy invites infection of the amnion and possible premature rupture of the membranes and preterm delivery'. Bobbit & Ledger[13] found monilial isolates with no other implicated organisms in amniotic fluid of women in PTL. Candidal chorioamnionitis diagnosed by amniocentesis has been reported in association with subsequent preterm delivery in 6 cases, though in three an intrauterine contraceptive device was in situ.[104] Many other common organisms or previously unsuspected pathogens have been implicated as a cause of chorioamnionitis in preterm delivery, including even *Lactobacillus* sp.[105] Genital microorganisms found in association with PTL and chorioamnionitis are shown in Table 9.1

Host defence mechanisms

In women with intra-amniotic infection, less than 5% of the neonates have clinically apparent sepsis. As a result of this low infection rate, a number of investigators have suggested that host defence mechanisms either prevent or attenuate development of intra-amniotic infections. A number of factors implicated in host defence are thought to be present in amniotic fluid, including polymorphonuclear leukocytes, lysozyme, betalysin, transferrin, immunoglobulins and an inhibitory factor which appears to be related to a

Table 9.1   Genital microorganisms found in association with 24 cases of histological chorioamnionitis following preterm delivery. *Lactobacillus* sp., *Diphtheroides* and *Staphylococcus epidermidis* have been excluded from the analysis[106]

Gram-positive cocci
Aerobic
Streptococcus viridans (2)
Streptococcus faecalis (3)
Beta-haemolytic streptococcus Group B (2)
Non-haemolytic streptococcus (2)

Anaerobic
Anaerobic streptococcus (2)
Microaerophilic streptococcus (4)

Gram-negative rods
Aerobic
Coliforms
   Escherichia coli (2)
   Klebsiella sp. (1)
   Proteus sp. (1)

Haemophilus sp.
   Haemophilus influenzae

Anaerobic
Bacteroides sp.
   Bacteroides fragilis (2)
   Bacteroides non-fragilis (9)

Gram-negative cocci
Neisseria gonorrhoeae (1)
Veillonella sp. (2)

Gram-variable cocci
Gardnerella vaginalis (1)

Yeasts
Candida albicans (2)

Others
Mycoplasma hominis (8)
Ureaplasma urealyticum (18)
Chlamydia trachomatis (1)

Numbers in brackets show the number of isolates.

zinc–peptide complex. This protective effect varies between individuals and at different stages of pregnancy. The capacity of amniotic fluid to inhibit bacterial growth increases as the life of the gestation increases and is diminished if meconium is present. It can also be overwhelmed by too large an inoculum of bacteria.

MECHANISM OF NORMAL LABOUR

Before it is possible to suggest a mechanism whereby bacteria may induce PTL, it is necessary to know the mechanisms of onset of normal labour.

Normal parturition requires the uterine cervix to change substantially to reduce resistance to the powerfully expulsive efforts of the uterine corpus, and prostaglandins (PGs) have an essential role in each of these processes.[107] This central role of PGs in human parturition has been well-documented:

1. There is a marked increase in the concentration of free arachidonic acid (AA), the obligate precursor of PG synthesis in the amniotic fluid (AF) of women in labour compared to women who are not in labour. The concentration of AA in AF continues to increase with increasing cervical dilation.[108]

2. The increase in free AA in AF during labour is disproportionately higher than that of any other free fatty acid.[109]

3. The introduction of AA into the AF of women in the second or third trimester of pregnancy where there has been intrauterine death is promptly followed by clinically normal labour and delivery.[109]

4. The high AA content of human amnion and chorion[110] is mainly sequestered in the phosphatidyl ethanolamine (PE) pool.[111,113] As labour progresses, there is a marked reduction in the AA content of PE.[112,124] The phospholipase A_2 (PLA_2) activity of human fetal membranes preferentially hydrolyses AA from the PE.[113]

5. Part of the PLA_2 activity of human fetal membranes is sequestered in the lysosomes[114] and an alteration in lysosomal activity can be demonstrated in amnions obtained from women in labour compared to amnions from non-labouring women.[115]

6. PG synthetase inhibitors such as indomethacin can inhibit uterine contractions in threatened PTL.[116]

7. The marked rise in AF levels of PGs during term labour and the rise in PG metabolites with advanced labour indicate that PGs participate in the mechanism of normal labour.

MICROORGANISMS AS A POSSIBLE TRIGGER FOR PRETERM LABOUR

PTL may be due to a normal signal occurring too early in pregnancy but is more likely due to an abnormal signal and there is increasing evidence that infection may be such a trigger.

There is a wide range of vaginal organisms present in women admitted in PTL. Almost 50% of women admitted in spontaneous early PTL have abnormal genital colonization compared to only 15% in a control group and in about half of these, anaerobic organisms were detected. Significantly more women were colonized by *Ureaplasma urealyticum* (86%) and high numbers of *Mycoplasma hominis* (18%). *Chlamydia trachomatis* was not found in the control group but in 8% of the women in PTL. The subsequent rate of chorioamnionitis (56%) and neonatal infection (23%) was significantly higher in the study group than in the control group (10 and 4% respectively).[46,83] With increasing gestation, the numbers of lactobacilli increase. This acidophilic commensal is thought to have the role of maintaining a significantly acid vaginal pH. At low pH, pathogens have a limited growth potential in vitro, and maintenance of a low vaginal pH may be protective against ascending infection. Women in PTL with intact membranes have a significantly higher mean vaginal pH.[117] If cervicovaginal pH is increased due to insufficient or poor-quality lactobacilli or other factors, this may lead to a proliferation of pathogens or an alteration in the balance of virulence of existing commensals .

Penetration of microorganisms through the cervix into the lower uterine segment

There are a number of ways in which microorganisms may initiate contractions after gaining access to the extraplacental membranes or the amniotic fluid.

Immunoglobulin A (IgA) secretory immunoglobulin is an important part of mucosal membrane defence which is present in cervical and vaginal fluid. Production of IgA-specific protease is considered an important feature of pathogenic strains of *Neisseria gonorrhoeae*[118] and has also been demonstrated in *Ureaplasma urealyticum*.[119] Mucin is a complex host molecule which contains considerable neuraminic acid. A number of genital tract microorganisms possess neuraminidase and mucinase activities.[120] Production of one or both of these enzymes has been considered helpful for gastrointestinal pathogens in gaining access to host cells. It is possible that mucinase and neuraminidase-producing cervicovaginal microorganisms may impair the defensive function of the occluding cervical mucous plug in pregnancy. Bacterial mucolytic action may further impair local cervical defence mechanisms, as the cervical mucous plug is initially displaced by uterine contractions, cervical ripening or obstetrical digital examination, all of which may take place during PTL.

Microorganisms release a large variety of proteases into their immediate environment. Bacterial proteases are often more powerful and not as specific in their hydrolytic abilities as mammalian proteases. Many different endogenous cervicovaginal organisms produce numerous proteases which are active on extracellular matrix substances, which give strength and substance to fetal membranes and cervical tissues.[120] These enzymes include collagenases and elastases as well as less specific proteases. Bacteria, and the collagenases which they produce, can clearly impair the structural integrity (tensile strength, elasticity, and work to rupture) of fetal membranes.[121] Similarly, hydrolytic enzymes contained within leukocytes also appear to weaken focally fetal membrane preparations. Endogenous or bacterial released PLA_2 may further reduce membrane tensile strength, probably by activating endogenous collagenase.[122] Elevated levels of nonspecific proteases in vaginal washings at 24 weeks' gestation have been found to be associated with subsequent occurrence of PPROM.[120] It is possible that bacterial and host proteases may be absorbed and induce collagenolysis in the cervix or lower uterine segment. However, it is more likely that endogenous fibroblasts produce collagenases which are released within these tissues as a result of prostaglandins. Such endogenous production of collagenases within the uterine structure is likely to account for the rise in serum collagenase observed during preterm and term parturition.[123]

Having gained access to the extraplacental membranes and decidua, cervicovaginal organisms may initiate or maintain labour in a number of different ways. Phospholipase-laden decidual cells are easily disrupted by various stimuli including infection and inflammation. This may result in release from the lysosomes of substances such as PLA_2 or phospholipase C which increase local concentrations of AA. In addition, many genital microorganisms themselves release PLA_2[124] or phospholipase C[121] which cleave AA from specific glycerophospholipids sequestered in the membranes. It has also been shown that amnion cells in tissue culture exposed to the intracellular or extracellular products of a wide range of bacteria produce increased amounts of PGE_2.[125,126]

The acute-phase reaction induced by such microbial infiltration may also result in elevated CRP levels which lower plasma zinc. This is reflected in lower zinc levels in AF, and a decrease in zinc-dependent antibacterial activity of AF may allow bacteria to proliferate in the liquor.

It is unlikely that bacteria themselves produce PGs since they do not appear to possess cyclooxygenase or lipoxygenase enzymes. Many Gram-negative organisms produce endotoxins or lipopolysaccharides which are components of the cell wall and these have been found in increased amounts in AF of women with intra-amniotic infection.[127] Endotoxins can stimulate PG production by several cell types such as macrophages[128] and human amnion and decidua,[31] which may contribute to the onset of labour. The quantity of endotoxins required to stimulate sufficient PG synthesis to initiate labour is not generally found in liquor so an additional mechanism must exist.

In search of an alternative mechanism (to a purely microbial-driven process) and to explain the increased bioavailability of PGs in infection associated with PTL, the similarities between fever and labour become apparent. Several substances, such as IL-1, tumour necrosis factor and platelet aggravating factor are secreted by macrophages or monocytes in response to stimulation by endotoxins. These intermediary substances of inflammation have multiple biological effects on several cell types, including macrophages, amnion and decidua[31,129-131] and drive the cascade of AA metabolism through lipoxygenase and cyclooxygenase pathways.[31,120,132-135]

The products of these pathways (PGE_2 $PGF_{2\alpha}$ leukotrienes, HETES) are responsible for inducing myometrial contractions and decreasing cervical resistance, the two processes essential for the progress of normal labour.[31,107,136-139] In this way, bacterial infiltration of the decidua and membranes may initiate and potentiate PTL. The mechanisms whereby

Table 9.2   Summary of evidence linking infection and preterm labour

1. Products of arachidonic acid metabolism are an essential part of normal parturition
2. Bacteria produce the enzyme phospholipase A_2[124]
3. Bacteria products increase prostaglandin E_2 production by amnion cells[125]
4. Bacteria produce proteases and other enzymes which may facilitate penetration of the cervical mucous plug and invasion of the membranes[120]
5. Endotoxins induce macrophages/monocytes to produce substances such as interleukin-1, tumour necrosis factor or platelet-aggravating factor which stimulate synthesis of prostaglandins[31]
6. In the amniotic fluid of women with intra-amniotic infection and preterm labour there are significantly increased levels of prostaglandins[31]
7. A wide range of microorganisms associated with preterm labour and chorioamnionitis cause an increase in prostaglandin E_2 production by amnion cells[126]

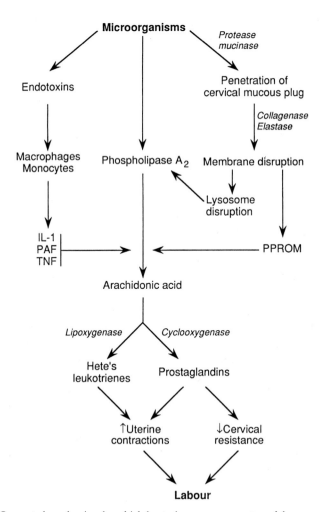

Fig. 9.1   Suggested mechanism by which bacteria may cause preterm labour.

microorganisms may initiate and potentiate PTL are summarized in Table 9.2 and shown in Figure 9.1.

Considerations

It is clear that many cases of PTL previously considered idiopathic are due to infection. While it may influence the use of tocolytics or steroids, the knowledge that infection is involved may be of limited help when a woman presents in PTL. By that time, substantive changes in the cervix may have taken place, rendering attempts to reverse the process unsuccessful. There is, however, one study where women admitted in PTL were randomized to a double-blind placebo-controlled trial of 7 days' oral treatment with erythromycin.[140] Overall, there was no statistically significant benefit in terms of birth weight, gestational age, prolongation of pregnancy, duration of tocolytics or hospitalization between erythromycin and placebo-treated groups. If, however, those women with cervical dilatation greater than 1 cm were examined, the erythromycin-treated group was found to be significantly associated with prolongation of pregnancy, the attainment of 37 weeks' gestation, increased birth weight and decreased duration of neonatal intensive care.

A high vaginal swab should be taken on admission,[141] though this may not alter obstetric management unless an organism such as gonococcus or GBS is isolated. The result may only have relevance in identifying sensitivities for organisms which are thought to be responsible for subsequent neonatal sepsis.

The knowledge that infection is associated with PTL may be of more help in its prediction and prevention. It has been shown that the carriage of *Trichomonas vaginalis* or *Ureaplasma urealyticum* or *Bacteroides fragilis* detected by high vaginal swab at 14–18 weeks' gestation is associated with a significantly increased incidence of PTL, preterm delivery or PPROM.[142] It may be possible to use a simple test such as a high vaginal swab in early pregnancy to detect an increase in vaginal pH, abnormal flora, presence of bacterial vaginosis or a marker organism such as *Mycoplasma hominis*. This information alone or in combination with existing scoring systems may improve the prediction and hence prevention of PTL. This hypothesis is currently being tested.

It is possible that in future pregnant women may be better identified as being at high risk of PTL from a combination of an early swab and existing scoring system. It may be necessary to advise the use of condoms during pregnancy or to recommend vaginal acid douches or gel to reduce vaginal pH. Antibiotics may also have a role in those women with abnormal genital tract flora in early pregnancy. Finally, a better understanding of the mechanisms whereby microorganisms may initiate PTL may lead to the development of more specific inhibitors of the lipoxygenase or cyclooxygenase enzyme pathways which may act as tocolytics.

REFERENCES

1. Lamont R F, Dunlop P D M, Crowley P, Elder M G. Spontaneous preterm labour and delivery at under 34 weeks gestation. Br Med J 1983; 286: 454–457
2. Rush R W, Keirse M J N C, Howat P et al. Contribution of preterm delivery to perinatal mortality. Br Med J 1976; 2: 965–968
3. Jones R A K, Cummins M, Davies P A. Infants of very low birthweight. A 15-year analysis. Lancet 1979; i: 1332–1335
4. Naeye R L, Kissane J M. Perinatal diseases, a neglected area of the medical sciences. In: Naeye R L, Kissane J M, Kaufman N, eds, Perinatal diseases. Baltimore, Md: Williams & Wilkins, 1980: pp 1–4.
5. Keirse M J N C, Rush R W, Anderson A B M, Turnbull A C. Risk of preterm delivery with previous preterm delivery and/or abortion. Br J Obstet Gynaecol 1978; 85: 81–85
6. Newcombe R, Chalmers I. Assessing the risk of preterm labor. In: Elder M G, Hendricks C H, eds. Preterm labor. Boston, Ma: Butterworths, 1981; pp 47–60
7. Fredrick J. Antenatal identification of women at high risk of spontaneous preterm birth. Br J Obstet Gynaecol 1976; 83: 351–354
8. Papiernik-Berkhauer E. Discussion in preterm labour. In: Anderson A, Bead R, Brudenell J M et al, eds. Proceedings of seventh Royal College of Obstetricians and Gynaecologists study group. London, RCOG: 1977: pp 29–39
9. Edmonds D K, Letchworth A T. The use of prophylactic oral salbutamol to prevent labour. Lancet 1982; i: 1310–1312
10. Lind T, Goderey K A, Gerrard J, Bryson M R. Continuous salbutamol infusion over 17 weeks to pre-empt premature labour. Lancet 1980; ii: 1165–1166
11. White B, Lamont R F, Letchworth A T. An approach to the problem of recurrent middle trimester abortion. J Obstet Gynaecol 1989; 10: 8–9
12. Hemminki E, Starfield B. Prevention and treatment of premature labour by drugs: review of controlled clinical trials. Br J Obstet Gynaecol 1978; 85: 411–417
13. Bobitt J R, Ledger W R. Unrecognised amnionitis and prematurity: a preliminary report. J Reprod Med 1977; 19: 8–12
14. Lauweryns J, Bernat R, Lerut A, Detourney G. Intrauterine pneumonia. An experimental study. Biol Neonate 1973; 22: 301–318
15. Miller J M, Hill G B, Welt S I et al. Bacterial colonisation of amniotic fluid in the presence of ruptured membranes. Am J Obstet Gynecol 1980; 137: 451–458
16. Cooperman N R, Kasin M, Rajachekaraiah K R. Clinical significance of amniotic fluid, amniotic membranes and endometrial biopsy cultures at the same time of caesarean section. Am J Obstet Gynecol 1980; 137: 536–541
17. Fox H. Pathology of the placenta. Philadelphia: W B Saunders, 1978
18. Pankuch G A, Applebaum P C, Lorenz R P et al. Placental microbiology and histology and the pathogenesis of chorioamnionitis. Obstet Gynecol 1984; 64: 802–806
19. Russell P. Inflammatory lesions of the human placenta. I. Clinical significance of acute chorioamnionitis. Am J Diagn Gynecol Obstet 1979; 1: 127–137
20. Naeye R L, Peters E C. Causes and consequences of premature rupture of fetal membranes. Lancet 1980; i: 193–194
21. Guzick D S, Winn K. The association of chorioamnionitis with preterm delivery. Obstet Gynecol 1985; 65: 11–15
22. Hillier S L, Martius J, Krohn M, Kiviat N, Holmes K K, Eschenbach D A. A case control study of chorionamnionic infection and histologic chorioamnionitis in prematurity. N Engl J Med 1988; 319: 972–978
23. Gibbs R S, Castillo M S, Rodgers P J. Management of acute chorioamnionitis. Am J Obstet Gynecol 1980; 136: 709–713
24. Daikoku N H, Kaltreider F, Khouzami V A. Premature rupture of membranes and spontaneous preterm labour: maternal endometritis risks. Obstet Gynecol 1982; 59: 13–20
25. Fisk N M. Modification to selective conservative management in preterm premature rupture of the membranes. Obstet Gynecol Surv 43: 328–334
26. Farb H F, Arnesen M, Geistler P et al. C-reactive protein with premature rupture of membranes and premature labor. Obstet Gynecol 1983; 62: 49–51

27. Ismail M A, Zinaman M J, Lowensohn R I, Moawad A H. The significance of C-reactive protein levels in women with premature rupture of the membranes. Am J Obstet Gynecol 1985; 151: 541–544

28. Hawrylyshyn P, Bernstein P, Milligan J E et al. Premature rupture of membranes: the role of C-reactive protein in the prediction of chorioamnionitis. Am J Obstet Gynecol 1983; 147: 240–246

29. Romem Y, Artal R. C-reactive protein as a predictor for chorioamnionitis in cases of premature rupture of the membranes. Am J Obstet Gynecol 1984; 150: 546–550

30. Fisk N M, Fysh J, Child A G, Gatenby P A, Jeffery H, Bradfield A H. Is C-reactive protein really useful in preterm premature rupture of the membranes? Br J Obstet Gynaecol 1987; 94: 1159–1164

31. Romero R, Mazor M, Wu Y K et al. Infection in the pathogenisis of preterm labour. Semin Perinatol 1988; 12: 262–279

32. Potkul R K, Moawad A H, Ponto K L. The association of subclinical infection with preterm labor. The role of C-reactive protein. Am J Obstet Gynecol 1985; 153: 642–645

33. Cammu H, Goosens A, Derde M P, Temmerman M, Foulon W, Amy J J. C-reactive protein in preterm labour; association with outcome of tocolysis and placental histology. Br J Obstet Gynaecol 1989; 96: 314–319

34. Hameed C, Tejani N, Verma U L, Archibald F. Silent chorioamnionitis as a cause of preterm labour refractory to tocolytic therapy. Am J Obstet Gynecol 1984; 149: 726–730

35. Larsen J W, Goldkrand J W, Hanson T M, Miller C R. Intrauterine infection in an obstetric service. Obstet Gynecol 43: 838–845

36. Bobitt J R, Ledger W R. Amniotic fluid analysis, its role in maternal and neonatal infection. Obstet Gynecol 1978; 51: 56–62

37. Garite T J, Freeman R K. Chorioamnionitis in the preterm gestation. Obstet Gynecol 1979; 54: 539–545

38. Miller J M, Pupkin M J, Hill G B. Bacterial colonisation amniotic fluid from intact fetal membranes. Am J Obstet Gynecol 1980; 136: 796–804

39. Garite R J, Freeman R K, Linzey E M et al. The use of amniocentesis in patients with premature rupture of the membranes. Obstet Gynecol 1979; 54: 226–230

40. Fisk N M. A dispstick test for infection in preterm premature rupture of the membranes. J Perinat Med 1987; 15: 565–568

41. Hoskins I A, Johnson T R B, Winkel C A. Leucocyte esterase activity in human amniotic fluid for the rapid detection of chorioamnionitis. Am J Obstet Gynecol 1987; 157: 730–732

42. Weible D R, Randall H W. Evacuation of amniotic fluid in preterm labor with intact membranes. J Reprod Med 1985; 30: 777–780

43. Romero R, Mazor M. Infection and preterm labor. Clin Obstet Gynecol 1988; 31: 553–584

44. Benirschke K. Routes and types of infection in the fetus and newborn. Am J Dis Child 1960; 99: 714–721

45. Romero R, Jimenez C, Lohda A K et al. (1990) Amniotic fluid glucose concentrations: a rapid and simple method for the detection of intra-amnionitis infection in preterm labour. Am J Obstet Gynecol 163: 968–974

46. Lamont R F, Taylor-Robinson D, Newman M et al. Spontaneous early preterm labour associated with abnormal genital bacterial colonisation. Br J Obstet Gynaecol 1986; 93: 804–810

47. Perkins R P, Zhou S, Butler C, Skipper B J. Histologic chorioamnionitis in pregnancies of various gestational ages: implications in preterm rupture of membranes. Obstet Gynecol 70: 856–860

48. Zaaijman J Du T, Wilkinson A R, Keeling J W et al. Spontaneous premature rupture of the membranes: bacteriology, histology and neonatal outcome. J Obstet Gynaecol 1982; 2: 155–160

49. Melingos S, Messinis I, Diakomanolis D et al. Influence of meteorological factors on premature rupture of the fetal membranes. Lancet 1978; ii: 435

50. Witter F R. The influence of the moon on deliveries. Am J Obstet Gynecol 1983; 145: 637–639

51. Marks J, Church C K, Benrubi G. Effects of barometric pressure and lunar phases on

premature rupture of the membranes. J Reprod Med 1983; 28: 485–488
52. Cederquist L L, Zervoudakis I A, Ewool E C, Litwin S D. The relationship between prematurely ruptured membranes and fetal immunoglobin production. Am J Obstet Gynecol 1979; 134: 784–788
53. Romem Y, Greenspoon J, Artal R. Clinical chorioamnionitis analysis of the incubation period in patients with preterm premature rupture of membranes. Am J Perinatol 1985; 2: 314–316
54. Gillibrand P N. Premature rupture of the membranes and prematurity. J Obstet Gynaecol Br Commonwith 1967; 74: 678–682
55. Nimrod C, Varela-Gittings F, Machin G et al. The effect of very prolonged membrane rupture on fetal development. Am J Obstet Gynecol 1984; 148: 540–543
56. Kappy K A, Cetrulo C L, Knuppel R A. Premature rupture of the membranes: a conservative approach. Am J Obstet Gynecol 1979; 134: 655–661
57. Varner M W, Galask R P. Conservative management of premature rupture of the membranes. Am J Obstet Gynecol 140: 39–43
58. Rush R W. The management of preterm rupture of the membranes. S Afr Med J 1980; 58: 690–691
59. Larsen B, Galask R P. Protection of the fetus against infection. Semin Perinat 1977; 1: 183–193
60. Pryse–Davies J, Hurley R. Infections and perinatal mortality. J Antimicrob Chemother 1979; 5 (suppl A): 59–70
61. Naeye R L, Peters E C. Amniotic fluid infections with intact membranes leading to perinatal death: a prospective study. Pediatrics 1978; 61: 171–177
62. Daikoku N H, Kaltreider F, Johnson T R B Jr et al. Premature rupture of the membranes and preterm labour: neonatal infection and perinatal mortality risks. Obstet Gynecol 1981; 58: 417–425
63. Toth M, Witkin S, Ledger W et al. The role of infection in the etiology of preterm birth. Obstet Gynecol 1988; 71: 723–726
64. Pugh W E, Fernandez N A. Coitus in late pregnancy. Obstet Gynecol 1953; 2: 636–642
65. Georgakopoulos P A, Dodos D, Mechleris D. Sexuality in pregnancy and preterm labour. Br J Obstet Gynaecol 1984; 91: 891–893
66. Zachau-Christiansen B, Ross E M. Babies: human development during the first year. London: John Wiley, 1975
67. Naeye R L, Kissane J M, Kaufman N. Common environmental influences on the fetus. Int Acad Pathol Monograph, No. 22 Perinatal diseases. Baltimore: Williams and Wilkins, 1981: pp 60–66
68. Naeye R L. Coitus and associated amniotic fluid infections. N Engl J Med 1979; 301: 1198–1200
69. Naeye R L, Ross S. Coitus and chorioamnionitis: a prospective study. Early Hum Dev 1982; 6: 91–97
70. Moghissi K S. Sperm migration through cervical mucus. In: Sherman A I, ed. Pathways of conception. The role of the cervix and oviduct in reproduction. Springfield, IL: Charles C Thomas, 1971: pp 214–236
71. Gnarpe H, Friberg J. T-Mycoplasmas on spermatozoa and infertility. Nature 1973; 254: 97–98
72. Fox C A, Wolff H S, Baker J A. Measurements of intravaginal and intrauterine pressures during human coitus by radiotelemetry. J Reprod Fertil 1970; 22: 243–251
73. Goodlin R C, Keller D W, Raffin M. Orgasm during late pregnancy. Possible deleterious effects. Obstet Gynecol 1971; 38: 916–920
74. Goodlin R C, Schmidt W, Crevy D C. Uterine tension and fetal heart rate during maternal orgasm. Obstet Gynecol 1972; 39: 125–127
75. Baird D. Infection of the urinary tract during pregnancy. Part IV. J Obstet Gynaecol Br Emp 1979; 42: 774–794
76. Kincaid-Smith P. Bacteruria and urinary infection in pregnancy. Clin Obstet Gynecol 1968; 11: 533–549
77. Galask R P, Varner M W, Petzold C R et al. Bacterial attachment to the chorioamniotic membranes. Am J Obstet Gynecol 1984; 148: 915–928
78. Levison M E, Corman L C, Carrington E R, Kaye D. Quantatitive microflora of the vagina. Am J Obstet Gynecol 1977; 127: 80–85

79. Lindner J G E M, Plantana F H F, Hoogkamp-Korstanje J A A. Quantitative studies of the vaginal flora of healthy women and of obstetric and gynaecologic patients. J Med Microbiol 1978; 11: 233–238

80. Goplerud C P, Ohm M J, Galask R P. Aerobic and anaerobic flora of the cervix during pregnancy and the puerperium. Am J Obstet Gynecol 1976; 126: 858–868

81. Moberg P, Eneroth P, Harlin J et al. Cervical bacterial flora in infertile and pregnant women. Med Microbiol Immunol 1978; 165: 139–145

82. Larsen, Galask R P. Vaginal microbial flora: practical and theoretical relevance. Obstet Gynecol 1980; 55 (suppl): 100S

83. Lamont R F, Taylor-Robinson D, Wigglesworth J S, Furr P M, Evans R T, Elder M G. The role of mycoplasmas, ureaplasmas and chlamydiae in the genital tract of women presenting in spontaneous early preterm labour. J Med Microbiol 1987; 24: 253–257

84. Anthony B F, Okada D M. The emergence of Group B streptococci in infections of the newborn infant. Annu Rev Med 1977; 28: 355–369

85. Regan J A, Chao S, James L S. Premature rupture of membranes, preterm delivery and group B streptococcal colonisation of mothers. Am J Obstet Gynecol 1981; 141: 184–186

86. Rothbard M J, Gregory T, Salerno L J. Intrapartum gonococcal amnionitis. Am J Obstet Gynecol 1975; 121: 565

87. Charles A G, Cohen S, Kass M B. Asymptomatic gonorrhoea in prenatal patients. Am J Obstet Gynecol 1970; 108: 595

88. Handsfield H H, Godson W A, Holmes K K. Neonatal gonococcal infection. I Orogastric contamination with *Neisseria gonorrhoeae*. JAMA 1973; 225: 697–701

89. Bobitt J R, Hayslip C C, Damato J D. Amniotic fluid infection as determined by transabdominal amniocentesis with intact membranes in premature labour. Am J Obstet Gynecol 1981; 140: 947–952

90. Evaldson G, Lagrelius A, Winiarski J. Premature rupture of the membranes. Obstet Gynecol Surv 1981; 36: 356

91. Wahbeh C J, Hill G B, Eden R B, Gall S A. Intra-amniotic bacterial colonisation in premature labor. Am J Obstet Gynecol 1984; 148: 739–742

92. Schwartz R H. Perinatal infections. In: Bolgnese J, Schwartz R H, Schneider J, eds. Perinatal medicine. Baltimore, Md: Williams & Wilkins, 1982: pp 313–335

93. Relier J P. Perinatal and neonatal infections. Listeriosis. J Antimicrob Chemother 1979; 5: 51–57

94. McCormack W M, Braun P, Lee Y-H et al. The genital mycoplasmas. N Engl J Med 1973; 288: 78–89

95. Taylor-Robinson D, McCormack W M. The genital mycoplasmas. Part I. N Engl J Med 1980; 302: 1003–1010

96. Taylor-Robinson, D McCormack W M. The genital mycoplasmas. Part II. N Engl J Med 1980; 302: 1063–1067

97. Shurin P A, Alpert S, Rosner B et al. Chorioamnionitis and colonisation of the newborn infant with genital mycoplasmas. N Engl J Med 1975; 293: 5–8

98. Kass E H, McCormack W M, Lin J et al. Genital mycoplasmas as a cause of excess premature delivery. Trans Assoc Am Phys 1981; 94: 261–266

99. Embree J E, Krause V W, Embil J A, Macdonald S. Placental infection with *Mycoplasma hominis* and *Ureaplasma urealyticum*: clinical correlation. Obstet Gynecol 1980; 56: 475–481

100. Blanco J D, Gibbs R S, Malkerbe H et al. A controlled study of genital mycoplasmas in amniotic fluid from patients with intra-amniotic infection. J Infect Dis 1983; 147: 650–653

101. Kundsin R B, Driscoll S G, Pelletier P A. *Ureaplasma urealyticum* incriminated in perinatal morbidity and mortality. Science 1981; 213: 474–476

102. Quinn P A, Shewchuk A B, Shuber J et al. (1983). Efficacy of amniotic therapy in preventing spontaneous pregnancy loss among couples colonised with genital mycoplasmas. Am J Obstet Gynecol 1983; 145: 239–244

103. Taylor E S. Sexually transmissable vaginal infections in pregnancy. Obstet Gynecol Surv 1980; 35: 21

104. Bruner J P, Elliott J P, Kilbride H W. Candida chorioamnionitis diagnosed by amniocentesis with subsequent fetal infection. Am J Perinatol 1986; 3: 213–218

105. Lorenz R P, Applebaum P C, Ward R M, Botti J J. Chorioamnionitis and possible neonatal infection associated with lactobacillus species. J Clin Microbiol 1982; 16: 558–561
106. Lamont R F. The role of infection in the aetiology of spontaneous early preterm labour. DM Thesis, University of Southampton
107. Lamont R F, Neave S, Baker A C, Steer P J. Intrauterine pressures in labours induced by amniotomy and oxytocin or vaginal prostaglandin gel compared with spontaneous labour. Br J Obstet Gynaecol 98: 441–447
108. Keirse M J N C, Hicks R B, Mitchell M D, Turnbull A C. Increase of the prostaglandin precursor arachidonic acid in amniotic fluid during spontaneous labour. Br J Obstet Gynaecol 1977; 84: 937–940
109. MacDonald P C, Schultz F M, Duenhoelter J H et al. Initiation of human parturition: I. Mechanisms of action of arachidonic acid. Obstet Gynecol 1974; 44: 629–636
110. Schwartz B E, Schultz F M, MacDonald P C, Johnston J M. Initiation of human parturition. III. Fetal membrane content of prostaglandin E_2 And F_{2a} precursor. Obstet Gynecol 1975; 46: 564–568
111. Okita J R, Okazaki T, MacDonald P C, Johnson J M. Alterations in phospholipid content of human fetal membranes during parturition. Proceedings of the Society For Gynecologic Investigation. San Diego, California, March 21–24. Abstr 188
112. Curbelo V, Bejar R, Benirschke K, Gluck L (1979) Premature labour: Placental arachidonic acid (20:4). Presented at the Proceedings of the Society for Gynaecological Investigations, San Diego, California. March 21–24 (abstr 144).
113. Okazaki T, Okita J R, MacDonald P C, Johnson J M. Initiation of human parturition X: substate specificity of phospholipase A2 in human fetal membranes. Am J Obstet Gynecol 1978; 130: 432–438
114. Schwartz B E, Schultz F M, MacDonald P C, Johnston J M. Initiation of human parturition. IV. Demonstration of phospholipase A_2 in the lysosomes of human fetal membranes. Am J Obstet Gynecol 1976; 125: 1089–1092
115. Schwartz B E, Macdonald P C, Johnston J M. Initiation of human parturition. XI. Lysosmal enzyme release in vitro from amnions obtained from laboring and non-laboring women. Am J Obstet Gynecol 1980; 133: 21–24
116. Zuckerman H, Reiss U, Rubinstein I. Inhibition of human premature labor by indomethacin. Obstet Gynecol 1974; 44: 787–792
117. Gleeson R P, Elder A M, Turner M J, Tutherford A J, Elder M G. Vaginal pH in pregnancy in women delivering at and before term. Br J Obstet Gynaecol 1979; 96: 183–187
118. Plaut A G. Microbial IgA proteases. Engl J Med 1978; 298: 1459–1463
119. Kapatais-Zoumbos K, Chandler D K F, Barile M F. Survey of immunoglobin A protease activity among selected species of ureaplasmas and mycoplasmas: specificity for host immunoglobin A. Infect Immun, 1985; 47: 704–709
120. McGregor J A, French J I, Lawellin D, Todd J K. Preterm birth and infection: pathogenic possibilities. Am J Reprod Immunol Microbiol 1988; 16: 123–132
121. McGregor J A, French J I, Lawellin D, Franco-Buff A, Smith B A, Todd J K. In vitro study of bacterial protease-induced reduction of chorioamniotic membrane strength and elasticity. Obstet Gynecol 1987; 69: 167–174
122. Sbarra A J, Selvaraj R, Cetrulo C L, Feingold M, Newton E, Thomas G B. Infection and phagocytosis as possible mechanism of rupture in premature rupture of the membranes. Am J Obstet Gynecol 1985; 153: 38–43
123. Rajabi M, Dean D D, Woessner J F Jr. High levels of serum collagenase in preterm labor – a potential biochemical marker. Obstet Gynecol 1987; 69: 179–186
124. Bejar R, Curbelo V, Davis C, Gluck L. Premature labor II. Bacterial sources of phospholipase. Obstet Gynecol 1981; 57: 479–481
125. Lamont R F, Rose M, Elder M G. Effect of bacterial products on prostaglandin E production by amnion cells. Lancet 1985; ii: 1131–1133
126. Lamont R F, Anthony R, Myatt L, Booth L, Furr P M, Taylor-Robinson D. Production of PGE_2 by human amnion in vitro in response to addition of media conditioned by microorganisms associated with chorioamnionitis and preterm labour. Am J Obstet Gynecol 1990; 162: 819–825
127. Romero R, Kadar N, Hobbins J C et al. Infection and labor: the detection of endotoxin in amniotic fluid. Am J Obstet Gynecol 1987; 157: 815–819

128. Kurland J I, Bockman R. Prostaglandin E production by human blood monocytes and mouse peritoneal macrophages. J Exp Med 1978; 147: 952–957
129. O'Flaherty J T, Wykle R L. Biology and biochemistry of platelet activating factor. Clin Rev Allergy 1983; 1: 353–367
130. Dinarello C A. Interleukin-1. Rev Infect Dis 1984; 6: 51–95
131. Dinarello C A. Clinical relevance of interleukin-1 and its multiple biological activities. Bull Inst Pasteur 1987; 85: 267–285
132. Nishihira J, Ishibashi T, Imai Y, Muramastu T. Mass spectrometric evidence for the presence of platelet-activating factor in human amniotic fluid during labor. Lipids 1984; 19: 907–910
133. Billah M M, Direnzo G C, Ban C, Anceschi M M, Bleasdale J E, Johnston J M. Platelet-activating factor metabolism in human amnion and the responses of this tissue to extracellular platelet-activating factor. Prostaglandins 1985; 30: 841–850
134. McGregor J A. Microorganisms and arachidonic acid metabolites in preterm birth. Semin Reprod Endocrinol 1985; 3: 273–278
135. Dinarello C A. An update of human interleukin-1 from molecular biology to clinic relevance. J Clin Immunol 1985; 5: 287
136. Carraher R, Hahn D W, Ritchie D M et al. Involvement of lipoxygenase products in myometrial contractions. Prostaglandins 1983; 26: 23–32
137. Ritchie D M, Hahn D W, McGuire J L. Smooth muscle contraction as a model to study the mediator role of endogenous lipoxygenase products of arachidonic acid. Life Sci 1984; 34: 509–513
138. Bennett P R, Elder M G, Myatt L. The effects of lipoxygenase metabolites of arachidonic acid on human myometrial contractility. Prostaglandins 1987; 33: 837–884
139. Romero R, Emamian M, Wan M et al. Increased concentrations of arachidonic acid lipoxygenase metabolites in amniotic fluid during parturition. Obstet Gynecol 1987; 70: 849–851
140. McGregor J A, French J I, Reller L B, Todd J K, Makowski E L. Adjunctive erythromycin therapy for idiopathic preterm labor: results of a randomised, double blinded, placebo-controlled trial. Am J Obstet Gynecol 1986; 154: 98–103
141. Lamont R F, Newman M J, Dunlop P D M, Elder M G. The use of high vaginal, endocervical and rectal swabs in the diagnosis of genital infection in association with preterm labour. Br J Clin Pract 1988; 42: 146–149
142. Minkoff H, Grunebaum A N, Schwarz R H et al. Risk factors for prematurity and premature rupture of membranes: a prospective study of the vaginal flora in pregnancy. Am J Obstet Gynecol 1984; 150: 965–972.

10. Failure to progress in labour

H. Gee   K. S. Oláh

The concept of an active approach to the management of labour was first introduced by O'Driscoll and colleagues in 1969.[1] By the regular assessment of cervical dilatation in labour and early correction of abnormal progress by oxytocin it has been suggested that the occurrence of prolonged labour in nulliparous patients can be 'virtually eliminated'[2] and the incidence of caesarean section can be dramatically reduced.[3-6] However, trends show that caesarean section rates are rising, often for those indications active management was meant to address,[7,8] and the expectations raised by the adoption of the principles of active management have hardly been fulfilled. Why have the results proved difficult to emulate despite apparent adherence to the principles advocated?

Central to active management is the use of oxytocin to control the powers of labour on the assumption that there is a direct relationship between uterine activity and progress. In order to avoid potentially harmful effects of oxytocin augmentation, measurement of uterine activity has been advocated.[9] However the clinical value of these measures has, also, not lived up to expectation.[10,11] Indeed, its quantification leads to paradoxes rather than solutions, namely:

1. Nulliparous labour is slower than multiparous labour yet uterine activity is greater in the former than in the latter.[12,13]

2. Poor progress in labour can be associated with high levels of uterine activity, as well as levels of uterine activity below the normal range.[14]

3. Precipitate labour can be associated with normal or low uterine activity.[13,15,16]

4. Premature labour leading to early delivery is often insidious with cervical dilatation taking place in the presence of little appreciable uterine activity.[17,18]

5. When uterine activity is normal, but progress slow, oxytocin augmentation may affect cervical dilatation but does not necessarily improve outcome.[19]

To address these paradoxes we make no apologies for critically reviewing even the most fundamental tenets regarding the physiology of the uterus

159

during the first stage of labour. Perhaps it is time to reflect on the whole of current management of labour, and to appraise critically the labour ward protocols that have been almost universally accepted.

ABNORMAL LABOUR PATTERNS

There is no doubt that the work of Friedman, dividing labour into phases according to rate of cervical dilatation (Fig.10.1) has been fundamental to a logical approach to labour management.[20,21] From the normal patterns it was possible to describe aberrant patterns, namely prolonged latent phase, primary dysfunctional labour and secondary arrest.[22] Because of the difficulty in identifying and defining the onset of labour, some of the definitions of the various abnormalities of labour progress originally described by Friedman have been altered, often arbitrarily, e.g.in the study by Cardozo

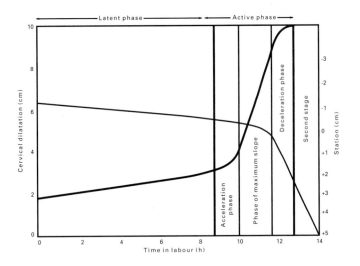

Pattern	Diagnostic criterion
Prolonged latent phase	Nulliparas 20 h or more
	Multiparas 14 h or more
Protracted active-phase dilatation	Nulliparas 1.2 cm/h or less
	Multiparas 1.5 cm/h or less
Protracted descent	Nulliparas 1 cm/h or less
	Multiparas 2 cm/h or less
Prolonged deceleration phase	Nulliparas 3 h or more
	Multiparas 1 h or more
Secondary arrest of dilatation	Arrest 2 h or more
Arrest of descent	Arrest 1 h or more
Failure of descent	No descent in decleration phase or second stage

Fig. 10.1 Friedman's partitioning of labour and normal limits for labour progress. From Friedman (1983)[78].

et al,[9] the time of admission in labour is taken as the start of the latent phase rather than the time of onset of regular purposeful contractions. The corruptions of the original definitions described by Friedman have become established in practice and the time limits imposed by these definitions have become accepted without any objective validation.

Prolonged latent phase

The whole concept of the latent phase is rather nebulous and difficult to define. It starts with the onset of painful, regular uterine contractions but the end can only be recognized retrospectively when the rate of cervical dilatation increases at the start of the active phase. A latent phase exceeding 6 hours in a primigravida or 4 hours in a multigravida is considered prolonged by some workers.[9,23] Friedman's original work suggested that the latent phase was less than 20 hours (mean 8.6 hours, s.d. 6 hours) in primigravidae and 14 hours (mean 5.3 hours, s.d 4.1 hours) in multiparae.[22] These limits have been criticized on the basis that his record of the onset of labour was retrospective, relying on the patient's memory, and from a dilatation of 0 cm which is rarely seen in patients admitted in labour.[24,25] However, the studies conducted by Friedman are the best statistical analyses of abnormal labour patterns to date. There is no validated evidence that the latent phase of labour should last less than 6 hours.

Primary dysfunctional labour

Primary dysfunctional labour has been described as the commonest abnormal labour pattern,[25] although the term is meaningless and the underlying pathology of the condition is not specified. All causes of slow labour that do not fit into the pattern of prolonged latent phase or secondary arrest are attributed to primary dysfunctional labour. The result is that the underlying cause of the pattern is varied. It is defined as a labour in which the active phase progresses at a rate of less than 1 cm/hour before a normal active-phase slope has been established.[22] The problem with this definition, when delay is apparent at lower dilatations, lies with the problem of prospectively defining the end of the latent phase.

Secondary arrest

Secondary arrest of cervical dilatation is relatively easy to define by comparison. It occurs when cervical dilatation ceases after a normal portion of active-phase dilatation. This pattern, although at one time considered to be entirely due to cephalopelvic disproportion, is often due to malposition or deflexion of the presenting part.

Friedman[26] described slow progress during the 7–10 cm interval as a prolonged decelerative phase and associated this pattern with an increased incidence of instrumental delivery. Davidson et al[27] not only agreed with this but also drew attention to the fact that the instrumentation was likely to be 'difficult' or 'moderately difficult'. They did not find oxytocin helpful in this situation. This pattern probably reflects borderline cephalopelvic disproportion and caution should be exercised in any subsequent instrumental vaginal delivery. This borderline state may be the most treacherous since severe cephalopelvic disproportion will have declared itself early and have been solved by caesarean section.

Cervicography

Based on the idea of graphic representation of cervical dilatation, a number of cervicograms have been produced.[3,28–30] Strictly speaking, all of these apply only to the active phase of dilatation. Beazley & Alderman[31] devised an Inductogram which plots a modified Bishop score against time for induced labour and applies to what is recognizable as the latent phase. This chart has not found as wide an application as the active-phase cervicograms.

Two problems arise: how is the clinician sure the active phase has been entered, i.e. are the criteria used for the cervicograms being used appropriately? Secondly, do the limits differentiate normal from abnormal? The first point will be addressed later. In answer to the second, the limits set are not the usual statistical limits to differentiate normal from abnormal populations. Philpott's cervicogram was devised to select those patients in a Third World practice who should be transferred for delivery to a properly equipped hospital. Studd's cervicogram was derived from Philpott's, and those patients crossing the nomogram line were found to have a threefold increase in instrumental delivery (from 17 to 53%). So, even when the nomogram line was crossed, there was still approximately a 50:50 chance of a normal delivery. Later, an arbitrary 'action line' 2 hours to the right of the line of 'normal' was adopted. Beazley & Kurjak[30] differentiated between 80 and 20% of *low-risk* outcome. A fundamental problem, which has never been addressed definitively by randomized trial, has been the efficiency with which the identification of these patterns, coupled with the principles of active management, could favourably affect outcome. To our knowledge only one study has approached this requirement.[32] This study demonstrates how difficult it is to avoid the introduction of bias and to obtain the desired end-points of outcome in terms of operative delivery and fetal well-being.

To be fair to cervicography, it is an aid to the management of labour, i.e. it detects signs of aberrance. Over time these patterns of cervical dilatation have assumed the role of diagnosis. The danger with this transformation is that therapy is instituted on the basis of patterns which may have several underlying causes. The therapy may be appropriate in some, but not all, cases.

Clinical implications

In prospective studies by Cardozo et al[9] in nulliparous labours and by Gibb et al[23] in multiparous labours, using specified definitions of the abnormal labour patterns, Studd's cervicogram and a protocol of active management, the following data were produced from an unspecified population in London.

Prolonged latent phase

The incidence in nulliparous women was 3.5%. The caesarean section rate for these women was 16.7% (compared to 1.6% for normal labour) and a low Apgar score ($\leq$6 at 5 min) occurred in 8.3% of neonates (compared with 2.6% after normal labour). The 37.5% incidence of an Apgar score $\leq$6 at 1 min was the highest found in the study and 4 babies (16.7%) in this group required endotracheal intubation (2.7% endotracheal intubations in those with normal patterns). Similarly, for multiparous women, the outcome is less favourable when the latent phase is prolonged, with caesarean section rates of 8.3% (0.5% for normal labour); Apgars $\leq$6 at 5 min in 8.3% (2.4% for normal labour) were reported.

It was suggested in conclusion to the study by Cardozo et al[9] that oxytocin may have been inappropriate in this condition. Friedman's advice was to sedate patients and prevaricate.[22] The proponents of active management advocate forewater amniotomy and oxytocin as soon as delay in labour is diagnosed.[5] The problem of prolonged latent phase is rare in O'Driscoll's population and we suspect that this is due to differences in the diagnosis of labour, i.e. labour is only recognized once the active phase has been properly entered. Recent work, which will be presented later, suggests that cervical response is different in the latent phase compared to the active phase. This has implications for the likely response to oxytocin administration.

Primary dysfunctional labour

Primary dysfunctional labour occurs in 26.3% of spontaneous nulliparous labours[9] and 8.1% of multiparous ones.[23]

Originally, Friedman was of the opinion that oxytocin did not help primary dysfunctional labour but subsequent studies have demonstrated a significant benefit from its use,[1,4,9,32,33] although one study has disagreed with this consensus.[34]

A total of 80% of nulliparous[9] and 90% of multiparous patients[23] will respond to oxytocin. The caesarean section rate in these responders is 5.4% for nulliparous and 0% for multiparous women. However, not all patients respond, and in these cases the picture is much different. In the study by Cardozo et al[9] the caesarean section rate was 77% in this group and there was a significantly increased fetal morbidity (intubation rate 20%, Apgar score ≤6 at 5 min, and admission to special care baby unit in 15%). In a prospective trial comparing oxytocin with placebo[32] progress could be improved but no conclusion could be drawn in terms of beneficial outcome.

Secondary arrest

Secondary arrest occurred in 6.3% of nulliparous and 2% of multiparous labours. Response to oxytocin occurred in 60% in the former and 70% of the latter. When response did not occur, caesarean section was required in 54% (11.6% for responders) and 70% (20% in responders) for nulliparous and multiparous patients respectively. These and other data have led to the assertion that secondary arrest is a more benign pattern than has hitherto been accepted.[32] The non-responders remain an unknown quantity. There may have been cephalopelvic disproportion since, in the series quoted above, birth weights were greater and maternal heights less in this group but, without appropriate data, this remains conjectural.

The main problem with interpreting the above data is that therapy was instituted only on cervimetric data. Uterine activity was not quantified, nor was pathology in the mechanism of labour specified. Bidgood & Steer[19,35] showed that in primary dysfunctional labour cervical dilatation could be speeded up by oxytocin but, paradoxically, outcome was not significantly improved. If uterine activity was already high, the response to oxytocin was limited.

THE MECHANISM OF LABOUR

Classically, progress in labour is described in terms of the 'powers', the 'passages' and the 'passenger'. Their interaction is complex and, though it may be simplistic to treat each one separately, it is difficult to see how any analysis can be made unless this is done initially. Even with the most favourable presenting part, namely a flexed head, a highly irregular shape is transmitted through the birth canal, undergoing a specific mechanism to succeed. Though moulding can permit some leeway, the passenger is the variable least open to manipulation of the three. This chapter will, therefore, concentrate primarily on an analysis of the other two, the powers and the passages.

THE POWERS

This section will concern itself primarily with the powers, though it must be recognized that flexion and rotation of the head, mechanisms which are essential to progress are, to some extent dependent on the other two

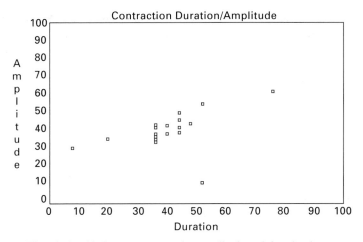

Fig. 10.2   The relationship between contraction amplitude and duration in a spontaneous multiparous labour.

variables, the passages and the passenger. Furthermore, there is no doubt that judiciously increasing the powers can encourage the correction of an abnormal mechanism in certain cases.

Assessment of uterine activity

Three main variables characterize uterine activity: repetition frequency, amplitude and duration. Resting tone is of importance but is difficult to measure. Other parameters such as the rate of pressure generation[36] and the offset[37] of the pressure waveform have theoretical attractions but little attention has been give to them.

In spontaneous labour, there is a relationship between duration and amplitude of contractions (Fig. 10.2) though some data suggest this relationship is not linear.[36] Therefore, palpation of contractions with timing of duration and repetition frequency can give an indication of uterine activity in spontaneous labour. Whether this is so when oxytocin is used is debatable.[14,38]

External guard ring tocodynamometry (EGT) is available on labour ward monitors. Its prime function is to relate events temporally in the heart rate trace with contractions. The tocodynamometer is sensitive to changes in the contour of the abdomen induced by changes in uterine wall curvature wrought by contractions. Its sensitivity will, therefore, be affected by the contour of the uterus and the thickness and contour of the maternal abdomen. It can only record repetition frequency accurately. No clinical comparison has been made between this form of monitoring and palpation, although EGT has been favourably compared to intrauterine pressure monitoring in augmented labour.[11] However, this may be seen as an indictment of intrauterine pressure monitoring rather than a vindication of

EGT. In the obese patient external detection of contractions may be fallacious by whatever technique.

Direct measurement of intrauterine pressure using various forms of catheter is the most accurate form of assessment of pressure generation within the uterus, although the clinical value of intrauterine pressure monitoring remains unclear.[10] The literature is replete with publications testifying to the merits of various derived units of uterine activity. Their authors all believe their unit has advantages over the others, although the benefits often seem marginal. This profusion of units (Montevideo units, Alexandria units, Uterine Activity Integral, Mean Active Pressure) coupled with their infrequency of employment clinically should lead us to question their true value.

The purpose of any derived unit is to combine the various parameters of the intrauterine pressure waveform into a single unit which has clinical, if not physiological, validity. Thus Montevideo units[39] include repetition frequency and average amplitude above basal tone. Alexandria units[40] include repetition frequency, average amplitude and average duration. Uterine Activity Integral[41,42] integrates area beneath the curve above basal tone. Mean Active Pressure[43] removes the time scale but still only measures activity above basal tone. The inclusion or omission of a variable, e.g. basal tone, seems arbitrary. However, this is not the case. Technological considerations have often been the determining factor. For example, the introduction of the transducer-tipped catheter obviated the need for painstaking calibration and clearing of the fluid-filled catheter to avoid artefact. However, baseline tone cannot be measured by this device because the hydrostatic pressure of liquor above the catheter tip cannot be measured.

Phillips & Calder[43] make an important point in their paper on units for the evaluation of uterine contractility. They state that 'the name given to a unit of measurement should describe the variable being measured'. This logic could be carried one step further, i.e. *the variable being measured should be defined and understood physiologically*. All derived units of uterine activity depend on the measurement of intrauterine pressure. Therefore, before their value can be judged, there must be a full comprehension of the mechanism of pressure generation.

Generation of intrauterine pressure

Intrauterine pressure is not an absolute index of myometrial activity. In the simplest of terms it depends upon the wall tension of the uterus and the radius of curvature of the wall (i.e. it is dependent on uterine size). The wall of the uterus has usually been considered only in terms of its muscle component, i.e. the myometrium. However, at term the 'lower segment' (the definition of which still defies precision) and the so-called 'passive' components of the cervix also make a significant contribution. These elements will 'give' when tension is applied by the muscular corpus. Therefore, they will attenuate the wall tension and hence the pressure recorded will be less.

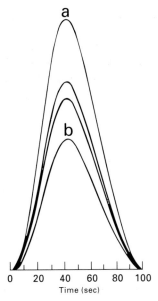

Fig. 10.3   The effect of changing cervical compliance on the computer-generated intrauterine pressure waveform. a = Minimum compliance; b = maximum compliance.

This effect can be modelled using a computer. While detailed modelling of biological systems is probably a vain hope, simple modelling to illustrate fundamental principles can be helpful in demonstrating the effect of individual variables — an impossibility in vivo.

Coren & Csapo[44] devised a simple model of the uterus to describe intra-uterine pressure generation which employed Laplace's law (which relates the tension in the wall of a vessel with its radius of curvature and the pressure within the vessel) and embodied contractile elements in series with elastic ones within the uterine wall. In their simulation they paid no attention to the effect on the wall tension of cervical compliance/elasticity. Addressing these factors[45] it can be shown that cervical compliance modulates wall tension, reducing the contraction amplitude while maintaining duration (Fig. 10.3). Repetition frequency, which is governed by other agencies, is not addressed in this model.

These simple predictions have enormous repercussions for the interpretation of intrauterine pressure waveforms.

The effects of changing cervical compliance. The cervix, though passive, has an effect on both intrauterine pressure and dilatation. This effect will be referred to as the cervical augmentation/attenuation of pressure (CAP) effect. The compliant cervix will permit rapid dilatation and progress in labour while attenuating wall tension and generating low intrauterine pressure. Therefore, one paradox — that of rapid progress with low uterine activity — is explained. Conversely, a non-compliant cervix will not dilate and will not modulate wall tension. The result will be an abrupt and rapid rise in pressure with high amplitude.[46] These circumstances set the scene

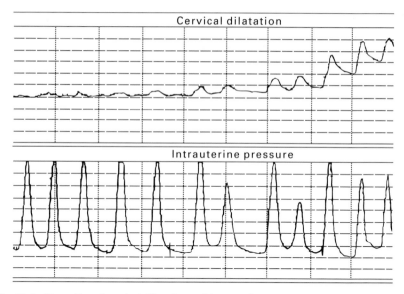

Fig. 10.4   Recording of cervical dilatation and intrauterine pressure over a 40-min period to demonstrate the CAP effect. Upper scale is 0–10 cm; lower scale is 0–100 mmHg.

not only for 'failure to progress' but also for poor placental perfusion due to high intrauterine pressure[47,48] and 'fetal distress'.[14]

The CAP effect suggests that rate of dilatation may not be directly dependent on pressure, but on myometrial wall tension. However, if the tension is modulated, e.g. by the cervix being compliant, the muscular activity will not be represented in pressure generation. With an infinitely compliant cervix there would be no pressure but immediate dilatation. This effect is not just theoretical. Figure 10.4 shows initially how contractions with high amplitudes have little effect on cervical dilatation. Later, there is rapid dilatation with a fall in pressure (it is interesting to note that not all contractions show the same magnitude of effect; the cause is obscure).

Spontaneous labour is mediated by agents, e.g. prostaglandins, which affect both myometrial activity and cervical compliance. Presumably, under ideal circumstances, these effects are balanced and hence uterine activity is optimally coupled with a cervix whose compliance is great enough to permit progress in labour while at the same time modulating intrauterine pressure, thus protecting the fetus against the potential problems of impaired placental perfusion resulting from high intrauterine pressures. The possible interactions regarding the balance between myometrial activity and cervical compliance are infinite and are represented in Figure 10.5. This spectrum of interaction explains the large range of normal variability seen for uterine activity in normally progressing labour.[7] However, two extremes can be postulated: line A represents a non-compliant cervix requiring high wall tensions and hence high intrauterine pressure to produce rates of dilatation consistent with normal cervico-

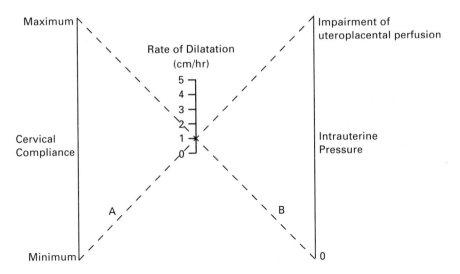

Fig. 10.5   Labour nomogram (see text for details).

graphy. At the same time, non-compliance of the cervix fails to modulate wall tension, generating high intrauterine pressure.[14] Thus the conditions of paradox 2 are explained.

The converse is high cervical compliance (line B) resulting in cervical dilatation with barely more than resting myometrial tone. At term this could result in precipitate labour once myometrial activity is generated, or preterm, would result in insidious progress with little appreciation of any uterine activity.[17,18] These are the features of paradoxes 3 and 4.

The effects of changing uterine dimension. As uterine size and hence radius of curvature of the uterine wall decrease, intrauterine pressure increases even though wall tension, and hence the force applied to the cervix remains constant. Modelling shows that this rise in amplitude is coupled with a reduction in duration (Fig. 10.6). Area beneath the curve is barely altered. Effects similar to these can be demonstrated in vivo. Caldeyro-Barcia et al[49] recorded uterine activity during reduction in uterine size as polyhydramnios was tapped, consistent with the theoretical prediction.

This effect could explain, at least in part, the abrupt rise in uterine activity seen towards the end of the first stage due to a decrease in uterine volume as fetal descent commences. The effect is more prominent when Montevideo units are used compared to Uterine Activity Integral[50] because Montevideo unit derivation depends on amplitude rather than area beneath the intrauterine pressure waveform. This may also partly explain the change in intrauterine pressure and apparent rise in uterine activity after amniotomy. In the past these phenomena have been attributed to endocrine effects.

The effects of oxytocin. Oxytocin increases amplitude, duration and frequency of weak contractions. Initially, the response is dose-dependent and

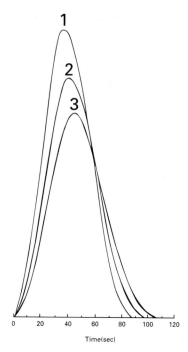

Fig. 10.6 The effect of changing uterine size on the computer-generated intrauterine pressure waveform (increasing uterine size from 1 to 3).

the effects are apparent whichever parameter of uterine activity is chosen. At higher dosages the response plateaus.[39] Hyperstimulation is evidenced by an increased repetition frequency and a rise in basal tone coupled with a reduction in pressure amplitude above basal tone, resulting in impaired placental perfusion[47] and limited ability to recover between contractions.

When poor progress results from suboptimal uterine activity, oxytocin is the logical and effective therapy. However, poor progress can be associated with uterine activity at, or above, the upper limits of normal.[14] The CAP effect could explain this finding. Increased myometrial tension without modulation by a compliant cervix would give rise to high-amplitude contractions of proportionately short duration (which would tend to be underestimated by palpation). When uterine activity is augmented with oxytocin from a relatively normal level, increased activity is achieved predominantly by an increased repetition frequency.[35]

Basal tone is not a component used by any of the units of uterine activity derived from intrauterine pressure measurement. Indeed, there has been a move away from the fluid-filled catheter systems to transducer-tipped catheters which are incapable of measuring tone. As hyperstimulation approaches, basal tone rises at the expense of amplitude above basal tone. Maximum recorded amplitude changes little. Thus, since derived units of uterine activity combine functions of amplitude above basal tone, and repetition frequency, their detection of overstimulation will, in effect, depend upon only one variable, repetition frequency. This could be measured more simply by palpation, explaining the favourable comparison of palpation with intrauterine pressure monitoring in oxytocin-induced labours.[38]

Clinical implications for assessment of uterine activity

When labour occurs spontaneously and progress is satisfactory, there seems little place for anything but palpatory assessment of contractions. Nevertheless, when oxytocin is employed there are good reasons to be cautious about overstimulation[14,51] and intrauterine pressure monitoring has been advocated.[9] However, even in complex obstetric practice, where the sophistication of intrauterine pressure monitoring may seem logical, there may be unexpected pitfalls unless the clinician understands what is being measured. In trial of scar, the fall in wall tension wrought by scar dehiscence can impart both a lack of tension to dilate the cervix and a fall in intrauterine pressure. These features may be interpreted as failure to progress due to poor uterine activity with the erroneous and, perhaps disastrous, consequence of prescribing oxytocin, thereby aggravating the scar rupture.[52] Though it may seem less accurate, simple palpation of repetition frequency and timing of duration has much to recommend it in this instance.

The lesson is that no single derived parameter is ideal and, in certain circumstances, intrauterine pressure monitoring may be no better than palpation and may even be misleading unless the system being monitored is understood. Furthermore, measuring the action without knowing the reaction gives only one side of a complex equation.

THE PASSAGES

The bony pelvis

The bony pelvis is often considered immutable, yet the ligamentous changes in pregnancy can permit an increase in dimension of several millimetres. The effect of posture, i.e. an upright squatting position, abducting the thighs, should increase space at the outlet by 'flaring out' the ischial tuberosities. Such a manoeuvre is used when shoulder dystocia is encountered, yet no formal investigation of the benefits of posture on the normal second stage has been published.

Pelvimetry, whether clinical or X-ray, has been disparaged since the outcome of labour depends upon additional factors such as flexion and moulding of the fetal head, stretching of ligaments and tissues of the pelvis which cannot be measured. In clinical practice, the progress of labour and descent of the head are the usual measures of cephalopelvic disproportion, i.e. performance of a trial of labour. Failure, however still leaves the vagaries of variables other than the pelvis. Many women who have patterns of progress consistent with cephalopelvic disproportion have normal X-ray and clinical pelvimetries and abnormalities of mechanism are often not substantiated, nor documented in reported series. The vague term 'dystocia' is all that is given. Furthermore, many women who have caesarean sections for abnormal cervimetric progress, whether coupled with fetal distress or not, go on to have normal vaginal deliveries in subsequent pregnancies, despite producing a larger baby than the first.

The soft tissues

The cervix is the primary soft tissue structure offering resistance to progress in the first stage. In the late first and second stages, when descent occurs, the tissues of the pelvic floor are encountered. The concept of pelvic resistance was developed by Crawford[16] who implied that rapid delivery could be a consequence of low resistance rather than high myometrial activity. This concept is consistent with the finding[15] that precipitate labour may be associated with low-normal levels of uterine activity. Arulkumaran et al[53] suggested that the total uterine activity throughout oxytocin-induced labour is indicative of the degree of cervical and pelvic tissue resistance, thus extending this precept. Lamont et al[54] found lower levels of uterine activity in nulliparous patients induced with prostaglandins compared with those who receive oxytocin. The levels of uterine activity in prostaglandin-induced labour resemble those in spontaneous labour. Pelvic resistance is a summation of all the soft tissue resistive factors in the pelvis. The study by Lamont et al would suggest the cervix is the major component and that it can be favourably manipulated.

The cervix in the first stage of labour

The cervix has conflicting demands placed upon it during pregnancy and labour. Prior to labour, it has to remain closed and continent. Its collagenous nature, with fibres tightly wound circumferentially round the canal[55] producing a tubular configuration, is ideally suited to its purpose of resisting dilatation. Interspersed between the collagen is a small amount of muscle which hitherto has been considered functionally insignificant.[55] At parturition the cervix has to allow the passage of the fetus without damaging its own architecture since it has to be able to repeat its pregnancy function within a matter of weeks. To achieve its second function, it undergoes a physicochemical change which is still poorly understood. The ground substance hydrates, coupled with changes in its glycoproteins, particularly an increased content of hyaluronidase. As a result the ground substance changes from a gel to a fluid medium, permitting dispersion of the collagen fibres,[56,57] altering its viscoelastic properties and permitting deformation of its structure.

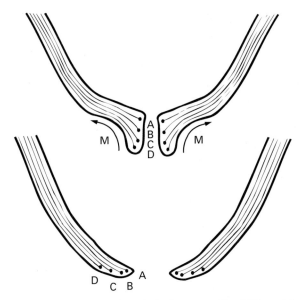

Fig. 10.7 Hypothetical mechanism of cervical effacement. M = Differential movement of tissue planes; A–D = Relative position of surface points relating to tissue planes before and after effacement.

The importance of this process has been acknowledged for the induction of labour but not for intrapartum progress. It is plausible that pathology in the ripening process could carry through to labour its pregnancy function of resisting dilatation. Recent biochemical data would add weight to this possibility.[58]

Effacement of the cervix and formation of the lower segment

To permit passage of the fetus the cervix has to dilate. As already stated, its tubular configuration is not conducive to this. Tissue has to be gradually removed to achieve a state in which tension from the myometrium can impart dilatation. This is the process of effacement. Obstetricians understand this process but cannot precisely describe it.

It has been suggested[15] that the cervix effaces as a result of differential movement of notional tissue planes in response to wall tension (Fig. 10.7). Although the tissue planes are not demonstrable histologically, the effect proposed may be viewed when the lower segment of the uterus is incised at caesarean section. Clinical evidence for this effect has been documented.[59] Hughesden[60] ascribed a similar process to the sparse muscle fibres found in the cervix but Danforth[55] argued that the strength of this muscle was not sufficient to achieve the proposed effect. Both may have been partially correct. The outer layers of the wall have a greater radius of curvature and for a given intrauterine pressure there will be more tension in the outer layers compared to the inner ones (Laplace's law). Even without the effect of intrinsic muscle activity, these forces would result in a shearing-off of tissue from the outside of the cervix, resulting in gradual effacement. This theoretical mechanism is contrary to the present teaching[5,61] but may explain some of the vagaries surrounding cervical continence. It is conventional teaching to ascribe continence to the internal os. In pregnancy, particularly in multiparous patients, the external os is often described as 'patulous', inferring continence of the upper canal while the external os lies loose. In the absence of frank cervical pathology, there is no evidence to suggest that multiparous patients develop cervical incompetence under these circumstances. At colposcopy, the external os tends to be 'flared open', making it easier to visualize the squamocolumnar junction than in non-pregnant patients. Cone biopsy of the cervix is associated with an increased incidence of premature delivery.[62] However, those procedures (i.e. loop excision) which do not impinge on the internal os have not been implicated with problems of this nature. The continence of the cervix would seem, therefore, to depend on the tissues that are found above the external os of the cervix.

The ground substance, composed as it is of glycoproteins, is the determining factor in the mechanisms concerning cervical change. In the fluid state, flow and deformation of architecture can take place. During effacement, the layers of the 'onion skin' can move one upon the other. As the layers move upward, the circumference of the collagen fibres must increase. Thus effacement and dilatation are different manifestations of the same process. Dispersion of the collagen reduces fibril–fibril interaction and permits distraction and dilatation. Activity of muscle cells, inserted into collagen fibres (some have suggested that the muscle cells secrete the collagen) would encourage this distraction. If however the fibres are 'glued' together, movement and distraction are not possible, effacement and dilatation cannot take place, there is no cervical modulation of wall tension and no response to it. On the contrary, any activity of the muscle in this state would increase tension in the collagen fibres which, unable to move one on the other, would impart tension to the cervix as a whole, producing constriction of the cervix not dilatation.

Management or delay in labour under these circumstances should be directed towards the physiochemical state of the cervix to improve its compliance, not towards myometrial force. This may take the form of timely non-intervention and sedation to allow natural 'ripening', as advocated by Friedman,[21] or it could be achieved pharmacologically. Unfortunately, presently used ripening agents also have uterotonic effects which are undesirable under these circumstances. Perhaps agents such as Relaxin could fulfil this role.

Measurement of cervical mechanics

Attempts to measure the resistive forces offered by the cervix have been made. Lindgren & Smyth[63] produced a triple transducer device which could be inserted between the fetal head and the cervix. A similar but improved device has been used more recently [64] and Gee[15] used fluid-filled balloons instead of transducers. A number of problems are encountered. It is difficult to standardize placement of the recording devices in relation to both head and cervix. Furthermore, since the orientation of the head changes with respect to the cervix and birth canal, reproduction and interpretation of recordings are difficult. Ideally, a system is required, possibly in the form of a 'skull cap', which contains multiple transducers to produce a simulation of the total force distribution around the fetal head. The placement of such a device carries with it obvious problems. Because of these limitations the measurement of head to cervix forces has found only research applications to date.

An alternative is to measure cervical response on a contraction cycle by cycle basis. The amount of dilatation in response to myometrial activity would index compliance while the recoil on removal of tension would reflect elasticity. Residual dilatation would represent plastic deformation, the summation of which equates with overall dilatation. At the present time the analysis of the data is simplistic and the use of the cervimeter[65] takes account of only two-dimensional response. Further work brings the prospect of three-dimensional analysis of cervical anatomy, and analysis of change with time would permit the derivation of viscoelastic function.

Clinical observations on the cervical response to myometrial activity

Studies conducted in pregnant women have shown that in the first and second trimesters the human cervix can contract in response to oxytocic agents[66,67] and, at term, the cervix can contract rhythmically, sometimes independently of the activity seen in the corpus.[68] Similar effects have been demonstrated in animals.[69–72] In human subjects it has always been assumed that the cervix responds passively in labour by dilating in response to contraction of the muscular corpus. However, when cervical dilatation is continuously monitored and recorded simultaneously with intrauterine pressure, the cervix has been noted to contract during myometrial activity, but only over the range of dilatations that correspond to the latent phase of labour (Fig. 10.8).[73] During the active phase of labour the cervix dilates in response to myometrial activity, as would be expected. Between the two phases, a transition or inflexion point has been noted, usually at 2–4 cm dilatation.[73]

Although generally a collagenous structure,[55,74] muscle tissue is present at the peripheral aspects of the cervix which is capable of contracting.[55,60] If the cervix effaces by the differential movement of tissue planes, as has been suggested,[15] the net result would be a taking up and thinning out of the cervix as a result of the greater movement of the outer layers. The effect would be to redistribute the muscle fibres, an effect which would explain the changing electromyographic pattern of the cervix noted in labour.[75]

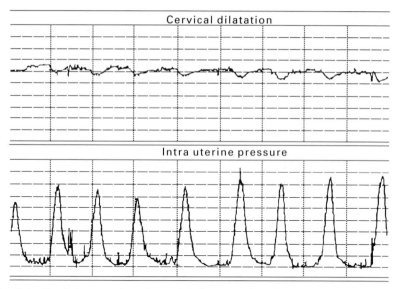

Fig. 10.8   Cervical contractions observed during a 30-min period in the latent phase of labour. Upper scale = 0–5 cm; lower scale = 0–100 mmHg.

The effect of an actively contracting cervix is obvious. Cervical compliance would decrease during contractions, and as a result of the CAP effect, higher pressures would be generated than if the cervix were passively compliant. The use of oxytocin would thus result in a high risk of fetal distress developing with no improvement in the rate of cervical dilatation. The logical approach to treatment would be a manipulation of the cervix to encourage 'ripening' and effacement without overstimulating the myometrium. Alternatively, a non-interventionist approach may be beneficial by allowing cervical change to occur spontaneously over a period of time. Certainly, Friedman[21] prescribed sedation to such women; its effect may have been to allow time for cervical change to occur.

Obviously, this would lead to prolongation of the labour which, by conventional teaching, would increase the likelihood of morbidity and mortality. However, if the hypoxic stress to the fetus could be alleviated by uterine relaxation, as practised by some workers,[76] the prolongation by itself would not be deleterious. Before the obsession with speed of labour, clinicians would sometimes allow 12 hours without oxytocin in those patients who had not responded. Normal progress took place thereafter.[77]

Implications for clinical practice.

Concern only with forces of labour without understanding the resistances gives only an incomplete concept of labour mechanisms. The apparent simplicity of the cervix belies its sophistication and crucial role in determining labour outcome. Observations, to date, have been concerned with its form rather than its behaviour. Until now the differentiation between latent and active phases of labour and the differences in response to oxytocin stimulation engendered by these two states have been imprecise. Measurement of cervical response to contractions offers the opportunity to differentiate the phases of labour on a functional basis. This function refers to the changing role of the cervix, i.e. from maintaining continence, its prime purpose during pregnancy, through a physicochemical transformation to a form which allows labour to proceed. This change in function can be recognized after the event by the inflexion in the dilatation curve but only prospectively by observing its functional response. Carrying through to the active phase its pregnancy function would lead to a less compliant and obstructive cervix. Despite Friedman's assertion that 'cervical dystocia is a rare condition', the abnormalities of function described here are being substantiated in biochemical terms[58] and in observations of cervical response during labour.

Use of tonic agents alone prior to this transition can result in cervical change due to force but the price is potential fetal compromise. A more logical approach would be to manipulate the cervical state, either pharmacologically or temporally. Manipulation of cervical ripeness is accepted practice for induction of labour and abnormal glycoprotein content of the cervix has been linked with aberrant cervical dilatation in labour.[58] Conversley, preterm labour may be a representation of pathological cervical change such that those cases which are most at risk progress insidiously with little apparent uterine activity. In these cases inhibition of the ripening process may bear more fruit than tocolysis alone.[17]

CONCLUSIONS AND THE FUTURE

1. There is substantial evidence to implicate a cervical component as a cause of delay in the progress of labour.

2. The cervical response to myometrial activity varies during the course of labour.

3. The response of the cervix to myometrial activity depends upon its physical state which, in turn, is determined by its biochemical state.

4. During the early part of labour and before the cervix is fully effaced the cervix may contract during myometrial activity.

5. Cervicography can identify delay but, by itself, is not diagnostic of underlying pathology, nor does it relate to the functional state of the cervix. However, the inflexion point between latent and active phases, which can only be recognized retrospectively, probably results from these functional changes.

6. Without knowledge of the cervical response to myometrial activity the functional state of the cervix is unknown. Recognition of the transition between the latent and active phase of labour is imprecise and can only be recognized retrospectively. Thus there is a danger of applying active-phase

limits to the latent phase. Active management as practised by O'Driscoll and colleagues takes care to avoid this pitfall by defining what they consider to be labour. Unless these definitions and practices are followed exactly, there is a danger that oxytocin will be used inappropriately. This could explain the inability to realize the expected results of active management.

7. The physical state of the cervix affects the generation of intrauterine pressure, such that a compliant cervix will attenuate the pressure, and a non-compliant cervix will augment generated pressure. This CAP effect explains certain paradoxes surrounding labour. It also limits the clinician's ability to drive cervical dilatation by increasing myometrial force.

8. Measurement of uterine activity gives only one side of a complex balance governing progress in labour in which the cervix has an effect on both sides. Thus, it is not suprising that quantification of uterine activity alone has failed to produce a commensurate increase in understanding and control, despite the application of increasingly sophisticated technology.

9. The logical approach to the management of cases that present with poor progress despite normal or high uterine activity may be manipulation of the cervix pharmacologically to improve the rate of dilatation. Should we choose to concentrate on manipulating cervical compliance, which is little more than an extension of the pharmacology familiar to us for ripening the cervix, there would be the prospect of selectively reducing cervical resistance resulting in the delivery of the fetus with the minimum of force — a medical caesarean section — an attractive option in those cases in which the fetus is already compromised.

REFERENCES

1. O'Driscoll K, Jackson R J H, Gallagher J T. Prevention of prolonged labour. Br Med J 1969; 2: 447–480
2. Duignan N. Active management of labour. In: Studd J, ed. The management of labour. Oxford: Blackwell Scientific Publications, 1985: pp 146–158
3. Philpott R H, Castle W M. Cervicographs in the management of labour in primigravidae. I. The alert line for detecting abnormal labour. Obstet Gynaecol Br Commonwlth 1972; 79: 592–598
4. Philpott R H, Castle W M. Cervicographs in the management of labour in primigravidae. II. The action line and treatment of abnormal labour. J Obstet Gynaecol Br Commonwlth 1972; 79: 592–598
5. O'Driscoll K, Meagher D. Active management of labour. London: Bailliere Tindall, 1986
6. Turner M J, Brassil M, Gordon H. Active management of labor associated with a decrease in the cesarean section rate in nulliparas. Obstet Gynecol 1988; 71: 150–154
7. Schifrin B S, Cohen W R. Labor's dysfunctional lexicon. Obstet Gynecol 1989; 74: 121–124
8. Kiwanuka A I, Moore W M. The changing incidence of caesarean section in the health district of Central Manchester. Br J Obstet Gynaecol 1987; 94: 440-444
9. Cardozo L, Gibb D M F, Studd J W W, Vasant R V, Cooper D J. Predictive value of cervimatric patterns in primigravidae. Br J Obstet Gynaecol 1982; 89: 33–38
10. Gordon A J. Measurement of uterine activity — a useful tool? Br J Obstet Gynaecol 1984; 91: 209–210

11. Chua S, Kurup A, Arulkumaran S, Ratnam S S. Augmentation of labour: does internal tocography result in better obstetric outcome than external tocography? Obstet Gynecol 1990; 76: 164–167

12. Al-Shawaf T, Al-Mogharaby S, Akiez A. Normal levels of uterine activity in primigravidae and mothers of high parity in spontaneous labour. J Obstet Gynaecol 1987; 8: 18–23

13. Turnbull A C. Uterine contractions in normal and abnormal labour. J Obstet Gynaecol Br Emp 1957; 64: 321–333

14. Gee H, Beazley J M. Uterine activity plotted on an inductograph as an aid to management of labour. Br J Obstet Gynaecol 1980; 87:115–121

15. Gee H. Uterine activity and cervical resistance determining cervical change in labour. M.D. thesis, University of Liverpool, England, 1981

16. Crawford J W. Computer monitoring of fetal heart rate and uterine pressure. Am J Obstet Gynecol 1975; 21: 342–350

17. Oláh K S, Gee H. The prevention of pre-term delivery — Can we afford to continue to ignore the cervix? Br J Obstet Gynaecol 1992; 99: 278–280

18. Pearce J M. Management of pre-term Labour. In Studd J, ed. The management of labour. Oxford: Blackwell Scientific Publications, 1985; pp 40–67

19. Bidgood K A, Steer P J. A randomized control study of oxytocin augmentation of labour. 1. Obstetric outcome. Br J Obstet Gynaecol 1987; 94: 512–517

20. Friedman E A. The graphic analysis of labor. Am J Obstet Gynecol 1954; 68: 1568–1575

21. Friedman E A. Primigravid labor. A graphicostatistical analysis. Obstet Gynecol 1955; 6: 567–589

22. Friedman E A, Sachtleben M R. Dysfunctional labor. I. Prolonged latent phase in the nullipara. Obstet Gynecol 1961; 17: 135–148

23. Gibb D M F, Cardozo L D, Studd J W W, Magos A L, Cooper D J. Outcome of spontaneous labour in multigravidae. Br J Obstet Gynaecol 1982; 89: 708–711

24. Hendricks C H, Brenner W E, Kraus G. Normal cervical dilatation pattern in late pregnency and labor. Am J Obstet Gynecol 1970; 106: 1065–1082

25. Cardozo L, Studd J. Abnormal labour patterns. In: Studd J, ed. The management of labour. Oxford: Blackwell Scientific Publications, 1985: pp 171–187

26. Friedman E A. Labor. Clinical evaluation and management. New York: Meredith 1967

27. Davidson A C, Weaver J B, Davies P, Pearson J F. The relation between ease of forceps delivery and speed of cervical dilatation. Br J Obstet Gynaecol 1976; 83: 279–283

28. Philpott R H. Graphic records in labour. Br Med J 1972; 4: 163–165

29. Studd J. Partograms and nomograms of cervical dilatation in management of primigravid labour. Br Med J 1973; 4: 451–455

30. Beazley J M, Kurjak A. Influence of a partogram on the active management of labour. Lancet 1972; II: 348–351

31. Beazley J M, Alderman B. The 'Inductograph' — a graph describing the limits of the latent phase of induced labour in low risk situations. Br J Obstet Gynaecol 1976; 83: 513–517

32. Cardozo L, Pearce J M. Oxytocin in active-phase abnormalities of labor: a randomized study. Obstet Gynecol 1991; 75: 152–157

33. Studd J W W, Cardozo L D, Gibb D M F. The management of spontaneous labour. In: Studd J, ed. Progress in obstetrics and gynaecology, vol 2. Edinburgh: Churchill Livingstone, 1982: p 60

34. Dryden P R. An evaluation of primary dysfunctional labour in primigravidae. Abstract. 23rd British Congress of Obstetrics and Gynaecology, pp. 99

35. Bidgood K A, Steer P J. A randomized control study of oxytocin augmentation of labour. 2. Uterine activity. Br J Obstet Gynaecol 1987; 94: 518–522

36. Seitchik J, Chatkoff M L. Intra-uterine pressure waveform characteristics of spontaneous first stage labour. J Appl Physiol 1975; 38: 443–448

37. Coren R L. Uterine contractions and intra-amniotic pressure. J Theor Biol 1965; 9: 1–15

38. Arulkumaran S, Ingemarsson I, Ratnam SS. Oxytocin titration to achieve pre-set active contraction area values does not improve outcome of induced labour. Br J Obstet Gynaecol 1987; 94: 242–248

39. Caldeyro-Barcia R, Sica-Blanco Y, Poseiro J J et al. A quantitative study of the action of synthetic oxytocin on the pregnant human uterus. J Pharmacol Exp Ther 1957; 121: 18–31
40. El Sahwi S E, Gaafar A A, Toppozada H K. A new unit for the evaluation of uterine activity. Am J Obstet Gynaecol 1967; 98: 900–903
41. Steer P J, Little D J, Lewis N L, Kelly M C M E, Beard R W. Uterine activity in induced labour. Br J Obstet Gynaecol 1975; 82: 433–441
42. Steer P J. The measurement and control of uterine contractions. In: Beard R W, Campbell S, eds. The current status of fetal heart rate monitoring and ultrasound in obstetrics. London: RCOG, 1977: pp 48–68
43. Phillips G F, Calder A A. Units for the evaluation of uterine contractility. Br J Obstet Gynaecol 1987; 94: 236–241
44. Coren R L, Csapo A I. The intra-amniotic pressure. Am J Obstet Gynecol 1963; 85: 470–483
45. Gee H, Taylor E W, Hancox R. A model for the generation of intra-uterine pressure in the human parturient uterus which demonstrates the critical role of the cervix. J Theor Biol 1988; 133: 281–291
46. Gee H. The interaction between cervix and corpus uteri in the generation of intra-amniotic pressure in labour. Eur J Obstet Gynecol Reprod Biol 1983; 16: 243–252
47. Janbu T, Neshein B. Uterine artery blood velocities during contractions in pregnancy and labour related to intra-uterine pressure. Br J Obstet Gynaecol 1987; 94: 1150–1155
48. Borell U, Fernstrom I, Ohlson L, Wiqvist N. The influence of uterine contractions on the utero-placental blood flow at term. Am J Obstet Gynecol 1964; 93: 44–48
49. Caldeyro-Barcia R, Pose S V, Alvarez H. Uterine contractility in polyhydramnios and the effects of withdrawal of the excess of amniotic fluid. Am J Obstet Gynecol 1957; 73: 1238–1254
50. Gibb D M F, Arulkumaran S, Lun K C, Ratnam S S. Characteristics of uterine activity in nulliparous labour. Br J Obstet Gynaecol 1984; 91: 220–227
51. Taylor R W, Taylor M. Misuse of oxytocin in labour. Lancet 1988; 1: 352
52. Beckley S, Gee H, Newton J R. Scar rupture in labour after previous lower uterine segment caesarean section: the role of uterine activity measurement. Br J Obstet Gynaecol 1991; 98: 265–269
53. Arulkumaran S, Gibb D M F, Ratnam S S, Lun K C, Heng S H. Total uterine activity in induced labour — an index of cervical and pelvic tissue resistance. Br J Obstet Gynaecol 1985; 92: 693–697
54. Lamont R F, Neave S, Baker A C, Steer P J. Intrauterine pressures in labours induced by amniotomy and oxytocin or vaginal prostaglandin gel compared with spontaneous labour. Br J Obstet Gynaecol 1991; 98: 441–447
55. Danforth D N. The distribution and functional activity of the cervical musculature. Am J Obstet Gynecol 1954; 68: 1261–1271
56. von Maillot K, Stuhlsatz H W, Mohanaradhakrishnan V, Greiling H. Changes in the glycosaminoglycans distribution pattern in the human uterine cervix during pregnancy and labour. Am J Obstet Gynecol 1979; 135: 503–506
57. Uldbjerg N. Cervical connective tissue in relation to pregnancy, labour and treatment with prostaglandin E₂. Acta Obstet Gynecol Scand suppl 148: 20–25
58. Granström L, Ekman G, Malmström A. Insufficient remodelling of the uterine connective tissue in women with protracted labour. Br J Obstet Gynaecol 1991; 98: 1212–1216
59. Oláh K S, Gee H, Brown J S. Measurement of the cervical response to uterine activity in labour and observations on the mechanism of cervical effacement. J Perinat Med 1991; 19 (suppl 2): 245
60. Hughesdon P E. The fibromuscular structure of the cervix and its changes during pregnancy and labour. J Obstet Gynaecol Br Emp 1952; 59: 763–776
61. Jeffcoate T N A. Physiology and mechanism of labour. In: Claye A, ed. British obstetric and gynaecological practice 3rd ed. London: Heinemann, 1963; p 159
62. Jones J M, Sweetnam P, Hibbard B M. The outcome of pregnancy after cone biopsy of the cervix: a case control study. Br J Obstet Gynaecol 1979; 86: 913–916
63. Lindgren C L, Smyth C N. Measurement and interpretation of the pressures upon the

cervix during normal and abnormal labour. J Obstet Gynaecol Br Commonwlth 1961; 68: 901–915
64. Gough G W, Randall N J, Dut G, Sutherland I A, Steer P J. Head-to-cervix forces and their relationship to the outcome of labor. Obstet Gynecol 1990; 75: 613–618
65. Richardson J A, Sutherland I A, Allen D W. A cervimeter for continuous measurement of cervical dilatation in labour — preliminary results. Br J Obstet Gynaecol 1978; 85: 178–184
66. Schild H O, Fitzpatrick R J, Nixon W C W. Activity of the human cervix and corpus uteri. Lancet 1951; i: 250–252
67. Mackenzie I Z. The effect of oxytocics on the human cervix during midtrimester pregnancy. Br J Obstet Gynaecol 1976; 83: 780–785
68. Karlson S. On the motility of the uterus during labour and the influence of the motility pattern on the duration of the labour. Acta Obstet Gynecol Scand 1949; 28: 209–250
69. Newton W H. Reciprocal activity of the cornua and cervix uteri of the goat. J Physiol 1934; 81: 277–282
70. Newton W H. The insensitivity of the cervix uteri to oxytocin. J Physiol 1937; 89: 309–315
71. Bonnycastle D D, Ferguson J K W. The action of pitocin and adrenalin on different segments of the rabbit uterus. J Pharmacol 1941; 72: 90–98
72. Adler J, Bell G H, Knox J A C. The behaviour of the cervix uteri in vivo. J Physiol 1944; 103: 142–154
73. Oláh K S, Gee H. Unpublished observations,1992
74. Danforth D N. The fibrous nature of the human cervix, and its relation to the isthmic segment in gravid and nongravid uteri. Am J Obstet Gynecol 1947; 53: 541–560
75. Pajntar M, Roskar D, Rudel D. Longitudinally and circularly measured EMG activity in the human uterine cervix during labour. Acta Physiol Hungarica 1988; 71: 497–502
76. Caldeyro-Barcia R. Intrauterine fetal reanimation in acute intrapartum distress. J Perinat Med 1991; 19 (suppl 2): 11
77. Whitely P F. Personal communication, 1989
78. Friedman E A. The management of labor. In: Cohen W R, Friedman E A, eds. Management of labor. Baltimore: University Park Press, 1983: pp 13, 15

11. Instrumental delivery: a lost art?

J. P. O'Grady   M. Gimovsky

More matter with less art. *Hamlet* II, ii, 95 — William Shakespeare (1564–1616)

The use of instruments to assist delivery has always been controversial. The history of labor management includes continuous and often acrimonious exchanges between minimalists preferring a natural approach versus interventionists favoring some type of assistance. The literature is replete with strongly worded opinions. Some counsel that there are minimal or rapidly diminishing indications for operative vaginal delivery while others with equally firm conviction suggest an ongoing role for instrumental assistance. We also face a difficult legal climate in the USA concerning birth injury where allegations of malpractice are often driven by maloccurrence, regardless of cause. This leaves clinicians justifiably concerned about the indications, risks and the defensibility of instrumentally assisted delivery procedures in modern obstetric practice. It is these issues that the current paper explores.

Cesarean section, the popular American response to possible difficult delivery, has not proven to be an entirely successful nor universally satisfactory remedy. The incidence of long-term neurological deficits in surviving neonates seems little changed even by very liberal use of cesarean delivery. As Green et al[1] point out, an increase from 22 to 94% in cesarean delivery for breech presentations made no impact on neonatal outcome. Such procedures also involve some measure of maternal risk and morbidity.[2,3] Other approaches are possible. The National Maternity Hospital group (Dublin) has presented impressive data concerning the active management of labor.[4,5] These data indicate a highly acceptable rate of perinatal mortality, accompanying a remarkably low incidence of cesarean delivery, with limited but continuing use of instrumental and/or assisted delivery. Active management focuses on the process of labor with careful attention to early diagnosis and prompt intervention. While there is quickening interest in active management techniques, American patterns of labor management and cesarean delivery have remained relatively stable for at least 10 years.

This paper does not intend to discuss the differences in labor management between European and American centres. Nor is it intended as a nostalgic review of obsolete techniques not applicable in modern practice.

183

Our aim is to provide a critique of the current status of instrumental delivery as practised for the most common indications of dystocia, presumed fetal jeopardy, and 'prophylaxis'. This will include discussions of clinical evaluation and delivery technique involving both forceps and the vacuum extractor. Our interest is in exploring both the techniques of assisted delivery as well as the obstetric decision-making process. The central question posed is the role of instrumental delivery in modern obstetric practice when fetal condition can be closely monitored, safe cesarean surgery is possible, and when there is great concern about traumatic delivery.

OPERATIONS

Definitions

In the effort to standardize reporting and practice, the American College of Obstetricians and Gynecologists (ACOG) periodically reviews obstetric procedures and issues guidelines. For the coding of forceps operations, the ACOG revised the definitions in 1989 and 1991[6,7] (Table 11.1). There are now three major subdivisions: mid forceps, low forceps, and outlet forceps operations. These new definitions for vaginal operative delivery have recently been validated as a reasonable reflection of both difficulty and fetomaternal risk.[8] While the ACOG guidelines were written for forceps operations, it seems reasonable to apply the same descriptions to vacuum extraction procedures. We have done so in this review.

Indications

The indications for operative vaginal delivery are either fetal or maternal.[7]

Table 11.1 ACOG 1989/1991[6,7] classification of forceps deliveries according to station and rotation

Type of procedure	Classification
Outlet forceps	The fetal head is at or on the perineum 1. Scalp is visible at the introitus without separating the labia 2. Fetal skull has reached the pelvic floor 3. Sagittal suture is in anteroposterior diameter or right or left occiput anterior or posterior position 4. Rotation does not exceed 45°
Low forceps	The leading point of the fetal skull is at station $\geq$ +2 cm*, but not on the pelvic floor 1. Rotation $\leq$ 45° (left or right occiput anterior to occiput anterior, or left or right occiput posterior to occiput posterior) 2. Rotation > 45°
Mid forceps	Station $\leq$ + 2 cm* station but the head is engaged
High forceps	Not included in classification

*Station is defined as the distance in *centimeters* between the leading bony portion of the fetal skull and the plane of the maternal ischial spines.
Modified with permission from ACOG.[6,7]

These include a *prolonged second stage of labor, indicated shortening of the second stage, and presumed fetal jeopardy.* The latter was coined as a non-specific descriptor for what was heretofore loosely termed fetal distress. The term 'presumed fetal jeopardy' requires documentation in the medical record. Evidence for distress might include abnormal fetal heart rate patterns, meconium passage, or abnormal scalp or cord pH values.

In situations of arrested descent or excessive prolongation of the second stage of labor special definitions apply. Second-stage labor of more than 2 hours *without* a regional or epidural anesthetic or 3 hours with such an anesthetic is considered prolonged for nulliparous women. For parous women the time intervals are 2 and 1 hour respectively.

Elective shortening of the second stage is an additional indication. Examples include individuals with cardiac, cerebrovascular, or neuro-muscular conditions where their medical condition makes voluntary expulsive efforts either contraindicated or impossible. Other situations might include maternal exhaustion, poor second-stage expulsive efforts due to limited ability to cooperate, excessive analgesia, or other clinical factors.

If a simple outlet procedure is possible, the second stage may also be terminated electively. This 'prophylactic' use of forceps was part of standard American practice for many years but is now undergoing critical re-evaluation.[9-14]

INSTRUMENTS AND OPERATIONS

A brief review of the major forceps types and vacuum extractor designs follows. Both the extractor and forceps have inherent advantages and disadvantages. Adequate education for practitioners in the correct use of these instruments is a continuing issue.

Forceps

While several hundred different forceps designs have been invented, several types are most popular in American practice. These are conveniently divided into classic instruments, modified classic instruments, specialized instruments, divergent blade instruments, and axis traction devices.[14]

Examples of the classic instruments are those originally invented by James Young Simpson and George L. Elliot Jr in the mid 19th century. These popular forceps are commonly chosen for outlet operations and low pelvic rotational deliveries. In experienced hands these blades can perform virtually all forceps operations.

The Tucker–McLane forceps, an Elliot-type design with overlapping, extended shanks and solid blades, is the most commonly applied modified classic instrument. Occasionally, the blades are pseudofenestrated (Luikart's modification). Tucker-McLane's are commonly used as mid pelvic rotators or outlet blades.

Specialized instruments include forceps designed for specific obstetric indications. Examples include the forceps of Barton, Keilland, and Piper. The appropriate use of each are, respectively, transverse arrest in a platypoid pelvis, mid pelvic rotation when correction of asynclitism is required, and delivery of the after-coming head in breech presentations.

Divergent or parallel blade instruments most likely to be encountered by clinicians are the designs of Laufe and Shute. These forceps were developed to limit fetal cranial compression by restricting the delivery forces by specialized design.[15,16]

Axis traction instruments are less commonly used in modern practice but were once quite popular. If axis traction is desired, it is easiest to attach a traction handle (Bill's handle) to a standard forceps. In some instruments, such as in the Hawk-Dennon and the DeWees forceps, axis traction is an integral part of the design.

Vacuum extractors

Vacuum extractors are of two general designs: rigid cup and flexible or soft cup. Rigid cup instruments include the metal vacuum cups of Malmström and the various modifications of Bird and others.[17] Soft cup instruments include the cone-shaped silastic cup (Kobayashi device) and various other, more conventional plastic cup designs (e.g. Mityvac, Softtouch cup, CMI cup, etc.).[18] Several modifications of vacuum cup design exist for deflexed or posterior-positioned fetal heads.[19] Most recent interest has centered upon the use of the disposable plastic cups due to their ease of application and lack of assembly requirements. Cup design and its relationship to maternal/fetal trauma and procedure success are addressed more extensively in the sections concerning technique.

Outlet and low pelvic operations

True outlet operations are commonly easy. These are performed with minimal analgesia and force.[14,18] While vacuum extractions at low station can be conducted with only local, or occasionally, no anesthesia, the use of forceps normally requires at least a pudendal block for patient comfort.[6,7,14]

Despite the simplicity of outlet procedures, the standard prerequisites for instrumental delivery apply: careful review of indication, adequate anesthesia or analgesia, accurate application, and the minimal use of force.

Traditionally, in American practice outlet and low forceps operations are performed with the forceps of Elliot or Simpson. However, any instrument with a pelvic curve will suffice in experienced hands. The Malmström vacuum extractor, one of the Bird modifications, or one of the newer disposable vacuum cup devices are also acceptable. The silastic extractor is less desirable as an outlet instrument as it frequently loses effective vacuum at the perineum due to cup buckling.

Mid pelvic operations

Mid pelvic operations are defined by the station of the fetal head and the degree of rotation required. The most important prerequisites for these more complex procedures are an adequately skilled surgeon, certain identification of the position, station, and attitude of the fetal skull, acceptable analgesia/anesthesia, and *the willingness to abandon the attempt promptly if the operation proves difficult.*[6,7,20]

Presumed fetal jeopardy, transverse arrests and failure of descent are the most frequent clinical problems associated with mid pelvic procedures. Mid pelvic arrest is usually related to failure of the powers, often combined with variations in pelvic architecture. True cephalopelvic disproportion (CPD) is uncommon. However, CPD needs to be carefully considered whenever the fetal head fails to descend beyond the mid-pelvis despite appropriate cervical dilation. Poor progress may have other causes, including platypoid or android pelves which predispose to transverse arrest, or epidural anesthesia. Transverse presentation also occurs as a transitional stage during spontaneous rotation from a posterior position or following delayed rotation of a normally aligned head, which fails to advance beyond the transverse. The latter circumstance is usually related to inefficient uterine activity and responds best to oxytocin stimulation.

The cardinal features of successful descent and rotation in mid pelvic forceps operations are accurate application, minimal force, and careful attention to the pelvic curve of the instrument used.[7,14,21] A correct application in mid pelvic procedures is governed by the location of the sagittal suture and the fontanelles. In general, mid pelvic application of the vacuum extractor is much easier than that for forceps as wandering or inversion of the instrument is not required.

When forceps are applied in the mid pelvis, asynclitism and deflexion often require correction. Rotation is generally performed *before* traction is applied[7] between contractions, with the mother cautioned not to bear down. In contrast, in vacuum extraction operations, rotation occurs spontaneously *while* traction is being applied and as the parturient bears down, as the device assists descent of the presenting part.[17] In some clinical services vacuum extraction has rapidly replaced forceps in trials of mid pelvic delivery due to its presumed greater safety, the ease of instrument application in the mid-cavity, and the difficulties in training new practitioners in the more demanding requirements of true mid-forceps applications.

Forceps versus vacuum extractor

Several factors influence which instrument to apply. Foremost is the experience and training of the accoucheur. Design features and potential complications of a given technique also guide the clinician's choice. No attempt should be made to use an unfamiliar instrument unless a qualified assistant or instructor is present. Unfortunately, the ease with which the vacuum extractor can be applied lends itself to use by the inexperienced.

Certain factors favor the use of the ventouse as the primary delivery instrument. The vacuum extraction cup can be inserted and traction applied with the use of minimal maternal analgesia.[19,22] This is particularly useful in settings where a regional anesthetic has failed or has only partially been successful, or when the mother has refused its administration. Also, the ventouse usually results in fewer maternal vaginal vault and perineal injuries than forceps.[23] Since the device is not applied between the fetal head and the vaginal side walls, when rotation occurs it does not cause the cup to come into contact with maternal tissues, thus minimizing vault injuries.[17,24,25] Vacuum extraction also reduces the risk for third- and fourth-degree perineal lacerations.[26–28] In addition, the likelihood of transitory or permanent fetal nerve injury is greater with forceps than with the vacuum extractor although these injuries are rare.

The vacuum extractor is not without risk and must be considered a surgical instrument. The successful use of the ventouse largely depends upon the clinician's[14,17,18] understanding of the physics of parturition and close adherence to protocol.[17,29] The ventouse is capable of exerting less immediate force than forceps and is thus less forgiving of lapses in traction technique.[22,25,27,30–35] Failure to time traction efforts carefully with contractions or performance of oblique pulls outside of the pelvic curve are common causes for vacuum extraction failure and predispose to injury.[17,36]

The problem of assuring rotation is frequently mentioned as a deficiency of the vacuum extractor in mid pelvic operations. However, with correct application of the vacuum cup and appropriate maternal coaching, the presenting part will rotate normally as the skull descends, faithfully reproducing the usual mechanism of labor.[14,17,24,36] The emphasis here is upon proper cup placement and verbal recruitment of maternal expulsive efforts to accompany uterine contractions. Clinicians should also recall that regardless of the cup type, traction can begin as soon as the working level of vacuum is reached, without waiting for a *chignon* to form.[35]

In deciding between forceps or the vacuum extractor in a given clinical setting, fetal safety is the central consideration. Since the use of vacuum extraction requires that force be applied to the soft tissues of the fetal cranium, fetal scalp injuries do occur and serious complications are possible, even if uncommon.[17] Minor skin ecchymoses or abrasions are usual with vacuum extraction but are of trivial clinical consequence (Table 11.2). With the use of a rigid cup instrument, the resultant *chignon* produces an unusual but temporary appearance of the fetal head. This often proves bothersome to clinicians and new parents and contributed to the initial slow acceptance of vacuum extraction in American practice. The *chignon* is less marked with the new soft cup designs and such complaints have largely disappeared.

Table 11.2 Perinatal complications: 256 vacuum extractions with Malmström-type rigid metal cup versus 300 forceps deliveries

	Vacuum extraction	Forceps	P
Cephalohematoma	10 (3.9%)	13 (4.3%)	NS
Neonatal jaundice	73 (28.5%)	51 (17%)	<0.01
Skin ecchymoses/abrasions	113 (44.1%)	89 (29.5%)	<0.001
Subconjunctival hemorrhage	4 (1.5%)	13 (4.3%)	NS
Shoulder dystocia	8 (3.1%)	1 (0.3%)	<0.01
Mortality	1 (0.4%)	1 (0.3%)	NS
Seizures	1 (0.4%)	2 (0.6%)	NS

NS = Not significant.
Reproduced with permission from Broekhuizen et al.[24]

Intracranial hemorrhage, skull fracture, cephalohematomas, and, uncommonly, subgaleal hemorrhage do occur with vacuum extraction.[27,37-39] However, these injuries are markedly infrequent and largely avoided by strict adherence to the protocols for correct use of the instrument. Minor neonatal jaundice and retinal hemorrhages are likely more common in vacuum-extracted neonates than in those delivered by forceps. Yet the evidence for an increased incidence of retinal hemorrhages with vacuum extraction versus forceps is equivocal, when comparable groups are closely studied.[17] It may be that such hemorrhages are more an indication of mild to moderate fetal asphyxia rather than a reflection of direct cranial trauma.

Results of comparative studies are mixed. Fetal scalp injuries and mild postnatal jaundice are more frequent with use of the vacuum extractor, while maternal perineal injuries are more likely with forceps deliveries. Such perineal damage is not inconsequential (Table 11.3).[22,26] Episiotomy,

Table 11.3 North Staffordshire/Wigan trial of perineal/vaginal trauma in a comparison of silicone vacuum extractor versus conventional forceps

Trauma	Silicone cup (n=132) n(%)	Forceps (n=132) n(%)
*Perineum**		
Intact	8 (6)	6 (5)
First-degree tear	11 (8)	2 (2)
Second-degree tear/cut	107 (81)	108 (82)
Third-degree tear		
Sphincter	6 (5)	13 (10)
Anal mucosa	0 (0)	3 (2)
*Vagina***		
No extension	97 (73)	76 (58)
Small extension	6 (5)	14 (10)
Extension to fornix	2 (2)	10 (8)
Not recorded	27 (20)	32 (24)

*P< 0.05; ** P< 0.005.
Reproduced with permission from Johanson et al.[25]

common or routine with forceps operations, predisposes to third-and fourth-degree perineal tears. Such injuries can result in long-term abnormalities in rectal sphincter function or, uncommonly, in fistula formation.[40-42]

There has been increasing experimentation in vacuum cup design with several novel devices described in recent years. New designs have entered the market much more rapidly than clinical studies can be performed to judge their performance in comparison to more conventional instruments. Despite this limitation, several randomized comparisons between instruments are available for review.[17,34,43,44] In comparing the polyethylene and silastic cups, the disposable extractor proved to be a more effective instrument, at least for outlet delivery.[45] When soft and metal cups have been compared, the flexible cup design has been associated with a higher incidence of failure but with less cosmetic injury to the fetus.[34,43,44,46] Higher failure rates for pliable silicone rubber cups have also been observed in randomized comparison to forceps.[25] Many practitioners experienced in vacuum extraction now favor one or more of the disposable polyethylene or polyethylene/silastic cup designs over the classic rigid metal cups due to their ease of use and possible lower incidence of fetal scalp injury. Determination of which instrument is best awaits well-conducted randomized studies. Clinicians should remain skeptical of extravagant claims of increased safety for newer cup designs until adequate comparative studies have been conducted.

Operator experience and the clinical setting are the principal determinates of the delivery instrument used. When an outlet procedure is performed, there is little to choose between the vacuum extractor and the forceps, assuming the presence of adequate analgesia.[14,23] If no anesthetic/analgesic is present, a pudendal block can be administered for forceps; this intervention can often be omitted for simple vacuum extraction. In terms of instrument, the newer disposable polyethylene devices or the classic Malmström–Bird cups are the best outlet devices. Direct occiput posterior presentations at low station are a special case. Vacuum extraction is most likely to fail in such applications due to difficulty in correctly applying the cup to the usually deflexed fetal head.[43,44,47] In experienced hands forceps are more useful in this setting, unless an occipitoposterior (OP) cup is available. Recent trials of new soft cup vacuum extractors suggest that there is a role for these vacuum cups in OP presentation but the extraction is usually more difficult.[25] Failure in extraction of posterior heads is largely due to cranial malpositioning and technical limitations of the application.

In instances of fetal distress at low station, most American practitioners prefer the use of forceps over the vacuum extractor, largely because of experience and training. Surprising to many traditionally trained practitioners, the objective data indicate that neither the ventouse nor forceps are superior in terms of fetal safety or speed.[13,23,25,27,45,48-50]

As a general rule, neither vacuum extraction nor forceps are to be applied at high station or used without full cervical dilation. A partial exception is fetal distress at advanced dilation or the extraction of a second twin. When fetal distress occurs in a multiparous patient with an adequate pelvis and advanced cervical dilation at low station, an experienced surgeon can apply the vacuum extractor in the effort to expedite delivery. The patient is instructed to push with contractions while simultaneous preparations are being made by the delivery room assistants for cesarean delivery. If station is not made immediately with the initial traction effort, or if the extraction is prolonged, the labor is terminated by cesarean section. It is well to re-emphasize that such procedures are to be attempted only by the most experienced, preferably in the operating room, while *simultaneous* preparations are under way for cesarean delivery.

In the management of second twins, the head of the second twin can often be grasped as soon as engagement occurs. The subsequent delivery is usually achieved promptly with minimal traction. Under these clinical circumstances it is best to use real-time ultrasound scanning to guide the fetal head into the pelvis, assure proper flexion, and monitor the fetal heart rate. As always, the rule of reasonable behavior prevails. The delivery room is no place for heroism. *Sang froid* and conservative efforts best characterize the obstetric surgeon.

The primary advantages of vacuum extraction over forceps are in potentially difficult mid pelvic procedures and in trials of instrumental delivery.[24,51] Highly experienced practitioners can perform mid pelvic rotations with Kielland or other forceps with success equal to practitioners utilizing the vacuum extractor.[52] However, such mid pelvic operations are increasingly infrequent and many younger practitioners have limited experience with such procedures. Further, even in experienced hands the likelihood for maternal injury is greater in mid-cavity forceps operations than with properly conducted vacuum extractions.[17,48,53,54] Thus, in true mid pelvic operations vacuum extraction is the procedure of choice for most, but not all, practitioners. Mid pelvic forceps procedures need not be abandoned by the experienced, but should *never* be attempted by the neophyte without immediate and skillful assistance.[55,56]

There are clinical settings in which the vacuum extractor should not or cannot be used. Applications to the after-coming head in breech presentations or to the fetal face are obvious examples. As previously discussed, vacuum extraction is generally contraindicated prior to full cervical dilation or at high station, although there are data concerning vacuum extraction during the first stage of labor and for extraction of a second twin.[48,57] While not subjected to any scientific study, most authorities caution against the use of the extractor for infants of less than 36 weeks' gestational age.[58] This restriction may be unnecessarily conservative. Vacuum extraction should also be performed with care if a prior scalp sample or samples were performed during labor.[59] Yet the risks of fetal hemorrhage if the ventouse is used following either scalp sampling or the application of a spiral scalp electrode is minimal at best.[25,60]

Other uses proposed for the vacuum extractor are less important. An example is the use of the ventouse for extraction of the fetal head at cesarean delivery. Such instrumentation is rarely necessary. With good anesthesia and an adequate incision difficult extractions at cesarean delivery are at best uncommon. In the unusual case an assistant can easily elevate the fetal head from below, assisting the efforts of the surgeons from above. If an instrumental assist from above is required, a Murless vectus or a modified forceps are much more convenient instruments to apply than the vacuum extractor.

A final point deserving emphasis is that formal training in vacuum extraction is frequently incomplete or deficient.[29] This is a particular challenge to teaching programs as minimization of risk in the use of vacuum extraction is dependent upon both adequate experience and strict adherence to technique.[17,19,61]

Documentation

Proper documentation is a critical part of the surgeon's responsibility in performing operative deliveries.[7,14,62] All operative or instrumental deliveries should be formally dictated into the medical record in the same fashion as any surgical procedure. This dictation includes a statement of the indications for the operation, the anesthesia used, the personnel involved, and an outline of the actual operation. Type of instrument, difficulties in insertion, and the station, position, and deflection of the fetal skull are reported along with a careful discussion of the reasons for the procedure and a review of the clinical setting. Additional comments about the difficulty of the extraction, the performance of rotation, and resulting maternal or fetal complications or injuries, their repair and an estimate of blood loss should be included. Such dictations assist in statistical analysis of instrumental deliveries and ultimately serve to protect both the institution and the surgeon in the event of subsequent and frequently delayed claims of maternal or fetal injury.

TECHNIQUE

An accurate application of the forceps or the vacuum extractor and close adherence to standard technique are essential to safe operations. Successful procedures and reduction of maternal and fetal injuries to the lowest possible level depend largely upon the care exercised by the surgeon.

Applications

A 'ghost' application of the forceps or the vacuum extractor should always occur *prior* to an attempt at insertion of the instrument. In ghosting, the

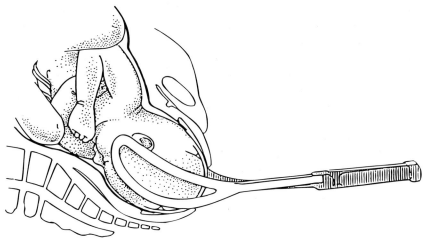

Fig. 11.1   Correct biparietal, bimalar, cephalic forceps application. Redrawn from Dennen.[21]

Table 11.4   Clinical checks for correct forceps application[7,14,21,63]

1. The sagittal suture lies in the midline of the shanks
2. The operator is unable to place more than a fingertip between the fenestration of the blade and the fetal head on either side
3. The posterior fontanelle of the fetal head is no more than one finger-breadth above the plane of the shanks of the forceps

* See Figure 11.1.

surgeon holds the forceps or the vacuum extractor in front of the perineum in the angle and position of the final application and mentally reviews the anticipated procedure. This is an additional check on fetal position, establishes the correct orientation of the instrument, and forces the surgeon to reconsider his or her intentions in the contemplated operation.[14,18,21]

In the case of forceps, the final position on the fetal head must result in a biparietal, bimalar application (Fig. 11.1). The application is judged by palpation of the sutures of the fetal head, determining the position of the instrument against these landmarks. The checks employed are the same for all vertex presentations regardless of the position or attitude of the fetal cranium (Table 11.4).

Special uses for forceps require modifications in application technique. For example, in the application of Piper forceps, fetal positioning precludes the usual techniques. After spontaneous delivery of the infant to the umbilicus, the fetal head occupies the direct occiput anterior position and cranial landmarks are not accessible to the surgeon.

As the long shanks of the Piper forcep are backward-curved, the handles are lower than the blades when the instrument is correctly applied. Thus the operator must insert these forceps from below, usually by dropping on

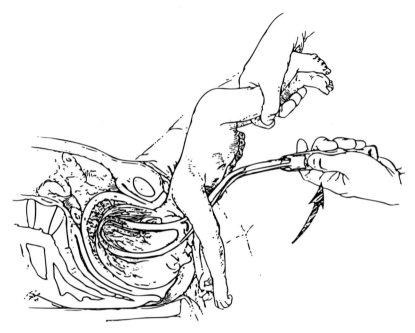

Fig. 11.2   Delivery technique: Piper forceps applied to the after-coming head in a breech delivery. The direction of traction is indicated. Reproduced with permission from Cunningham.[64]

one knee during their application, as the usual cranial landmarks cannot be palpated. Thus, the application is pelvic, not cephalic. The forceps exert a class 1 lever effect, with the fulcrum as the posterior aspect of the symphysis pubis, and little traction is required for delivery of the after-coming head (Fig. 11.2). Due to the arc transversed by the blades, this procedure is best accompanied by a generous episiotomy, particularly in nulliparae.

Correct application of the vacuum extraction is important to both success and safety.[14,17,18] Once the vacuum cup has been tentatively located on the fetal head an initial suction is applied, just sufficient to fix the device to the fetal scalp. Next, special checks of application are made. When correctly placed, a 50 mm vacuum cup is positioned midline over the sagittal suture with its *center* lying 6 cm behind the anterior fontanelle. This means that the cup *edge* lies 3 cm from the border of the fontanelle.

Table 11.5   Clinical checks for correct vacuum extractor placement[14,17,19]

---

1. The vacuum port of a Bird-design cup or the handle of a plastic soft cup extractor is directed toward the fetal occiput
2. No maternal tissue is included under the cup margin
3. The cup is mid sagittal, with the edge of a 50 mm cup 3 cm from the anterior fontanelle

---

* See Figure 11.3.

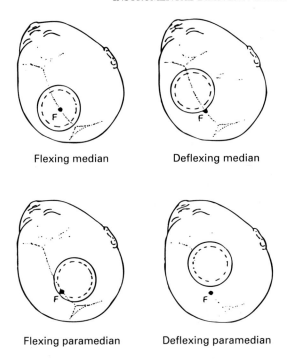

Flexing median

Deflexing median

Flexing paramedian

Deflexing paramedian

Fig. 11.3 Correct and incorrect vacuum extractor cup applications to the fetal head. Point F marks the flexing point of the skull 6 cm from the anterior fontanelle. The surrounding circles indicate the inner and outer diameters of a 50 mm Malmström-design vacuum cup. Traction at point F in a flexing median application promotes cranial flexion and synclitism; other applications do not. Extraction failure rates are: flexing median 4%, deflexing median 29%, flexing paramedian 17% and deflexing paramedian 35%. Reproduced with permission from Vacca.[17]

Traction is not applied until a correct application of the instrument is assured and full vacuum has been developed (Fig. 11.3; Table 11.5).

When the vacuum cup application is correct, full suction is applied. Traction follows, coordinated with maternal contractions and her voluntary bearing-down efforts. The operation is aided by placing the surgeon's non-dominant hand within the vagina, palpating the fetal scalp with one or more fingers and placing a thumb on the extractor cup to provide counter-pressure and noting the relative position of the cup edge to the scalp.[14,19,36] In this position the clinician can judge descent of the presenting part and early cup separation. This reduces the risk of sudden cup displacement. When either a soft or rigid metal cup type is applied, full suction and traction may immediately follow a correct application without waiting an arbitrary period of time for the development of a *chignon*.[17,35]

Immediately prior to any attempt at traction the surgeon needs to repeat a final series of checks (Table 11.6). Failure to achieve an appropriate application demands immediate reassessment of the contemplated operation.

Table 11.6 Events requiring immediate reassessment of an attempted instrumental delivery

1. Operator is uncertain of fetal position
2. Palpation indicates heavy cranial moulding and fetal station is uncertain or thought to be high
3. The cervix is incompletely dilated
4. Inadequate anesthesia is present
5. The operator cannot articulate or lock the forceps
6. The operator cannot insert or successfully wander a forceps blade
7. The operator cannot correctly orient the vacuum cup on the fetal scalp
8. The fetal head is dislodged to a higher station during the attempted application

Use of force

The control and direction of applied force are curiously underemphasized in discussions of instrumental delivery. Much maternal/fetal trauma and many failed procedures are related to inappropriately timed or directed traction efforts. Simplistically, descent of the presenting part depends upon both overcoming maternal soft tissue resistance and achieving cranial rotation. However, if the vector of force is angled either too anteriorly or too posteriorly, the traction is directed toward either the pubic symphysis or the posterior perineum. If this occurs, progress will be difficult or impossible. No instrument can overcome the fixed resistance of the bony pelvis. Alternatively, excessive posterior pressure risks potentially avoidable perineal injury.

In considering techniques of assisted delivery, particular attention is necessary to the *attitude* of the fetal head. If the fetal head is not firmly flexed, a larger diameter is presented to the birth canal. Any attempted instrumental delivery in the face of such uncorrected cranial extension simply increases the degree of the dystocia and fetal and maternal risk.[14,17,66] Cranial flexion is fairly easily judged if forceps have been applied, as the location of the posterior fontanelle with respect to the shank of the blades is one of the cardinal checks (Table 11.4). Thus, if the blades are correctly applied, deflexion is immediately obvious. With the vacuum extractor, the situation is more complex. The ventouse cup covers a large proportion of the area of the fetal scalp, and correct positioning to maintain flexion rather than promote extension is not as easy to judge, especially if molding or caput is present. Incorrect vacuum cup applications are more frequent depending upon the position of the fetal head. Not surprisingly, fewer correct applications occur in occipitolateral and posterior positions (Fig. 11.2). Vacuum extraction procedure failures are more often related to incorrect cup positioning or poor traction technique than to the existence of true CPD.

Excessive force is a risk to both mother and baby. The greatest fetal risk for intracranial injury from forceps and the vacuum extractor results from compression or distortion of the fetal head.[14, 37,39] For classic cross-bladed

Table 11.7 Number of tractions required in vacuum extraction and forceps deliveries*

Number of traction efforts	Malmström vacuum extractor (n = 433)	Forceps (n = 555)
1–2	296 (68.4%)	213 (38.4%)
3–4	108 (24.9%)	270 (48.6%)
˜ 5	29 (6.7)	72 (12.9%)

* Neonates <600 g are excluded; other exclusions include breech presentations, cesarean deliveries, transverse lies, and multiple gestations. Twins were included if >600 g and one was delivered spontaneously, by vertex.
Modified with permission from Sjostedt.[66]

forceps, cranial compression is proportional to the amount of traction applied at the handles.[63] While the amount of force is difficult to control, some guidance can be given. More than 85% of ultimately successful deliveries occur with four traction efforts or less (Table 11.7). A critical point is that *descent of the fetal head should commence with the initial traction effort by either forceps or the vacuum extractor.* Failure of immediate descent is grounds for abandoning the procedure, unless there has been a technical failure. Also, if the vacuum extractor has initially failed to achieve descent despite correct application and technique, forceps should be applied only with great care.

Forceps traction is applied using the two-handed Saxtorph–Pajot maneuver[14,18,21] (Fig. 11.4). There are several simple additional precautions to be taken. The surgeon is best seated. One hand pulls horizontally while the second adds downward force over the lock. This assures that the traction force vector follows the natural pelvic curve (curve of Carus) as

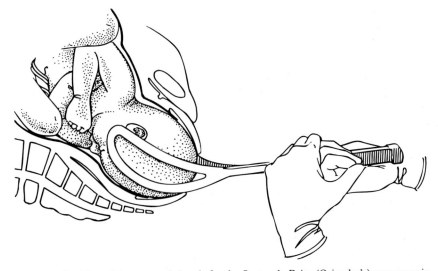

Fig. 11.4 Position of the surgeon's hands for the Saxtorph–Pajot (Osiander's) maneuver in occipitoanterior position for an outlet forceps operation. Reproduced with permission from O'Grady.[14]

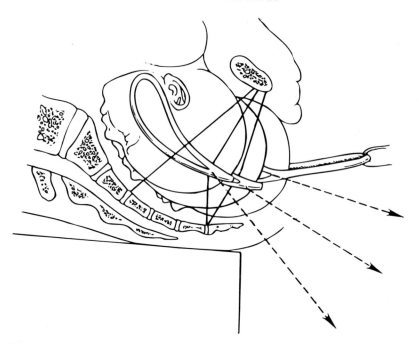

Fig. 11.5 Lateral pelvic view of the course of the fetal head through the curve of Carus (pelvic curve) during a forceps operation. The pelvic transit of the fetal head is similar in vacuum extraction procedure. See text for details. Modified with permission from Dennen.[21]

descent occurs (Fig. 11.5). A folded towel can be placed between the handles of the forceps to reduce compression. The amount of force used should never be greater than that which can be applied by the operator flexing his or her forearm. Bracing of the operator's feet should not be necessary. As always, the higher the station of the fetal head, the more posteriorly is the vector of force directed. Traction technique for the vacuum extractor is exactly similar.

With vacuum extraction, excessive operator effort or efforts not co-ordinated closely to uterine contractions usually result in prompt cup displacement and predispose to fetal scalp injury. Bird[19] especially cautions against what he has termed negative 'traction'. By this he means force applied to the fetal scalp with no corresponding advancement of the fetal head. Such traction has the potential to injure bridging scalp vessels and probably predisposes to cephalohematomas and subgaleal hemorrhages. With the ventouse, the cup should not be in place for more than 20 minutes and only four traction efforts or two cup displacements are permitted during any delivery.

CLINICAL ISSUES

Other important clinical issues affect the likelihood of assisted delivery. These include use of anesthesia/analgesia, maternal positioning, practices of membrane rupture, and the techniques for use of oxytocin. The primary clinical concerns are the evaluation of and response to CPD or failure to progress and the use and abuse of epidural anesthesia/analgesia.

Cephalopelvic disproportion

The process of labor remolds the relatively plastic fetal head into the classic elongate shape, better fitting the architecture of the birth canal but also distorting cranial landmarks. Evaluation of progress in labor, the appropriateness of operative intervention as well as the correct application of instruments depend upon a correct diagnosis of the station, attitude, and position of the fetal head.

Dystocia, including CPD and failure to progress in labor, results either from true or relative disparity between the maternal pelvis and the fetal head, or from a combination of conditions.[69] In most instances, failure to progress or *relative* CPD arises from inadequate uterine powers, ineffectual maternal bearing-down efforts, or a complex of fetal malpositioning, maternal soft tissue dystocia, and other factors.[4,69] In current practice a true contracted pelvis with an average-sized fetus is a rare cause of CPD. A more common problem is a macrosomic fetus in an average-sized pelvis or the malpresentation of an average-sized fetus in an otherwise adequate pelvis.[70,71]

In establishing the correct diagnosis, close analysis of the course in labor is helpful. Protraction or arrest disorders are common with dystocia and cessation of progress is associated with obstructed or more difficult deliveries.[72-76] In a poorly progressing labor the risk of oxytocin labor augmentation — even with the resumption of normal progress — is additive with epidural anesthesia and results in a higher incidence of instrumental delivery.[77]

Labors complicated by secondary arrest of cervical dilation require careful evaluation before potentially difficult operative deliveries are contemplated. Fortunately, approximately two-thirds of cases of dystocia respond to oxytocin stimulation, ambulation, or aminorrhexis.[72]

The classic clinical evidence for CPD is progressive molding during labor *unaccompanied* by true descent of the presenting part. If CPD is present, vaginal delivery proves impossible. The disproportion between the fetal head and the maternal pelvis precludes a successful cranial transit of the pelvis. However, because of progressive molding of the fetal cranium and the development of caput succedaneum, the presenting part progresses deeper into the maternal pelvis. This confuses the clinician into believing that actual descent of the fetal head has occurred and that appropriate progress is being made.

If advancement of the fetal head has ceased following adequate stimulation, maternal encouragement, and positioning, the clinician must decide between modes of operative delivery — either cesarean delivery or a trial of instrumental delivery. In the face of apparently adequate uterine activity —

with or without oxytocin stimulation — but inadequate progress, more detailed clinical pelvimetry is required. This meticulous re-examination excludes the rare misshapen pelvis, and judges general pelvic architecture and gauges the fetopelvic relationship.[17] Knowledge of pelvic architecture assists in deciding if instrumental delivery is desirable and which procedures are technically possible. For example, a persisting occiput transverse position in a platypoid pelvis contraindicates a trial of Kielland forceps. A deeply engaged, partially deflexed occiput posterior in an android pelvis is not one in which rotation to anterior is desirable or even possible and one in which vacuum extraction is most likely to fail.

Initially, it is prudent to perform Leopold's maneuvers by abdominal palpation as well as the Muller–Hillis maneuver during a careful pelvic examination.[78] This assists the clinician in judging the degree of cranial molding and rough fetopelvic capacity. If on vaginal bimanual examination the presenting part fails to descend with fundal pressure and especially if marked cranial molding is present, pelvic capacity is suspect. If so, any effort at instrumental delivery must proceed with great circumspection.

The important issue is the true position of the midpoint of the fetal head (biparietal diameter). If heavy cranial molding is present, station cannot be accurately judged based solely on palpation of the leading edge of the presenting part.[14,21,69] In such cases, other clinical findings are important. Failure of the fetal head to fill the posterior hollow of the sacrum is a strong suggestion that the head lies higher than expected and has not negotiated the mid-pelvis. Similarly, failure easily to palpate the fetal ear also suggests high station.[79] Careful estimation of the extent of the fetal head abdominally is also useful.[80] In this technique, the extent of cranial descent into the pelvis is estimated in fifths. Engagement of the fetal head has occurred when no more than one-fifth of the fetal head remains palpable abdominally. Obviously, anesthesia, patient habitus, and compliance relate to the success and accuracy of such examinations.

Philpott[71] and Vacca[17] describe an additional technique of gauging the extent of disproportion. In this method, the degree of cranial molding is estimated by judging the overlap of the bones of the fetal skull at the occipitoparietal and parietal–parietal junctions. The extent of this overlap and the ease of reduction by simple digital pressure are noted. If the bones are in apposition and cannot be easily separated by simple digital pressure, molding is advanced or extreme and disproportion is likely. Instrumental deliveries are to be avoided under such circumstances.

In cephalic presentations, radiographic pelvimetry has little, if any role to play in evaluating labor progress or the possibility of CPD.[4,64,69] In contrast, in breech presentation there are reasonable data that pelvic measurement by computed tomography (CT) pelvimetry assists in deciding which patients are appropriate for trials of safe vaginal delivery.[73, 81, 82]

Unfortunately and unexpectedly, ultrasonic estimation of fetal weight or ratios between specific fetal measurements has not proven to be of use in judging relative fetopelvic size. This is largely due to the relative inaccuracy of this method in estimating the bulk of precisely those infants of greatest interest to the clinician — the large ones — and our ability to relate these measurements to pelvic capacity. Similarly, there is limited utility in clinical pelvimetry as usually practised in deciding which patients should either have a trial of labor or receive oxytocin stimulation, except in extreme cases.

In cephalic presentations as long as absolute disproportion or malpresentation is not present the best measure of pelvic adequacy is a trial of labor under close observation.[4] If true CPD is absent by examinations previously discussed, uterine activity is suboptimal and progress is desultory, oxytocin should be given in the effort to strengthen contractions and achieve progress. Bottoms and co-workers[72] have shown that 71% of arrest disorders unresponsive to amniotomy, ambulation, and other simple measures improve with oxytocin stimulation, resulting in either spontaneous or low forceps deliveries. Oxytocin can safely be administered to nulliparae by standard protocols. Special care needs to be taken in cases of dystocia in multiparous patients as the risks of oxytocin stimulation are greater.[5,83]

Trials of labor require close attention to possible maternal and fetal distress.[73] Adequate uterine activity can be documented by continuous monitoring of uterine activity using a pressure catheter or transducer.[69,84,85] However, such invasive monitoring may not be required in all cases. In any event, close clinical observation is essential. Labor progress is judged by serial vaginal examinations with careful recording of cervical dilation, station, and position of the fetal head. While close surveillance is prudent in pregnancies complicated by arrest disorders, Bottoms et al[72] observed neither a higher incidence of depressed infants (based on Apgar scores) nor increased perinatal mortality when these labors were monitored by modern techniques.

Anesthesia/analgesia

In most obstetrical services a regional blockade is the anesthetic of choice when pain relief during labor is necessary. Yet it is generally concluded that there is an association between the use of epidural anesthesia and the likelihood of instrumental delivery.[14,63,77,86–90] A study of this issue reveals the complex nature of obstetric decision-making and the interrelationship between management choices and the incidence of assisted delivery.

The literature on this subject is largely unsatisfactory.[91] Studies reviewing epidurals and labor progress often fail to distinguish between difficult labors utilizing epidural anesthesia for pain relief and/or oxytocin augmentation from those less intense labors which do not. The latter group has fewer complications, specifically a lower incidence of dystocia, and are less likely to require or request a major anesthetic or need assisted delivery. Also, in many studies it is difficult to distinguish between cases of indicated vaginal instrumental deliveries versus elective procedures.[91]

Despite these limitations, several facts are clear. Epidurals have physiologic effects that potentially alter the course of labor. Vasodilation can lead to maternal hypotension. The usual brachial artery blood pressure determinations do not reflect the extent of this underperfusion. Adverse consequences are avoided by continuous attention to adequate maternal hydration and lateral recumbency positioning.

When aortocaval compression and occult or overt hypotension are avoided, the fetus easily tolerates the second stage under epidural blockade.[77] With adequate maternal hydration and proper positioning, intervillus blood flow is generally improved and the fetal heart tracing remains unchanged.[92] Adequate maternal pain relief also enhances cooperation, prevents maternal exhaustion, and tends to reduce the stress-related elevations in catecholamines that accompany labor.[93] Effects upon the neonate are minimal.[91] The major adverse effects of epidural blockade on parturition result from interference in maternal muscle tone and reflex arcs that potentially interfere with the second stage of labor. Epidurals reduce the force of the spontaneous uterine contractions only transiently and prolong first-stage labor slightly, even when oxytocin is administered. However, this effect is generally of minor consequence.[94,95] The second stage of labor is the more important issue.

Poor progress under epidural blockade is not related to malpresentation alone.[88] Epidurals interfere with voluntary expulsive efforts by the mother, and with the bearing-down reflex. Normally, uterine contractions increase in strength with cranial descent as the second stage progresses (transition phase). Especially marked in unmedicated labors, those more intense uterine contractions occur at or near full dilation, usually rapidly followed by the mother's spontaneous urge to bear down. This effect is believed due to stimulation of sensory output by the pelvic autonomic nerves and endogenous release of oxytocin.[95,96] Epidural anesthesia interferes with this process by blockade of nerve transmission. The more profound the motor and sensory blockade, the greater is the likelihood of inhibiting this bearing-down reflex arc.[97] The result is prolongation of the second stage, interference with cranial descent/rotation, and an increased likelihood of instrumental delivery.

It is not clear that consistently effective analgesia can be provided throughout the second stage of labor without some increase in the incidence of instrumental delivery and possibly in cesarean section.[89,91,98,99] However, there is a strong suggestion that different management protocols for oxytocin and epidural use make it possible to provide adequate analgesia for most labors, and to permit near normal labor progress.[84,99] Anesthetic techniques combining various opioids with local anesthetics and administering these agents by continuous peridural infusion result in an overall reduction in the amount of the local anesthetic administered. This decreases the extent of motor block, and reduces the risk of side-effects. More dilute solutions are also safer, particularly if an inadvertent intravascular injection occurs. While yet untested in prospective and randomized studies, clinical experience suggests that these techniques provide adequate pain relief for both delivery and vaginal instrumentation, with minimal effect on second-stage labor.[91, 100, 101]

Positioning, adequate prehydration to help avoid hypotension and aortocaval compression, and active management of the second stage are key if an epidural is administered. However, other techniques to encourage spontaneous delivery in individuals receiving epidurals may prove counterproductive. The epidural blockade is frequently permitted to wear off in the second stage of labor. Unfortunately, the rapid return of pain in a previously pain-free patient results in prompt elevation of plasma catecholamines, contributing to dysfunctional labor.[93] Also, the swift return of discomfort after a prolonged period of absence is not favorably received and reduces the likelihood of patient cooperation.[87] This technique is unnecessary with informed obstetric and anesthetic management.

Coaching, administration of oxytocin and extension of the second stage are helpful in promoting either spontaneous delivery or in achieving a lower station of the fetal head prior to an instrumental delivery.[14,77,102,103] Voluntary bearing down in the second stage is best deferred until spontaneous descent occurs. This more closely simulates normal second-stage progression. Squatting or partial upright positioning is also beneficial in gaining station.[104,105] By initiating such practices, needlessly prolonged and exhaustive maternal expulsive efforts are avoided.[103,106]

With these changes in both obstetrical and anesthesia management, many potential mid pelvic procedures are converted into simple low pelvic or outlet operations.[97] In sum, the focus for both the obstetrician and the anesthesiologist must be on providing *analgesia* for labor, not surgical *anesthesia*. Surgical anesthesia is unnecessary for labor pain control and invites poor labor progress. As Bailey and co-workers have shown,[107,108] when appropriate alterations in both obstetric and anesthesia management are made, initiation of an epidural service need not be associated with major changes in the rate of either assisted delivery or cesarean section (Fig. 11.6).

RISKS AND BENEFITS

Instrumental delivery has never been without critics and is not without risk.[14,18,39,53,65,108–115] Both intrapartum asphyxia and, to a much lesser degree, intrapartum trauma contribute to neonatal morbidity. However, abnormal fetal growth, prematurity, intrauterine infection, and chromosomal and other non-genetic congenital abnormalities far outweigh both intrapartum asphyxia and injury as contributors to permanent neonatal brain damage and poor long-term neonatal development.[116–118]

The question remains of the safety of instrumental assistance. All

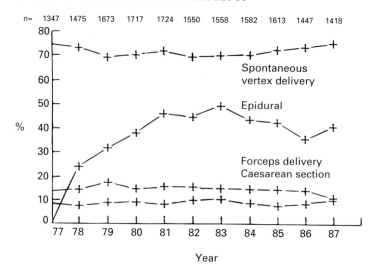

Fig. 11.6   Delivery type and the effects of the introduction of an epidural service at the Dorcaster Royal Infirmary, 1977–1987. From Bailey.[107]

clinicians agree that injuries to mother and rarely to the fetus are possible with a complicated or poorly conducted instrumental delivery.[13,90,119,120] Most obstetric trauma occurs in premature infants (<1500 g) or those born of difficult or breech deliveries.[121] Injuries also result from unanticipated shoulder dystocia, difficult applications, inadequate anesthesia, poor technique, or simply bad luck. Under all but unusual circumstances most immediate injuries are neither severe nor life-threatening and the vast majority prove to be of only trivial clinical consequence.

Against this record of risk must be weighed the enormous clinical experience of successful atraumatic delivery with reductions in maternal and fetal distress using forceps or the vacuum extractor.[12,14,17,18,122–124]

Information derived from several large follow-up studies of instrumentally delivered infants is generally reassuring.[125–128] These data reinforce the idea that long-term neonatal outcome has more to do with pregnancy *antecedents* rather than delivery events. However, long-term outcome studies of infants subjected to either vacuum extraction or forceps delivery are not *sans tache*. Cases are inevitably lost to follow-up, and adequate controls are not always provided. Despite these limitations, permanent neurological sequelae are rare except when trauma has been combined with birth asphyxia.[129] The best available follow-up data comparing infants born by vacuum extraction versus forceps[17,130] or vacuum extraction versus spontaneous delivery[124,125,131] or assisted delivery, cesarean section, and spontaneous delivery[126,128] indicate little if any long-term adverse effects of instrumental assistance.

In a more restricted analysis Dierker and co-workers[111,112] noted similar outcomes for mid-forceps delivery versus cesarean section infants when cases were carefully matched for multiple confounding variables, the most important being fetal condition at the time of instrumentation.

Despite the general reassurance provided by these data, there remains a degree of hazard in instrumental delivery.[114] At issue is which procedures or clinical settings increase risk and whether the acceptable alternatives are better or worse.

Interpreting the data, the consensus of opinion seems to be that properly conducted *outlet* operations result in unmeasurable fetal risk.[75,132,133] However, these operations are associated with an increased incidence of perineal trauma. This is most marked for forceps operations, but less true for vacuum extractor procedures.[10,13,23,49] The use of forceps in assisted breech delivery is another area of general consensus.[81,134] Instrumental assistance probably reduces the likelihood of birth or delivery trauma in this setting.

In specific relation to breech presentation, Milner[127] reported a substantial decrease in neonatal death rates when forceps were used to assist delivery. (Table 11.8). In theory, Piper forceps maintain a strictly flexed attitude of the fetal head during the delivery process. This avoids hyperextension of the after-coming head, minimizing the risks of manipulations which may injure the fetus.[81,135] However, Milner's data were not collected in a random study, are dated and potentially flawed by selection bias. Since management of breech labor and delivery is especially dependent on the skill of the operator, it is possible that in his series the more skilled operators tended to use forceps and thus had the better results. Despite their inherent limitations, these data *suggest* an improvement in outcome if forceps are applied. Such information is the justification that many clinicians employ for the routine use of Pipers in breech delivery.[81]

The situation for the more complex low pelvic rotational and mid pelvic operations is highly controversial and there is little consensus and much argument.[109,111,112,114,136-138] In reviewing the literature it is evident that not all mid-cavity procedures are necessarily hazardous nor contraindicated. Most experienced clinicians agree that a place remains for judiciously chosen operations.[14,18,21,112]

The literary controversy concerning mid pelvic procedures contains

Table 11.8 Vaginal breech delivery: impact of the use of forceps to the after-coming head

Birth weight (g)	Neonatal deaths (%)	
	No forceps	Forceps
1500–1999	22.3	11.0
2000–2499	7.8	0.0
2500–2999	3.5	0.5

Reproduced with permission from Milner (1975).[127]

much that sparks more of simple velitation than common sense. With modern management and liberal use of oxytocin, true mid-cavity operations are increasingly uncommon. In Dierker's reviews[111,112] such procedures represented less than 1% of all deliveries. If all of these procedures had gone to cesarean delivery the impact on the overall operative delivery rate would have been minimal. The reason why the controversy persists is because the prohibitions against mid-cavity operations are continually extended to less complex extractions, tending toward a blanket prohibition against *any* assisted delivery procedure.

There are several important issues to consider. In modern obstetric practice, even extensive reliance on abdominal delivery has not resulted in a disappearance of maternal or fetal trauma.[90,139] The cynic will also observe that the very liberal use of cesarean delivery for dystotic labor and presumed fetal distress has had little, if any, discernible impact on the incidence of cerebral palsy and other long-term neurological deficits, let alone perinatal mortality rates.[116,138,140] Many of the traumatic fetal injuries seen with vaginal delivery also occur during cesarean section, albeit at a lower incidence.[139] Thus, even if cesarean delivery was resorted to for all obstetric complications, malpresentations, and occurrences of dystocia, maternal and some fetal injuries would still occur and certainly not all neonates would prove normal.

As we have attempted to review in this paper, important considerations precede the performance of any vaginal operative procedure. Initially, the clinician should consider alternatives, especially in issues of mid pelvic arrest. Careful examination is required to exclude disproportion, either relative (and thus potentially treatable) or absolute. Whenever possible, use of uterotonics, maternal repositioning, encouragement, judicious use of continuous-infusion, low-dose, mixed-agent epidural anesthesia, and time should be used to promote delivery or, minimally, descent of the fetal head. When progress ceases, or fetal problems ensue, neither cesarean delivery nor instrumental delivery should be looked upon as a panacea. At this time, careful abdominal-pelvic re-examination is necessary with consideration of all alternatives. Poor progress is not an immediate indication for either a cesarean delivery or a trial of forceps/vacuum extractor *if the fetal condition remains good.*[72,142] It is, however, a time to reconsider management, and to establish a plan for how to proceed.

Assistance in the birth process may be desirable, can be life-saving, and should be always available. Even when protocols for the active management of labor are aggressively pursued, a need remains for instrumental delivery.[4] Thus, there is a continuing role for the judicious use of instrumental assistance in modern obstetric management.[7,14,18,20,21,24,63,79,136] What is demanded of practitioners is that they make choices carefully and proceed with meticulous attention to detail and *sang froid.* Even a simple vacuum extraction on the perineum is a surgical procedure, and as such demands the same attention to detail, recording and reporting as any other surgical endeavor.

We must also have the courage of our convictions. While we continue to perform indicated vaginal operative procedures we must also accept the responsibility for the correct tutoring of new clinicians in the appropriate use of *all* obstetric operative techniques. This includes forceps/vacuum extraction operations and cesarean sections. Combining our knowledge of labor physiology, fetal monitoring, patient management, and surgery into comprehensive obstetric management is the best way to inject science into instrumental delivery — the classic art of the accoucheur.[14,143]

REFERENCES

1. Green J, McLean F, Sauth L et al. Has an increased cesarean section rate for term breech reduced the incidence of birth asphyxia and death? Am J Obstet Gynecol 1981; 142: 643–648
2. Rydhstrom H. Prognosis for twins with birth weight < 1500 grams: the impact of cesarean section in relation to fetal presentation. Am J Obstet Gynecol 1990; 162: 528–533
3. Bowes W A, Bowes C. Current role of the midforceps operation. Clin Obstet Gynecol 1980; 23: 549–557
4. O'Driscoll K, Foley M, MacDonald D. Active management of labor as an alternative to cesarean section for dystocia. Obstet Gynecol 1984; 63: 485–490
5. O'Driscoll K, Meagher D. Active management of labour. 2nd ed. London: Baillière Tindall, 1986
6. American College of Obstetricians and Gynecologists Committee on Obstetrics: Maternal and Fetal Medicine. Obstetric forceps. Committee opinion #71. Washington DC: American College of Obstetricians and Gynecologists, 1989
7. American College of Obstetricians and Gynecologists. Operative vaginal delivery. Technical bulletin #152. Washington DC: American College of Obstetricians and Gynecologists, 1991
8. Hagadorn-Freathy A S, Yeomans E R, Hankins G D V. Validation of the 1988 ACOG forceps classification system. Obstet Gynecol 1991; 77: 356–360
9. DeLee J. The prophylactic forceps operation. Am J Obstet Gynecol 1920; 1: 34–44
10. Niswander K R, Gordon M. Safety of the low-forceps operation. Am J Obstet Gynecol 1973; 117: 619–630
11. Schwartz D B, Miodovnik M, Lavin J P. Neonatal outcome among low birth weight infants delivered spontaneously or by low forceps. Obstet Gynecol 1983; 62: 283–286
12. Bishop E H, Israel S L, Briscoe L C. Obstetric influences on the premature infant's first year of development. Obstet Gynecol 1965; 26: 628–635
13. Yancey M K, Herpolsheimer A, Jordan G D, Benson W L, Brady K. Maternal and neonatal effects of outlet forceps delivery compared with spontaneous vaginal delivery in term pregnancies. Obstet Gynecol 1991; 78: 646–650
14. O'Grady J P. Modern instrumental delivery. Baltimore: Williams & Wilkins, 1988
15. Seidenschnur G, Koepcke E. Fetal risk in delivery with the Shute parallel forceps. Am J Obstet Gynecol 1979; 135: 312–317
16. Spencer-Gregson N. Experience in the use of the Shute's parallel forceps. Br J Clin Pract 1966; 20: 629–634
17. Vacca A. The place of the vacuum extractor in modern obstetric practice. Fetal Med Rev 1990; 2: 103–122
18. Laufe L E, Berkus M D. Assisted vaginal delivery. New York: McGraw-Hill, 1992
19. Bird G C. The use of the vacuum extractor. Clin Obstet Gynaecol 1982; 9: 641–661
20. Paintin D B. Commentary: Mid-cavity forceps delivery. Br J Obstet Gynaecol 1982; 89: 495–496

21. Dennen P C. Dennen's forceps deliveries 3rd ed. Philadelphia: F A Davis, 1989
22. Vacca A, Grant A, Wyatt G, Chalmers I. Portsmouth operative delivery trial: a comparison of vacuum extraction and forceps delivery. Br J Obstet Gynaecol 1983; 90: 1107–1112
23. William M C, Knuppell R A, O'Brien W F et al. A randomized comparison of assisted vaginal delivery by obstetric forceps and polythylene vacuum cup. Obstet Gynecol 1991; 78: 789–794
24. Broekhuizen F F, Washington J M, Johnson F, Hamilton P R. Vacuum extraction versus forceps delivery: indication and complications, 1979–1984. Obstet Gynecol 1987; 69: 338–342
25. Johanson R, Pusey J, Livera N, Jones P. North Staffordshire/Wigan assisted delivery trial. Br J Obstet Gynaecol 1989; 96: 537–544
26. Combs C A, Robertson P A, Laros R K Jr. Risk factors for third-degree and fourth-degree perineal lacerations in forceps and vacuum deliveries. Am J Obstet Gynecol 1990; 163: 100–104
27. Keirse M J N C. Vacuum extraction vs forceps delivery. In: Chalmers I, ed. Oxford database of perinatal trials. Oxford: Oxford University Press, 1988
28. Meyer L, Mailloux J, Marcoux S, Blanchet P, Meyer F. Maternal and neonatal morbidity in instrumental deliveries with the Kobayashi vacuum extractor and low forceps. Acta Obstet Gynecol Scand 1987; 66: 643–647
29. Iffy L, Lancet M, Kessler I. The vacuum extractor. In: Iffy L, Charles D, eds. Operative perinatology: invasive obstetric techniques. New York: Macmillan Publishing, 1984: pp 582–593
30. Svigos J M, Cave D G, Vigneswaran R, Resch A, Christiansen J. Silastic cup vacuum extractor or forceps: a comparative study. Asia-Oceanic J Obstet Gynaecol 1990; 16: 323–327
31. Duchon M A, DeMund M A, Brown R H. Laboratory comparison of modern vacuum extractors. Obstet Gynecol 1988; 71: 155–158
32. Saling E, Hartung M. Analyses of tractive forces during the application of vacuum extraction. J Perinat Med 1973; 1: 245–251
33. Moolgaoker A S, Ahamed S O S, Payne P R. A comparison of different methods of instrumental delivery based on electronic measurements of compression and traction. Obstet Gynecol 1979; 54: 299–309
34. Hofmeyr G J, Gobetz L, Sonnendecker E W W, Turner M J. New design rigid and soft vacuum extractor cups: a preliminary comparison of traction forces. Br J Obstet Gynaecol 1990; 97: 681–685
35. Svenningsen L. Birth progression and traction forces developed under vacuum extraction after slow or rapid application of suction. Eur J Obstet Gynecol Reprod Biol 1987; 26: 105–112
36. Malmström T, Jansson I. Use of the vacuum extractor. Clin Obstet Gynecol 1965; 8: 893–913
37. Hanigan W C, Morgan A M, Kokinski L, Stahlberg L K, Hiller J L. Tentorial hemorrhage associated with vacuum extraction. Pediatrics 1990; 85: 534–539
38. Lahat E, Schiffer J, Heyman E, Dolphin Z, Starinski R. Acute subdural hemorrhage: uncommon complication of vacuum extraction delivery. Eur J Obstet Gynecol Reprod Biol 1987; 25: 255–258
39. Hall S L. Simultaneous occurrence of intracranial and subgaleal hemorrhages complicating vacuum extraction delivery. J Perinatol 1992; 12: 185–187
40. Gass M S, Dunn C, Stys S J. Effect of episiotomy on the frequency of vaginal outlet lacerations. J Reprod Med 1986; 31: 240–244
41. Thorp J M, Bowes W A, Brame R G, Cefalo R. Selected use of midline episiotomy: effect on perineal trauma. Obstet Gynecol 1987; 70: 260–262
42. Haadem K, Dahlstrom J A, Ling L, Ohrlander S. Anal sphincter function after delivery rupture. Obstet Gynecol 1987; 70–53–56
43. Cohn M, Barclay C, Fraser R et al. A multicentre randomised trial comparing delivery with a silicone rubber cup and rigid metal vacuum extractor cups. Br J Obstet Gynaecol 1989; 96: 545–551
44. Hammarstrom O, Czemiczky G, Belfrage P. Comparison between the conventional Malmström extractor and a new extractor with silastic cup. Acta Obstet Gynecol Scand 1986; 65: 791–792

45. Fall O, Ryden G, Finnstrom K, Finnstrom O, Liejon I. Forceps or vacuum extraction? A comparison of effects on the newborn infant. Acta Obstet Gynecol Scand 1986; 65: 75–80
46. Barclay C M, Barclay C, Fraser R et al. A multicentre randomised trial comparing delivery with a silicone rubber cup and rigid metal vacuum extractor cups. Br J Obstet Gynaecol 1989; 96: 545–551
47. Bird G C. The importance of flexion in vacuum extractor delivery. Br J Obstet Gynaecol 1976; 83: 194–200
48. Chalmers J A, Chalmers I. The obstetric vacuum extractor is the instrument of first choice for operative vaginal delivery. Br J Obstet Gynaecol 1989; 96 : 505–506
49. Punnanen R, Avo P, Kuukankorpi A, Pystynen P. Fetal and maternal effects of forceps and vacuum extraction. Br J Obstet Gynaecol 1986; 93: 1132–1135
50. Lasbrey A H, Orchard C D, Crichton D. A study of the relative merits and scope for vacuum extraction as opposed to forceps delivery. S Afr J Obstet Gynaecol 1964; 2: 1–3
51. De Jonge E T M, Lindeque B G. A properly conducted trial of a ventouse can prevent unexpected failure of instrumental delivery. S Afr Med J 1991; 79: 545–546
52. Herabutya Y, O-Prasertsawat P, Boonrangsimant P. Kielland's forceps or ventouse — a comparison. Br J Obstet Gynaecol 1988; 95: 483–485
53. O'Driscoll K, Meagher D, MacDonald D, Geoghegan F. Traumatic intracranial haemorrhage in firstborn infants and delivery with obstetric forceps. Br J Obstet Gynaecol 1981; 88: 577–581
54. Baerhlein W C, Sangithan M, Stinson S K. Comparison of maternal and neonatal morbidity in midforceps delivery and midpelvis vacuum extraction. Obstet Gynecol 1986; 67: 594–597
55. Bashore R A, Phillips W H Jr, Brinkman C R. A comparison of the morbidity of midforceps and cesarean delivery. Am J Obstet Gynecol 1990; 162: 1428–1435
56. Cibils L A, Ringler G E. Evaluation of midforceps delivery as an alternative. J Perinat Med 1990; 18: 5–11
57. Chalmers J A, Prakash A. Vacuum extraction initiated during the first stage of labour. J Obstet Gynaecol Br Commonwlth 1971; 78: 554–558
58. Rosemann GWE. Vacuum extraction of premature infants. S Afr J Obstet Gynaecol 1969; 7: 10–12
59. Roberts I F, Stone M. Fetal hemorrhage: complication of vacuum extractor after fetal blood sampling. Am J Obstet Gynecol 1978; 132: 109
60. Thiery M. Fetal hemorrhage following blood samplings and use of vacuum extractor. Am J Obstet Gynecol 1979; 134: 231
61. Plauche W C. 1979 Fetal cranial injuries related to delivery with the Malmström vacuum extractor. Obstet Gynecol 1979; 53: 750–757
62. Pearse W H. Forceps versus spontaneous vaginal delivery. Clin Obstet Gynecol 1965; 8: 813–821
63. Laufe L E, Compton A A, Dilts P V Jr. Forceps and vacuum delivery. In: Dilts P V Jr, Sciarra J J, eds. Gynecology and obstetrics, vol 2. Philadelphia: J B Lippincott, 1990: 1–25
64. Cunningham F G, MacDonald P C, Gant N F. Williams' obstetrics. 18th ed. Norwalk, C T: Appleton & Lange, 1989
65. Taylor E S. Can mid-forceps operations be eliminated? Obstet Gynecol 1953; 2: 302–307
66. Sjostedt J E. The vacuum extractor and forceps in obstetrics: a clinical study. Acta Obstet Gynecol Scand 1967; 46 (suppl 10): 3–208
67. O'Grady J P, Moskovitz H F. Vacuum extraction and intracranial hemorrhage. J Mat Fet Med 1993; in press
69. American College of Obstetricians and Gynecologists. Technical bulletin #137. Dystocia. Washington DC: American College of Obstetricians and Gynecologists, 1989
70. Phillips R D, Freeman M. the management of the persistent occiput posterior position: a review of 552 consecutive cases. Obstet Gynecol 1974; 43: 171–177
71. Philpott R H. The recognition of cephalopelvic disproportion. Clin Obstet Gynaecol 1982; 9: 609–624

72. Bottoms S F, Hirsch V J, Sokol R J. Medical management of arrest disorders of labor: a current overview. Am J Obstet Gynecol 1987; 156: 935–939
73. Bowes W A Jr. Clinical aspects of normal and abnormal labor. In: Creasy R K, Resnik R, eds. Matenal-fetal medicine: principles and practice. 2nd ed. Philadelphia: W B Saunders, 1989: pp 510–546
74. Friedman E A. Patterns of labor as indicators of risk. Clin Obstet Gynecol 1973; 16: 172–183
75. Friedman E A, Acker D B, Sachs B P. Obstetrical decision making. 2nd ed. Philadelphia: B C Decker, 1987: 240–241
76. Davidson A C, Weaver J B, Davies P. The relation between ease of forceps delivery and speed of cervical dilatation. Br J Obstet Gynaecol 1976; 83: 279–283
77. Studd J W W, Crawford J S, Duignan N M, Hughes A O. The effect of lumbar epidural analgesia on the rate of cervical dilatation and the outcome of labour of spontaneous onset. Br J Obstet Gynaecol 87: 1015–1021
78. Hillis D S. Diagnosis of contracted pelvi. Il Med J 1938; 74: 131–134
79. Compton A A. 1990 Avoiding difficult vaginal deliveries. In: Dilts P V Jr, Sciarra J J, eds. Gynecology and obstetrics, vol 2. Philadelphia: J B Lippincott, 1990: 1–8
80. Crichton D. A reliable method of establishing the level of the fetal head in obstetrics. S Afr Med J 1974; 48: 784–787
81. Gimovsky M L, Petrie R H. Breech presentation. In: Evans M I, Fletcher J C, Dixler A O, Schulman J D, eds. Fetal diagnosis and therapy. Philadelphia: J B Lippincott, 1989
82. Gimovsky M L, Paul R H. Singleton breech presentation in labor — experience in 1980. Am J Obstet Gynecol 1982; 143: 733–739
83. American College of Obstetricians and Gynecologists. Induction and augmentation of labor. Technical bulletin #110. Washington DC: American College of Obstetricians and Gynecologists, 1987
84. Neuhoff D, Burke M S, Porreco R P. Caesarean birth for failed progress in labor. Obstet Gynecol 1989; 73: 915–920
85. Hauth J C, Hankins G D V, Gilstrap L C, Strickland D M, Vance P. Uterine contraction pressures with oxytocin induction/augmentation. Obstet Gynecol 1986; 68: 305–309
86. American College of Obstetricians and Gynecologists. Obstetric anesthesia and analgesia. Technical bulletin #112. Washington DC: American College of Obstetricians and Gynecologists, 1988
87. Reynolds F. Pain relief in labour. In: Studd J, ed. Progress in obstetrics and gynaecology, vol. 9. Edinburgh: Churchill Livingstone, 1991: pp 131–148
88. Kaminski H M, Stafl A, Aiman J. The effect of epidural analgesia on the frequency of instrumental obstetric delivery. Obstet Gynecol 1987; 69: 770–773
89. Thorp J A, Parisi V M, Boylan P C, Johnston D A. The effect of continuous epidural analgesia on cesarean section for dystocia in nulliparous women. Am J Obstet Gynecol 1989; 161: 670–675
90. Cyr R M, Usher R H, McLean C M. Changing pattens of birth asphyxia and trauma over 20 years. Am J Obstet Gynecol 1984; 148: 490–498
91. Chestnut D H. Epidural anesthesia and instrumental vaginal delivery. J Anesthesiol 1991; 74: 805–808
92. Reynolds F. Epidural analgesia in obstetrics: pros and cons for mother and baby. Br Med J 1989; 299: 751–752
93. Shnider S M, Abboud T K, Artal R, Henriksen E H, Stefani S J, Levinson G. Maternal catecholamines decrease during labor after lumbar epidural anesthesia. Am J Obstet Gynecol 1983; 147: 13–15
94. Johnson W L, Winter W W, Eng M et al. Effect of pudendal, spinal, and peridural block anesthesia on the second stage of labor. Am J Obstet Gynecol 1972; 113: 166–175
95. Bates R G, Helm C W, Duncan A, Edmonds D K. Uterine activity in the second stage of labour and the effect of epidural analgesia. Br J Obstet Gynaecol 1985; 92: 1246–1250
96. Goodfellow C R, Hull M G R, Swaab D, Dogtero M J, Bvijs R M. Oxytocin deficiency at delivery with epidural analgesia. Br J Obstet Gynaecol 1983; 90: 214–219

97. Doughty A. Selective epidural analgesia and the forceps rate. Br J Anaesth 1969; 41: 1058–1062
98. Phillips K C, Thomas T A. Second stage of labour with or without extradural analgesia. Anaesthesia 1983; 38: 972–976
99. O'Grady J P, Youngstrom P. Must epidurals always imply instrumental delivery? Contemp Ob/Gyn 1990; 35: 19–27
100. Youngstrom P, Sedensky M, Frankmann D. Continuous epidural infusion of low-dose bupivacaine-fentanyl for labor analgesia. Anesthesiology 1988; 69: A686
101. Vertommen J D, Vandermeulen E, Van Aken H, Vaes L, Soetens M, Van Steenberge A. The effects of the addition of sufentanil to 0.125% bupivacaine on the quality of analgesia during labor and on the incidence of instrumental deliveries. J Anesthesiol 1991; 74: 809–814
102. Drife J O. Kielland or Caesar? Br Med J 1983; 287: 309–310
103. Crawford J S. The stages and phases of labour: an outworn nomenclature that invites hazard. Lancet 1983; ii: 271–272
104. Gardosi J, Hutson N, B-Lynch C. Randomised, controlled trial of squatting in the second stage of labour. Lancet 1989; ii: 74–77
105. Russell J G B. Moulding of the pelvic outlet. J Obstet Gynaecol Br Commonwlth 1969; 6: 817–820
106. Maresh M, Choong K H, Beard R W. Delayed pushing with lumbar epidural analgesia in labour. Br J Obstet Gynaecol 1983; 90: 623–627
107. Bailey P W. Epidural anesthesia and instrumental delivery. Anaesthesia 1989; 44: 171–172
108. Bailey P W, Howard F A. Epidural analgesia and forceps delivery: laying a bogey. Anaesthesia 1983; 38: 282–285
109. Robertson P A, Laros R K Jr, Zhao R L. Neonatal and maternal outcome in low-pelvic and mid-pelvic operative deliveries. Am J Obstet Gynecol 1990; 162: 1436–1444
110. Friedman E A, Neff R K. Labor and delivery; impact on offspring. Littleton, MA: PSG Publishing, 1987
111. Dierker L J Jr, Rosen M G, Thompson K, Debanne S, Linn P. The midforceps: maternal and neonatal outcomes. Am J Obstet Gynecol 1985; 152: 176–182
112. Dierker L J, Rosen M G, Thompson K, Lynn P. Midforceps deliveries: long-term outcome of infants. Am J Obstet Gynecol 1986; 154: 764–768
113. Varner M W. Neuropsychiatric sequelae of midforceps deliveries. Clin Perinatol 1983; 10: 455–460
114. Friedman E A. Midforceps delivery: no? Clin Obstet Gynecol 1987; 30: 93–105
115. Danforth D N, Ellis H. Midforceps delivery — a vanishing art? Am J Obstet Gynecol 86: 29–37
116. Sunshine P. Epidemiology of perinatal asphyxia. In: Stevenson D K, Sunshine P, eds. Fetal and neonatal brain injury: mechanisms, management, and the risks of practice. Philadelphia: B. C. Decker, 1989: 2–10
117. Illingworth R S. Why blame the obstetrician? A review. Br Med J 1979; 1: 797–801
118. Nelson K B, Ellenberg J H. Antecedents of cerebral palsy. N Engl J Med 1986; 315: 81–86
119. Newton E R. Complications of operations and procedures for labor and delivery. In: Newton M, Newton E R, eds. Complications of gynecologic and obstetric management. Philadelphia: W B Saunders, 1988; 11: 315–384
120. Falco N A, Eriksson E. Facial nerve palsy in the newborn: incidence and outcome. Plast Reconstr Surg 1990; 85: 1–4
121. Painter M J, Bergman I. Obstetrical trauma to the neonatal central and peripheral nervous system. Semin Perinatol 1982; 6: 89–104
122. Hayashi R H. Midforceps delivery: yes? Clin Obstet Gynecol 1987; 30: 90–92
123. Berkus M D, Ramamurthy R S, O'Connor P S, Brown K, Hayashi R H. Cohort study of silastic obstetric vacuum cup deliveries: I. Safety of the instrument. Obstet Gynecol 1985; 66: 503–509
124. Blennow G, Svenningsen N W, Gustafson B, Sunden B, Cronquist S. Neonatal and prospective follow up study of infants delivered by vacuum extraction. Acta Obstet Gynecol Scand 1977; 56: 189–194
125. Bjeer I, Dahlin K. The long term development of children delivered by vacuum extraction. Dev Med Child Neurol 1974; 16: 378–381

126. McBride W G, Black B P, Brown C J, Dolby R M, Murray A D, Thomas B D. Method of delivery and developmental outcome at five years of age. Med J Aust 1979; 1: 301–304

127. Milner R D G. Neonatal mortality of breech deliveries with and without forceps to the aftercoming head. Br J Obstet Gynaecol 1975; 82: 783–785

128. Seidman D S, Laer A, Gale R, Stevenson D K, Mashiach S, Danon Y L. Long-term effects of vacuum and forceps deliveries. Lancet 1991; 337: 1583–1585

129. Bryce R, Stanley F, Blair E. The effects of intrapartum care on the risks of impairments in childhood. In: Chalmers I, Enkin M, Keirse M J, eds. Effective care in pregnancy and childbirth. Oxford: Oxford University Press, 1989: 1313–1321

130. Nilsen S T. Boys born by forceps and vacuum extractor examined at 18 years of age. Acta Obstet Gynecol Scand 1984; 63: 549–554

131. Ngan H Y S, Miu P, Ko L, Ma H K. Long-term neurological sequelae following vacuum extractor delivery. Aust NZ J Obstet Gynaecol 1990; 30: 111–114

132. Gilstrap LC III, Hauth J C, Schiano S, Connor K D. Neonatal acidosis and method of delivery. Obstet Gynecol 1984; 63: 681–685

133. Nyirjesy I, Pierce W E. Perinatal mortality and maternal morbidity in spontaneous and forceps vaginal deliveries. Am J Obstet Gynecol 89: 568–578

134. Piper E B, Bachman C. The prevention of fetal injuries in breech deliveries. JAMA 1929; 92: 217–221

135. Brenner W E, Bruce R D, Hendricks C H. The characteristics and perils of breech presentation. Am J Obstet Gynecol 1974; 118: 700–712

136. Richardson D A, Evans M I, Cibils L A. Midforceps delivery: a critical review. Am J Obstet Gynecol 1983; 145: 621–632

137. Friedman E A, Sachtleben-Murray M R, Dahrouge D, Neff R K. Long-term effects of labor and delivery on offspring: a matched pair analysis. Am J Obstet Gynecol 1984; 150: 941–945

138. Verma U L 1990 A critical analysis of the long-term sequelae of midcavity forceps delivery. In: Tejani N, ed. Obstetrical events and developmental sequelae. Boca Raton: CRC Press, 1990: pp 161–179

139. Bell D, Johansson D, McLean F H, Usher R H. Birth asphyxia, trauma, and mortality in twins: has cesarean section improved outcome? Am J Obstet Gynecol 1986; 154: 235–239

140. Opit L J, Selwood T S. Caesarean section rates in Australia. Med J Aust 1979; 2: 706–709

141. Catamanchi G R, Tamaskar V, Egel R T et al. Intrauterine quadraplegia associated with breech presentation and hyperextension of the fetal head: a case report. Am J Obstet Gynecol 1981; 140: 831–833

142. Cohen W R. 1977 Influence of the duration of second stage labor on perinatal outcome and puerperal morbidity. Obstet Gynecol 1977; 49: 266–268

143. Healy D L, Laufe L E. Survey of obstetric forceps training in North America in 1981. Am J Obstet Gynecol 1985; 151: 54–58

12. Delivery following previous caesarean section

F. P. Meehan   N. M. Rafla   I. I.Bolaji

Cragin's 'once a caesarean, always a caesarean'[1] must be abandoned and replaced by 'once a caesarean, always a hospital delivery'. Patients with previous caesarean section now represent a relatively large proportion of the obstetric population. In the USA, more than 6% of all obstetric patients had at least one caesarean section, and no other single indication exceeded that of previous caesarean section as an indication for repeat surgery.[2] In Galway, Ireland, patients with previous caesarean section formed 3.42% of the obstetric population (Table 12.1). Watchful waiting has always been an essential virtue in obstetric management and should not be replaced by hopeful expectancy. This aspect of the art of obstetrics would appear to require rejuvenation if we are to stem the rising tide of caesarean section.[3]

HISTORY OF CAESAREAN SECTION

The term 'caesarean section' is considered to have come from Roman law, entitled *lex regia*. This law is alleged to have ordered that a dead or dying pregnant woman should have an abdominal delivery to preserve her child for the state. *Lex regia* eventually became known as *lex caesarica*. Hippocrates, Galen or Soranus made no reference to the procedure, but deep in the folklore of lay and scholarly writings of Egyptian, Greek, and Roman, it is obvious that the technique was known and practised in their time.[4]

The first recorded caesarean section on a living woman occurred in 1500, and was performed by a Swiss man, Jacob Nufer, on his wife.[5] In the UK, the first recorded caesarean section on a living woman was performed in Edinburgh by Robert Smith in 1737.[6] Munro Kerr established the low transverse incision in England and it was not until the late 1940s at the 12th British Congress of Obstetrics and Gynaecology that the lower segment operation at last received universal acceptance.[7]

Initially the introduction of caesarean section was an attempt to improve maternal mortality. In 1962 the maternal mortality from caesarean section in the UK (3.5 per 1000 births) was 10 times that of the overall maternal mortality.[8] This figure had fallen to 0.52 per 1000 for the period 1979–1981[9] and 0.37 per 1000 for the period 1982–1984.[10]

Table 12.1 Caesarean section in Galway (1973–1989)

Year	Total patients delivered	Caesarean section		Primary LSCS			Repeat LSCS		
		n	%	n	Total sections %	Total deliveries %	n	Total sections %	Total deliveries %
1973	2292	139	6.06	82	58.99	3.58	57	41.01	2.49
1974	2487	144	5.79	75	52.08	3.02	69	47.92	2.77
1975	2544	156	6.13	94	60.26	3.69	62	39.74	2.44
1976	2586	166	6.42	103	62.05	3.98	63	37.95	2.44
1977	2797	208	7.44	116	55.77	4.15	92	44.23	3.29
1978	2773	206	7.43	124	60.19	4.47	82	39.81	2.96
1979	2946	293	9.95	200	68.26	6.79	93	31.74	3.16
1980	2972	268	9.02	159	59.33	5.35	109	40.67	3.67
1981	2872	297	10.34	193	64.98	6.72	104	35.02	3.62
1982	3122	271	8.68	165	60.89	5.29	106	39.11	3.40
1983	2948	303	10.28	170	56.11	5.77	133	43.89	4.51
1984	2788	296	10.62	181	61.15	6.49	115	38.85	4.12
1985	2600	279	10.73	181	64.87	6.96	98	35.13	3.77
1986	2640	277	10.49	177	63.90	6.70	100	36.10	3.79
1987	2643	269	10.18	172	63.94	6.51	97	36.06	3.67
1988	2399	263	10.96	171	65.02	7.13	92	34.98	3.83
1989	2097	251	11.97	165	65.74	7.87	86	34.26	4.10
Total	45506	4086	8.98	2528	61.87	5.56	1558	38.13	3.42

LSCS = Lower segment caesarean section.

CAESAREAN SECTION RATE

USA

When caesarean section rate (CSR) is debated, we are compelled to ask not only 'How high is too high?', but also 'How low is too low?'[11] It was on the North American continent that the most dramatic increase in caesarean section incidence was noted. In over 30% of caesarean sections performed in the USA in 1982, the sole indication was previous caesarean birth.[12] Neuhoff et al[13] reported the CSR in 1985 at 22.7% and suggested that at the end of the decade one in four infants in the USA will have been born by caesarean section. As of 1986, 23 hospitals in Southern California (Los Angeles area) had CSR of 33% or greater; five of these had rates of 37–39%.[14]

The rising trend is extensive, affecting hospitals and patients in all parts of the country and the CSR has increased about threefold from 5.5% in 1970 to 15.2% in 1978. The state with the highest rise was California. During the years 1960 to 1975, the rate had risen from 4.8% to 12.75%; most of this rise occurred from 1969 onwards. The hospital with the highest CSR in 1960 was 6.5% and with the highest rate in 1975 was 28%.[15] Those figures found in California in 1975 are now widespread across the USA, with rates ranging between 25 and 30%, according to Flamm et al.[16] In Canada the CSR more than doubled from 6 to 13.9% during the 1970s, according to Wadhera & Nair.[17]

Europe

The rising CSR is a worldwide phenomenon, more apparent in the developed than the developing countries. In Sweden the incidence of caesarean section has increased more than 10-fold over the past three decades: 0.87% (1946–1950) to 11.9% in 1976.[18] In Norway, it increased from 2% in 1967 to 8% in 1979.[19] In England and Wales the incidence was 3.1% in 1963 and increased to 7.5% by 1978.[20] In the period 1982–1984, the incidence increased to 10.1%.[10]

Developing countries

In the underdeveloped countries the CSR is low; in Guyana, for example, it is about 3% and is comparable to that found in other hospitals in the West Indies.[21] However, maternal mortality from caesarean section is much higher in the developing countries. Fortney et al[22] reported that 5% of all maternal mortality in Menoufia, Egypt was from caesarean sections. Ojo et al,[23] in a retrospective analysis of 27 maternal deaths after caesarean section over 5 years in Nigeria, found that the CSR was 4.1%. Maternal mortality rate (MMR) following caesarean section was 18.1 per 1000 (81.5% because of sepsis), while that following vaginal delivery was 1.89 per 1000.

Ireland

In the Coombe Maternity Hospital, Dublin, the CSR was reported at 7% by Feeney.[24] In our unit, the mean CSR for the period 1973–1989 was 8.98% (Table 12.1). There is one institution which shines like a beacon in having controlled its CSR between 4 and 6%, while maintaining a perinatal result equal to and better than most reported series, and that is the National Maternity Hospital, Dublin.[25] However, Leveno and his colleagues[11] challenged this, stating that this low CSR could not be achieved in Parkland Memorial Hospital, USA where population and infant outcome differences precluded such a low rate of caesarean section.

Galway

The figures for caesarean section in University College Hospital, Galway are shown (Table 12.1, Figs 12.1 and 12.2). It is evident that our CSR is also rising, having almost doubled from 1973 to 1988.[3,26] There were 4086 caesarean sections performed between the years 1973 and 1989, giving a mean CSR of 8.98 over the 17-year period. Of these, 61.87% were primary and 38.13% were repeat operations (Table12.1).

In the 17 years studied (1973–1989) the section rate increased from 6.06% in 1973 to 11.97% in 1989 (Table 12.1, Fig. 12.3). However, with the mean repeat caesarean section incidence at 38.13% for the 17-year period (Table 12.1), it would appear that we are controlling the overall CSR in this unit with our policy of attempted vaginal delivery following a caesarean section. The increase in CSR is caused mainly by an increase in the primary sections.[27] The uncorrected perinatal mortality rate (PMR) in Galway has improved over the last 17 years from 3.32% in 1973 to 1% in 1989 (Table 12.2). These are the lowest reported figures in this country and yet the yearly CSR has never gone beyond 12%. It is obvious that the rise in the CSR in Galway was not associated with a similar corresponding drop in the PMR, as reported by Meehan et al[28] (Fig. 12.2).

CAUSES AND EFFECTS OF INCREASED CAESAREAN SECTIONS

In seeking an explanation for the tripling of the incidence of caesarean section in the USA during the past decade, one must consider the medicolegal influence as a possible cause. Although Caesarean Birth Task Force[29a] did not accept fear of litigation and the possible consequent practice of 'defensive medicine' as a major cause of the increased caesarean birth rate, an obstetrician has only to look at his or her annual malpractice insurance premium to recognize the existence of this social force and to feel the personal vulnerability. Essentially, every American obstetrician has come to recognize that physicians are almost never sued for

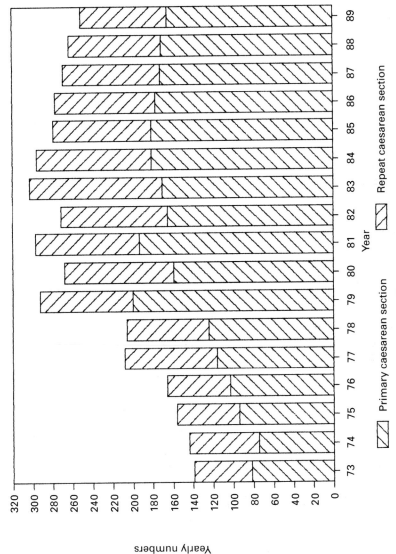

Fig. 12.1 Primary and repeat caesarean section in Galway (1973–1989).

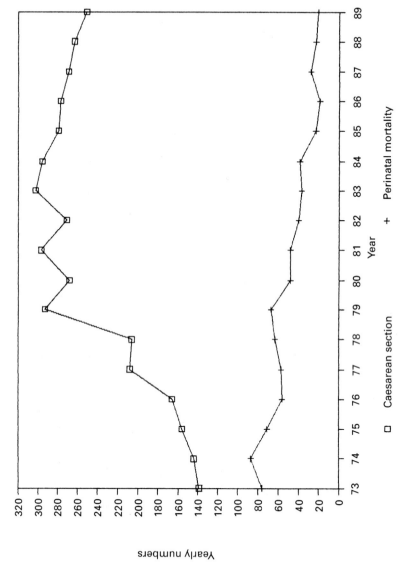

Fig. 12.2 Perinatal mortality and caesarean section in Galway (1973–1989).

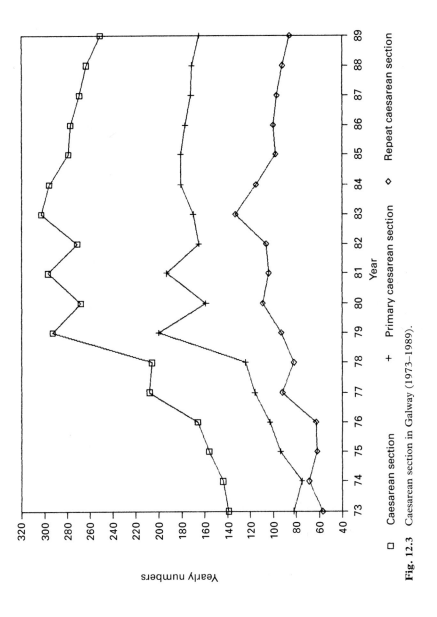

Fig. 12.3   Caesarean section in Galway (1973–1989).

Table 12.2 Perinatal mortality in Galway (1973–1989)

Year	Total patients delivered	Perinatal deaths		Stillbirths			Neonatal deaths		
		n	%	n	Total perinatal deaths %	Total deliveries %	n	Total perinatal deaths %	Total deliveries %
1973	2292	76	3.32	40	52.63	1.75	36	47.37	1.57
1974	2487	87	3.50	39	44.83	1.57	48	55.17	1.93
1975	2544	71	2.79	34	47.89	1.34	37	52.11	1.45
1976	2586	56	2.17	29	51.79	1.12	27	48.21	1.04
1977	2797	57	2.04	36	63.16	1.29	21	36.84	0.75
1978	2773	63	2.27	28	44.44	1.01	35	55.56	1.26
1979	2946	67	2.27	37	55.22	1.26	30	44.78	1.02
1980	2972	48	1.62	28	58.33	0.94	20	41.67	0.67
1981	2872	48	1.67	25	52.08	0.87	23	47.92	0.80
1982	3122	40	1.28	29	72.50	0.93	11	27.50	0.35
1983	2948	37	1.26	25	67.57	0.85	12	32.43	0.41
1984	2788	39	1.40	22	56.41	0.79	17	43.59	0.61
1985	2600	23	0.88	11	47.83	0.42	12	52.17	0.46
1986	2640	19	0.72	7	36.84	0.27	12	63.16	0.45
1987	2643	28	1.06	16	57.14	0.61	12	42.86	0.45
1988	2399	23	0.96	10	43.48	0.42	13	56.52	0.54
1989	2097	21	1.00	14	66.67	0.67	7	33.33	0.33
Total	45506	803	1.76	430	53.55	0.94	373	46.45	0.82

performing unnecessary caesarean sections. This fact compounds the problem, and more sections will be performed as we establish new indications.[3]

Complacency regarding the safety of caesarean section and fear of litigation have been instrumental in effecting change in our practice habits and have influenced our obstetric decisions. Where doubt arose, caesarean section became the answer. Berkowitz et al[29b] found that older, more experienced physicians performed significantly fewer caesarean sections for dystocia and a higher percentage of forceps deliveries and breech extractions. The CSR has increased to astronomical proportions in a relatively short time without due regard to the recent advances, e.g. ultrasonics, intrapartum monitoring and neonatology, and the contribution they could have made in their own right, if correctly applied, without resorting to caesarean section.[3,27,30]

Maternal mortality following caesarean section

The study of maternal mortality is important in evaluating the quality of obstetric care, the training of obstetricians who care for pregnant women, and the improvement in the safety of childbirth. In England and Wales the confidential inquiry into maternal death is an invaluable exercise determining the standards of different obstetric practices.[9,10,20] It is not dependent on death certificates as the principal source of information, as happens in the USA. Rubin et al[31] have shown that the record linkage procedure which they have adopted in Georgia, USA, enabled them to identify 45% more maternal deaths after a caesarean section delivery than the death certificate reporting system. There is therefore a great need for a standardized professional medical audit on maternal mortality in the USA, akin to the confidential inquiries into maternal deaths in England and Wales.

In England and Wales, there were 69 deaths amongst women delivered by caesarean sections during 1982–1984, 44 of which were direct deaths. The proportion of all direct deaths having a caesarean section has risen from 24% in 1970–1972 to 32% during the period 1982–1984. The commonest immediate cause of death in association with caesarean section was pulmonary embolism, hypertensive disease, followed by anaesthesia. Seven per cent of maternal deaths associated with caesarean section had a prior section.[10]

There were 87 deaths in women delivered by caesarean section during 1979–1981 in England and Wales; 59 were direct maternal deaths, 25 were indirect and 3 were fortuitous.[9] The fatality rate for caesarean section in National Health Service hospitals was 0.37 per 1000 in 1982–1984 compared with 0.5 per 1000 in 1979–1981 and 1 per 1000 in 1970–1972. The number of caesarean sections performed annually has risen from 42 000 in 1978 to 57 000 in 1981, increasing the proportion from 7.5% of the total number of deliveries to 10% in 1981. Obstetricians should review their practice regularly and attempt to balance the relative risks to mother and child.[9]

Obstetric outcome of patients with more than one previous section

Novas et al[2] reviewed the records of 69 patients with more than one previous section: 36 underwent trial of labour, and 80% achieved a vaginal delivery. Twenty of these patients had three or more previous caesarean sections and concluded that trial of labour in patients with more than one previous caesarean section did not result in deleterious outcome. Lawson [32] also reported on vaginal delivery following three previous sections with no maternal or fetal morbidity.

Unknown uterine scar and trial of labour

Pruett et al[33] reviewed 393 patients undergoing trial of labour after one or more previous section. In this study, 300 patients had an unknown type of uterine scar: the rate of vaginal delivery and maternal and fetal morbidity was no different in those patients with an unknown prior uterine incision compared with those having a known prior low cervical transverse incision. Similar findings have been noted in our unit.

INDICATIONS FOR PRIMARY CAESAREAN SECTION AND TRIAL OF LABOUR IN THE SUBSEQUENT BIRTH

'The rising Caesarean section birth rate has become of increasing concern to the obstetric profession and the public'.[29b] The major obstetric indications responsible for the rising rate are dystocia, fetal distress, breech presentation, very low birth weight, multiple pregnancies and previous caesarean birth.

Cephalopelvic disproportion (CPD)

Failure to progress in labour or dystocia is a leading indication for primary caesarean section and has major impact on escalating CSR in the USA.[13] Recent literature indicates that the diagnosis of CPD has no prognostic value from one pregnancy to the next and generally should not exclude a patient from a trial of labour.[16] Meier & Porreco[34] studied 230 trials of labour and found that, of 107 patients whose primary section was for CPD, 67.3% were delivered vaginally — 31% of which were larger than the one they had by caesarean section. These authors also found that, of 83 women whose first pregnancy ended by caesarean section for CPD, 78% were delivered vaginally following trial of labour.

Breech presentation

Breech babies are often subjected to birth injuries and intrauterine hypoxia. Kubli et al[35] found that fetal acidosis were much more common in breech than cephalic presentations and concluded that all breeches should be delivered by caesarean section. However, Schutte et al[36] and O'Driscoll & Foley[25] showed that breeches could be allowed to deliver vaginally. In Galway we allow breeches to deliver vaginally on the basis of the following:

1. Anticipated fetal weight is 3.500 kg or less by ultrasound examination.
2. Normal pelvic shape and dimensions by lateral X-ray pelvimetry.
3. Frank breech presentation with flexed head.
4. The presence of an experienced obstetrician to conduct the delivery.

In patients who had a primary caesarean section for breech presentation, 93.4% were delivered vaginally following trial of labour. However in patients having breech presentation with previous caesarean section scar, the consensus is that they should have a repeat caesarean section. Paul et al[37] examined 72 patients with breech presentation and found that vaginal delivery was achieved in 46% of 18% allowed a trial of labour.

Multiple pregnancy

In a retrospective study by Gilbert et al,[38] it was shown that a transverse low uterine segment scar does not present a risk because of uterine distension secondary to a twin pregnancy. Strong et al[39] studied the pregnancy outcome of 56 women with twin gestation and a previous section birth. In these patients, 31 (55%) underwent an elective repeat caesarean delivery and 25 (45%) attempted a vaginal delivery. In the latter 18 (72%) were vaginally delivered of both infants. The dehiscence rate among women with twin pregnancies who attempted a trial of labour was 4% compared with 2% in women with a singleton pregnancy.

Fetal distress in labour

Although this is an acceptable indication for caesarean section, identification of the fetus at risk from hypoxia is not always easy. The diagnosis of hypoxia based on cardiotocography alone has led to an increase in CSR. In France, Peter et al [40] found that fetal distress was the cause of one-quarter of caesarean sections in their study. Ayromlooi & Garfinkel[41] found that fetal blood sampling has helped reduce CSR. MacDonald et al,[42] however, have shown that electronic fetal monitoring did not influence the number of caesarean sections in low-risk pregnancies at the National Maternity Hospital, Dublin.

Very low birth weight babies

It is now the practice of many hospitals to perform caesarean section for very low birth weight infants to reduce the incidence of long-term handicap. Haesslein & Goolin[43] found that the incidence of interventricular haemorrhage in cephalic presentation is markedly reduced after caesarean section. However, Lamont et al[44] recommended caesarean section only in breech presentation.

MANAGEMENT OF TRIAL OF SCAR (TOS) IN GALWAY

The perinatal mortality rate for patients with previous section is higher than the rest of the population, and the need for antenatal surveillance is emphasized. We believe that trial of labour is as safe for the fetus as elective repeat section. In our unit the following rules are applied in the management of TOS:[45]

1. We use continuous cardiotocography throughout labour without intrauterine pressure monitoring. These devices are commonly recommended for the management of trial of labour patients, but they are invasive and therefore not without inherent risks. Our data demonstrate that they are not absolutely necessary.

2. Oxytocin is administered when required, by automatic pump to a maximum of 12 mU/min, but may be increased to 40 mU/min upon a consultant decision. Induction of labour is associated with high success rates and does not increase the true uterine rupture, provided proper patient selection is made and induction performed and supervised correctly.[27] We believe the use of artificial rupture of the membranes and intravenous oxytocin for induction is safe, when properly managed. Prostaglandin has proved safe in our unit with proper monitoring. MacKenzie et al[46] used prostaglandins on 143 patients with previous scars and no true rupture or bloodless dehiscence was observed.

3. Automatic monitoring of maternal blood pressure and pulse recordings should be made at 15-min intervals.

4. Epidural analgesia for TOS: we demonstrated that epidural analgesia for patients undergoing TOS is safe for mother and fetus in properly conducted trial of labour.[45] Patients are often having their first vaginal delivery and require more pain relief. An increased instrumental delivery rate can be anticipated in patients with trial of labour and a further 15–20% may require termination of trial by caesarean section. Both procedures are often easier and safer under regional analgesia.[47]

5. Anaesthetic and paediatric staff are informed of the trial.

6. Compatible cross-matched blood should always be available.

7. A midwife is in attendance at all times.

8. The '6-hour rule' is observed — the trial of labour is terminated after 6 hours of active labour if delivery is not imminent.

9. Caesarean section theatre is available.

Trial of labour following previous section is associated with little risk of true rupture, and with no added risk to the fetus. Our policy and management have helped maintain over the past 5 years an overall CSR of 10–11%.[26] Over the same period, the vaginal delivery rate was 82%; no perinatal death was associated with delivery and there was total elimination of true rupture.[45]

SOLUTION

The problem of the high CSR will have to be attacked on two fronts: firstly, by reducing the primary section rate, and secondly, by attacking the repeat section incidence. The more primary caesarean sections performed, the more repeat caesarean sections that are likely to follow, as shown by Sehgal.[48] He discussed the changing rates and indications for caesarean section, showing levels of 4.4% in 1972, which had risen to 8.8% in 1975 and 17.2% in 1979. Repeat caesarean section was the indication for 30.3% of all sections performed in his series. In over 30% of caesarean sections undertaken in the previous 3 years, the sole indication was previous caesarean birth in the series reported by Taylor et al.[49]

That 37% of the indications for caesarean section were repeat caesarean operations in Graham's unit[50] is an indication of the problem to overcome. He estimated that if the trial of labour had been contemplated for all suitable patients in his series, even with a 50% success rate, it would have reduced the caesarean section incidence from 19 to 15%. Many other reports in recent years — the most notable being that of Lavin et al[51] and Flamm[52] — have confirmed the safety of vaginal delivery following caesarean section and have dispelled the myth of scar dehiscence following this procedure. Yetman & Nolan,[53] however, found that infants with birth weights >3720 g were less likely to deliver vaginally. They urged that fetal weight estimation at term should be a part of the decision-making process before vaginal birth after caesarean section is attempted.

CONCLUSIONS

It is sad but true that defensive obstetrics is practised more often today. The National Institutes of Health (NIH) consensus committee on caesarean section[54] recommends that hospitals with appropriate facilities, service and staff for prompt emergency caesarean birth in a proper selection of cases should permit a safe trial of labour and vaginal delivery for women who have had a previous lower segment caesarean section. It also supports the belief held by Lavin[55] that the physician who opts to allow appropriately selected patients to undergo a trial of labour, while following the well-established guidelines for management of such patients, would be subjected to a very low risk of a successful suit for malpractice. Because the medical profession is vulnerable, it must be prepared to fight back against the litigious urge and the small groups of unprincipled lawyers who bring discredit to the legal profession, unnecessary anxiety to the doctor, and inflict hardship, not to mention possible dangers, on the unfortunate and unsuspecting patient. What better way to do this than follow through with what we believe to be the correct management in a given circumstance and so obviate this growing cancer within our specialty known as defensive obstetrics.[3]

In managing patients with prior caesarean section, it must be realized that intensive antenatal surveillance is required. In our unit we demonstrated that perinatal mortality associated with delivery following previous caesarean section is increased irrespective of the method of delivery.[27] The risk of true uterine rupture is extremely low with modern obstetric practice. In Galway the incidence of true rupture in the last 5 years was 0.2%.[27] and hence it must not be retained as the excuse for choosing elective repeat caesarean delivery.

REFERENCES

1. Cragin E B. Conservatism in obstetrics. NY Med J 1916; 104: 1–3
2. Novas J, Myers S A, Gleicher N. Obstetric outcome of patients with more than one previous cesarean section. Am J Obster Gynecol 1989; 160: 364–367
3. Meehan F P. Delivery following prior Cesarean section: an obstetrician's dilemma? Obstet Gynecol Surv 1988; 43: 582–589
4. Meehan F P. Caesarean section — past, present and what of the future? J Obstet Gynaecol 1988; 8: 201–205
5. Young J H. Caesarean section: the history and development of the operation from the earliest times. London: Lewis, 1944
6. Naqvi N H. James Barlow (1767–1839): operator of the first successful Caesarean section in England. Br J Obstet Gynaecol 1985; 92: 468–472
7. Marshall C M, Cox L W. Transactions of XIIth British Congress of Obstetrics and Gynaecology. Bourne A W, Nixon W C W, eds. London: Astral Press, 1949
8. Peel J. Caesarean section in modern obstetric practice. J Obstet Gynaecol India 1962; 125: 535–548
9. DHSS. Report on confidential enquiries into maternal death in England and Wales 1979–1981, vol 29. London: HMSO, 1986: pp 76–82
10. DHSS. Report on confidential enquiries into maternal death in England and Wales 1982–1984, vol 34. London: HMSO, 1989: pp 87–95
11. Leveno K J, Cunningham G, Pritchard J A. Caesarean section: the house of horne revisited. Am J Obstet Gynecol 1989; 160: 78–79
12. Shiono P H, McNellis D, Rhoads G G. Reasons for the rising cesarean delivery rates: 1978–1984. Obstet Gynecol 1987; 69: 696–700
13. Neuhoff D, Burke M S, Porreco R P. Cesarean birth for failed progress in labor. Obstet Gynecol 1989; 73: 915–920
14. Flamm B L. Personal communication, 1989
15. Petitti D, Olson R, Williams R. Caesarean section rates. Am J Obstet Gynecol 1979; 133: 391–397
16. Flamm B L, Dunnett C, Fischermann E et al. Vaginal delivery following cesarean section: use of oxytocin augmentation and epidural anesthesia with internal tocodynamic and internal fetal monitoring. Am J Obstet Gynecol 1984; 148: 759–763
17. Wadhera S, Nair C. Trends in Caesarean section deliveries Canada 1968–1977. Can J Public Health 1982; 73: 47–54
18. Nielsen T F, Hokegard K. The course of subsequent pregnancies after previous cesarean section. Acta Obstet Gynecol Scand 1984; 63: 13–16

19. Nilsen S T, Bergsjo P, Lokling A et al. A comparison of cesarean section frequencies in two Norwegian hospitals. Acta Obstet Gynecol Scand 1983; 62: 555–561
20. DHSS. Report on confidential enquiries into maternal death in England and Wales 1976–1978, VOL 26. London: HMSO, 1982: p 67
21. Rohra S, Bacchus M J. A review of caesarean sections performed at the Georgetown Hospital Guyana. W Ind Med J 1983; 32: 91–96
22. Fortney J A, Susanti I, Gadalla S, Saleh S, Feldblum P J, Potts M. Maternal mortality in Indonesia and Egypt. Int J Gynecol Obstet 1988; 26: 21–32
23. Ojo V A, Adetoro O O, Okwerekwu F E O. Characteristics of maternal deaths following cesarean section in a developing country. Int J Gynecol Obstet 1988; 27: 171–176
24. Feeney J. There are seldom absolute indications for caesarean section, but demand for it is increasing. Ir Med Times 1982; Vol 3, September 10th: 38–39
25. O'Driscoll K, Foley M. Correlation of decrease in perinatal mortality and increase in cesarean section rates. Obstet Gynecol 1983; 61: 1–5
26. Meehan F P, Burke G. Trial of labour following prior section; a 5 year prospective study (1982–1987). Eur J Obstet Gynecol Reprod Biol 1988; 31: 109–117
27. Meehan F P, Burke G, Kehoe J T. Update on delivery following prior Cesarean section: a 15-year review 1972–1987. Int J Gynecol Obstet 1989; 30: 205–212
28. Meehan F P, Burke G, Casey C, Sheil J G. Delivery following Cesarean section and perinatal mortality. Am J Perinatol 1989; 6: 90–94
29a. National Institutes of Health (NIH) Consensus development on Caesarean births: the Caesarean Birth Task Force.Obstet Gynecol 1981; 57: 537–545
29b. Berkowitz G S, Fiarman G S, Mojica M A et al. Effect of physician characteristics on the Cesarean birth rate. Am J Obstet Gynecol 1989; 161: 146–149
30. Meehan F P. Trial of scar with induction/oxytocin in delivery following prior section. Clin Exp Obstet Gynecol 1988; XV: 117–123
31. Rubin G L, Peterson H B, Rochat R W et al. Maternal death after cesarean section in Georgia. Am J Obstet Gynecol 1981; 139: 681-685
32. Lawson G W. Vaginal delivery after 3 previous caesarean sections. Aust N Z J Obstet Gynecol 1987; 27: 115–116
33. Pruett K M, Kirshon B, Cotton D B. Unknown uterine scar and trial of labor. Am J Obstet Gynecol 1988; 159: 807–810
34. Meier P R, Porreco R P. Trial of labor following cesarean section: a two-year experience. Am J Obstet Gynecol 1982; 144: 671–678
35. Kubli F, Boss W, Ruttgers H. Caeserean section in the management of singleton breech presentation. In: Rooth G, Bratteby L E eds. Perinatal medicine. Stockholm: Almqvist & Wiksell, 1976: pp 69–75
36. Schutte M F, van Hemel O J C, van de Berg C, van de Pol A. Perinatal mortality in breech presentations as compared to vertex presentations in singleton pregnancies: an analysis based upon 57 819 computer-registered pregnancies in the Netherlands. Eur J Obstet Gynecol Reprod Biol 1985; 19: 391–400
37. Paul R H, Phelan J P, Yen S. Trial of labor in the patient with a prior cesarean birth. Am J Obstet Gynecol 1985; 151: 297–304
38. Gilbert L, Saunders N, Sharp F. The management of multiple pregnancy in women with a lower-segment caesarean scar. Is a repeat caesarean section really the "safe" option? Br J Obstet Gynaecol 1988; 95: 1312
39. Strong T H, Phelan J P, Ahn M O, Sarno A P. Vaginal birth after Cesarean delivery in the twin gestation. Am J Obstet Gynecol 1989; 161: 29–32
40. Peter J, Martaille A, Roynaytte D et al. Les indications de la cesarienne. A propos de 1000 cas. Rev Fr Gynecol Obstet 1982; 77: 175–182
41. Ayromlooi J, Garfinkel R. Impact of fetal scalp blood pH on incidence of Caesarean section performed for fetal distress. Int J Obstet Gynecol 1980; 17: 391–392
42. MacDonald D, Grant A, Pereira M et al. The Dublin randomised controlled trial of intrapartum electronic fetal heart rate monitoring. Am J Obstet Gynecol 1985; 154: 524–539
43. Haesslein H C, Goolin R C. Delivery of the tiny newborn. Am J Obstet Gynecol 1979; 134: 192
44. Lamont R F, Dunlop P D M, Crowley P, Elder M G. Spontaneous preterm labour and delivery under 34 weeks' gestation. Br Med J 1983; 286: 454–457
45. Meehan F P, Rafla N M, Burke G. Regional epidural analgesia for labour following

previous caesarean section. A 15 year review, 1972–1987. J Obstet Gynaecol 1990; 10: 312–316

46. MacKenzie I Z, Bradley S, Embrey M P. Vaginal prostaglandins and labour induction for patients previously delivered by caesarean section. Br J Obstet Gynaecol 1984; 91: 7–10

47. Meehan F P, Moolgaoker A S, Stallworthy J. Vaginal delivery under caudal analgesia after Caesarean section and other major uterine surgery. Br Med J 1972; 2: 740–742

48. Sehgal N N. Changing rates and indications of Cesarean sections at a community hospital from 1972 to 1979. J Community Health 1981; 7: 33–46

49. Taylor E, Petitti D, Olsen R et al. Comment. Obstet Gynecol Surv 1982; 37: 530–532

50. Graham A. Trial of labour following repeat Cesarean section. Am J Obstet Gynecol 1984; 149: 35–45

51. Lavin J P, Stevens R J, Miodovnik M et al. Vaginal delivery in patients with a prior Cesarean section. Obstet Gynecol 1982; 59: 135–148

52. Flamm B L. Vaginal birth after Cesarean section: Controversies old and new. Clin Obstet Gynecol 1985; 28: 735–744

53. Yetman T J, Nolan T E. Vaginal birth after Cesarean section: a reappraisal of risk. Am J Obstet Gynecol 1989; 161: 1119–1123

54. National Institutes of Health consensus development task force statement on caesarean childbirth. Am J Obstet Gynecol 1981; 139: 902–906

55. Lavin J P. Vaginal delivery after cesarean birth: frequently asked questions. Clin Perinatol 1983; 10: 439–453

PART TWO

Gynaecology

13. HIV infection in women

S. Norman   M. Johnson   J. Studd

The description of a new disease is an unusual event and the arrival of a disease, manifest as a pandemic, transmitted by a variety of routes including normal sexual activity, with no cure and an apparently universally fatal outcome is very rare indeed. Human immunodeficiency virus (HIV), the cause of acquired immune deficiency syndrome (AIDS), is a retrovirus which may have been active for three decades, although the syndrome was only described in 1981.[1,2] Since then it has become the leading cause of death amongst urban women of reproductive age in many areas of both the developed and developing world. Worldwide the major risk factor for acquisition is simple, unprotected vaginal intercourse.

The average interval between infection and the onset of clinical disease is 10 years. During this period sexually active women will consult their general practitioners and specialists concerning family planning, antenatal care, menstrual difficulties, fertility and eventually the menopause. Inevitably obstetricians and gynaecologists will be required to deal increasingly with the consequences of HIV infection in their patients.

This article considers the extent of HIV infection amongst women and the risk to as yet uninfected, sexually active women. It considers the effects of pregnancy on HIV infection, the effect of HIV on pregnancy, the part that HIV plays in the aetiology of gynaecological disease and the risks to both the unborn child of the HIV seropositive patient and the health care workers who undertake the care of such women.

THE EPIDEMIOLOGY OF HIV

Estimates of the number of women infected with HIV are open to sampling bias, with wide variations in seroprevalence amongst samples drawn from different geographical and demographic areas and different hospital populations. Unlinked anonymous testing reveals different levels of infection from figures gained by screening women with acknowledged risk factors.[3] Table 13.1 summarizes a few of the studies of seroprevalence.

HIV in the developing world

The World Health Organization (WHO) classifies much of the developing

231

Table 13.1   HIV seroprevalence amongst various populations

Country	Sample population	Seroprevalence (%)	Date	Reference
East Africa	Lorry drivers	35.2	1989	12
Kenya	Rural antenatal	0.5	1989	6
		2.2	1990	
Kenya	Urban prostitutes	66	1986	11
Kenya	Urban antenatal	2.6	1986	7
		5.5	1990	
Kenya	Urban antenatal	2.6	1990	60
Uganda	Rural population	2.9–8.8	1991	5
Uganda	Semirural population	24	1990	13
Uganda	Urban antenatal	28	1990	4
Ivory Coast	Urban antenatal	9.1	1991	8
	STD clinic (male)	7.0	1988	
		13.9	1990	
	TB sanatorium	16	1988	
		31	1990	
Italy	Urban antenatal	0.16	1991	85
Italy	Urban antenatal and termination clinic	1	1991	86
Italy	Urban antenatal	0.3	1990	87
	Urban termination clinic	1.5		
France	Urban antenatal	0.4	1991	88
	Urban parturients	0.3		
	Spontaneous abortion	0.5		
	Urban termination clinic	0.7		
UK	Urban infant survey	0.02	1990	19
Scotland	Urban infant survey	0.03	1991	20
USA	Urban infant survey	0.21	1987	89
	National infant survey	0.14	1988	90
	New York City	0.58		
	Washington DC	0.55		
	New Jersey	0.49		
	Florida	0.45		

STD = Sexually transmitted diseases; TB = tuberculosis.

world as a pattern II zone for HIV transmission, where transmission of HIV is essentially heterosexual. It is in these areas that the highest seroprevalence of HIV is found. In Kampala up to 45% of 22-year-olds attending for care are infected.[4] If such figures can be dismissed as a sampling bias from an underprivileged area with a high prostitution rate, less comfort can be gained from reports of a seroprevalence of 8.8% in other areas.[5] In rural Kenya the current seroprevalence is 2.2%, a rate which has quadrupled in 2 years.[6] In urban Kenya antenatal clinics the rate has doubled to 5.5% over 4 years.[7] A similar situation prevails in West Africa with 9% of antenatal patients seropositive for HIV.[8] As one would expect, seroprevalence rates are higher in clinics for sexually transmitted disease (14%) and in tuberculosis sanatoria (31%).[9]

In Africa sexually transmitted disease, particularly ulcerative disease, has been proposed as a co-factor in the transmission of HIV and is much more widespread than in the west, especially amongst pregnant women. Active syphilis is seen in nearly 3% of pregnant women who are HIV-positive in Kinshasa compared to 1.3% in HIV-negative women.[10] Certainly the majority of urban Kenyan prostitutes, in whom genital ulcerative disease is common, are infected with HIV with the highest seroprevalence rates seen in prostitutes of low socioeconomic standing.[11] The chain of infection may thus be maintained by the high incidence of sexually transmitted disease and prostitution, compounded by population movement during political turmoil and by the more mundane, but equally effective efforts of travellers such as East African lorry drivers where apparently 35% are infected.[12] Until recently heterosexual spread appeared to have generated a 1:1 male to female ratio in Africa. However, evidence is now appearing in population-based serosurveys that the sex ratio has changed to 1:1.4 to the detriment of women.[13] Such observations may reflect a longer survival amongst infected women or there may be more efficient transmission in sexual encounters when a woman is initially seronegative when compared to liaisons between seropositive women and seronegative men. Any concentration of the HIV virus amongst women will have enormous implications for child care in the developing world.

In some areas where HIV prevalence has been low in the past and the primary mode of transmission not clear, the situation has changed rapidly. In Thailand a 2% seroprevalence for HIV amongst (male) army recruits has risen to 6% within 6 months and a 50% carriage rate has been observed in some urban prostitute populations.[14] The situation in the Far East has the same potential for sexual spread as in Africa, with the added complication that drug use is established in these areas. The rapid changes in seroprevalence mean that worldwide an estimated 600 000 women infected sexually will contract AIDS by 1992 with a further 4 000 000 seropositive but asymptomatic. As a consequence up to 600 000 children will develop AIDS and 1 000 000 will become seropositive. There will be a further 3 000 000 HIV-seronegative orphans.[15]

HIV in the developed world

In the developed world (pattern I areas) the spread of HIV has been dominated by homosexual contact and intravenous drug use. Estimates of seroprevalence in the heterosexual population are much lower than in Africa and are more susceptible to sampling bias. The UK lies tenth in seroprevalence ranking of the 31 European countries for which data are collected, with a cumulative incidence of AIDS cases twice as high in Spain and Italy and four times in Switzerland and France.[16] In the UK 11% of registered HIV-seropositive patients are female — about 1700 women. The female to male ratio of HIV infection has risen from 1:48 in 1985 to 1:7 recently.[17] Figures show that 36% of new cases amongst women were registered in the last 2 years compared to only 28% amongst men. About 40% of women are infected by sexual contact — a figure very similar to that seen amongst American women.[18] Of those sexually infected, 70% follow contact with a high-risk male, whether bisexual, an intravenous drug user or an individual from a pattern II area.

Nationally two large serosurveys of neonatal blood taken for metabolic testing show that the number of women infected amongst the antenatal population is 0.02% in the London region[19] and 0.03% in Scotland.[20] Although such surveys suffer an implicit bias by excluding women who elect not to become pregnant (possibly because they are HIV-positive), who are infertile, or who refuse sampling, they do sample large numbers of sexually active women inexpensively.

Isolated reports of a 0.44% carriage rate in some UK clinics are difficult to interpret since unlinked anonymous surveys from a single site with only a few thousand parturients and a handful of seronegative patients are likely to be heavily biased by migration from high-risk areas.[21]

GYNAECOLOGY IN HIV INFECTION

As yet there are no AIDS-defining diseases unique to women and the majority of symptomatic women in developed countries present with opportunistic infections in similar proportions to those reported in men. There is some evidence that women may have a poorer prognosis than men but this observation may be due to late presentation. There has been pressure for gynaecological conditions to be accepted as part of the spectrum of HIV infection, with likely first candidates for AIDS-defining conditions of recurrent vaginal monilia infection and abnormally aggressive or progressive dysplastic or neoplastic lesions of the cervix, with or without human papillomavirus (HPV) infection. The incidence of menorrhagia and amenorrhoea and the other common gynaecological complaints has not been systematically studied. However, preliminary reports from the USA indicate that menstrual abnormalities are significantly more common in HIV-positive intravenous drug users compared to matched controls.[22]

Cervical disease

The association of HPV, cervical intraepithelial neoplasia (CIN), cancer of the cervix and HIV was noted in 1987[23] and since then many studies have reproduced data to support the observation. The majority of studies are cross-sectional, often uncontrolled, use data gathered from heterogeneous populations of HIV-seropositive women and frequently rely on smear rather than biopsy results to screen for cervical abnormalities. There are few properly controlled longitudinal trials investigating the incidence of HIV on cervical disease. The reason for this is probably the complexity of organizing such trials, involving, as they must, repeated examinations over several years in seropositive and seronegative women. Cervical abnormalities and gynaecological infection rates are high amongst such patients and changes in lifestyle over time are confounding factors in any investigation. Matching of controls for sexual and social risk factors is a formidable task and ensuring follow-up in such a mobile population of young people is equally daunting. However, it is abundantly clear from almost all cross-sectional reports that HIV seropositivity is a powerful predictor of cervical abnormality[24] and cervical HPV infection.

Vermund et al[25] have demonstrated a 70% carriage rate of HPV amongst symptomatic HIV patients in New York compared to a background rate of 22% amongst asymptomatic HIV- positive women and controls. Fifty-two per cent of women who are both HIV- and HPV-positive have dysplasia on smear compared to only 9% in the control group. Maiman and colleagues[26] have supported such findings, using biopsy-proven CIN as a measure of abnormality. Only 5 of their 32 HIV-positive group had normal biopsies, but 78% had completely normal smears, suggesting that studies relying on Papanicalaou smearing alone may underestimate the extent of cervical disease. Several studies have found a correlation of frequency and severity of dysplasia with falling measures of immunity and that patients symptomatic of HIV suffer a higher rate of HPV infection and more severe dysplastic abnormalities.[27,28] The above observations derive from the west, but similar observations have been made in Africa.[29]

These results invite the presumption that HIV immunosuppression (possibly) allows HPV-generated cervical abnormalities to develop at an accelerated rate in HIV-infected women. Such a hypothesis would fit well with observations in other immunocompromised groups such as renal transplant patients.[30] However, it would be incorrect to make this assumption on purely cross-sectional data since most reports derive from areas where a comparison of dysplasia in HIV-positive and -negative women is also implicitly a comparison of sexual lifestyles, itself a powerful determinant of dysplastic risk. The correlation of cervical abnormalities with impaired immune response may only reflect a longer duration of infection during which time the patient has been exposed to more factors which predispose to cervical abnormalities, independent of her HIV status. Nevertheless, Conti et al[31] have made a cross-sectional comparison between groups of intravenous drug users matched for drug use and sexual exposure, but discordant for HIV infection. They showed a relative risk of 4 and 6 for HPV and CIN respectively in the HIV-positive group.

Longitudinal controlled trials are in their infancy and suffer from the fact that the finding of an abnormality naturally necessitates treatment which will alter the natural progression of the disease, as will encouraging the use of condoms. One report from Milan appears to have allowed longitudinal untreated follow-up in 62 HIV-positive and 110 HIV-negative control women, all with HPV infection.[32] Initially 73% of HIV-seropositive women had CIN compared to 30% of seronegatives. Over about 12 months CIN lesions progressed in about 35% and regressed in 30% amongst HIV-positive women, corresponding figures being 10% and 60% in the HIV-seronegative women. More extensive HPV infection was seen in 70% of the HIV-seropositive women but only 10% of HIV-seronegative women. The cumulative probability over 2 years of progression to a more severe HPV infection was estimated at 60% and 24% in the seropositive and seronegative groups.

Whatever the aetiology of cervical dysplasia in HIV-seropositive women, research has identified HIV-positive women to be at risk of cervical abnormality. The corollary of this observation is of course that cervical abnormality is, especially if persistent, a marker of HIV infection and HIV screening should be extended from antenatal and sexually transmitted disease clinics to colposcopy clinics. This hypothesis has only been addressed briefly by Maiman[33] who found a 10.6% carriage rate of HIV in his colposcopy population. This sample was collected from a hetero-geneous population in New York City where background seroprevalence is high. Nevertheless, rates amongst colposcopy patients were five times and three times higher than that found in antenatal and sexually transmitted disease clinics respectively in the same geographical area. Such investigations are being repeated urgently in the UK, but our initial results indicate a very low incidence of seropositivity in women with severe dysplasia of the cervix.

Gynaecological infections

Gynaecological infections such as candida, herpes virus and chronic pelvic inflammatory disease are associated with HIV infection, as they are with all forms of sexually transmitted disease. Recchia et al[34] emphasize the rule that the discovery of one sexually transmitted disease should initiate the search for others, including HIV. In general it is difficult to assess whether the association of sexually transmitted disease and HIV infection is a casual or causal association, for the same reasons that complicate the issue of cervical abnormalities and HIV. Most publications describe uncontrolled cross-sectional studies which point to a strong association, particularly of genital ulcerative disease and risk of HIV seroconversion. They focus on sexually transmitted disease facilitating the transfer of virus between sexual partners, rather than the issue of whether such disease is more common in HIV-seropositive individuals. The implication is that coincident sexually transmitted disease, which damages epithelial barriers, allows a more efficient passage of HIV.

There is evidence that candidiasis and herpes simplex infections are more common in HIV- infected women. Naiyer et al[35] have demonstrated that amongst a group of 66 HIV-positive women, 50% had new or repeated vaginal candidal infections in the absence of serological evidence of immune depression. In 50% of those infected, the candida attacks started well before diagnosis of HIV infection, although oesophageal candidiasis was only manifest in those who suffered marked immune deficiency. Repeated vaginal candidiasis may thus be an early marker of HIV risk. Anderson et al[36] have confirmed these observations and added herpes simplex virus to the genital infections seen in HIV-seropositive women. Although an uncontrolled study, it did demonstrate a relationship between immune status and herpes simplex virus infection, which was only found in women with CD4 lymphocyte counts less than 200/ml.

PREGNANCY AND HIV INFECTION

Women in both the developed and developing world continue to conceive despite knowing that they are HIV-positive. Anderson et al[36] noted that amongst his high-risk population in Baltimore, 14% became sexually abstinent following diagnosis with 72% continuing to have intercourse. Half of these had intercourse without a condom. Sunderland et al[37] found that nine of 11 HIV-positive women became pregnant following diagnosis of HIV seropositivity. Five of these women already had an AIDS-affected child.

The initial impression from uncontrolled studies was that pregnancy might lead to progression of disease in asymptomatic HIV-positive women and this led to the recommendation that infected women should avoid pregnancy. Studies now suggest that a less dogmatic approach to pregnancy in HIV-seropositive women is warranted. Women infected with HIV who are considering pregnancy want to know the effect of HIV on pregnancy, the effect of pregnancy on their own disease and the risks to their pregnancy in terms of vertical transmission. Many will wish to know if doctors can predict the risk of passing HIV to their unborn child.

The risk to the child

The vertical transmission rate of HIV is the focus of intense research since the efficiency with which young women can pass the virus to their offspring will be a major determinant of the paediatric medical load in the next decade. In the west the best estimates are provided by the European Collaborative Study (1991) which indicates that 12.9% of infants will be infected.[38] In Africa the situation appears different, with higher rates of perinatal infant transmission recorded. Hira et al[39] report a 39% vertical transmission rate in Zambia and rates of 19–27% are seen in Burkino Faso[40], 36% in Kampala,[41] and 21% in Kinshasa.[42] The explanation of this difference in transmission rates between Africa and the west is not understood, but a preliminary report from Nairobi using polymerase chain reaction techniques suggests that perinatal infection is only 10% but increases to 38% after 12 months.[43] The implication is that post-natal infection, probably through breast-feeding, is responsible for the apparently higher transmission rate. In the west, HIV mothers should be encouraged to use artificial feeds as there are reports of babies infected postnatally by mothers infected after transfusion with contaminated blood following postpartum haemorrhage. It is of note that the European Collaborative Study found no cases of seropositivity once an uninfected infant had cleared the HIV antibody gained passively from its mother, despite 390 infant years of close living. Presently the promotion of artificial feeding in Africa as a preventive measure will certainly cause an increase in infant mortality due to infection.[44]

HIV and termination of pregnancy

The significant risk to the fetus of the HIV-positive mother and the conflicting evidence on the effect of pregnancy on the mother's health mean that the requirements for legal abortion in the UK are certainly met in a woman who does not wish to continue her pregnancy. However, knowledge of HIV status and risk does not appear to be a central consideration in women requesting termination of pregnancy.[37] Many HIV-positive women who choose to continue their pregnancy cite religious beliefs, family pressure and their own desire for a family as important factors in decision-making.[45] High rates of termination amongst HIV-positive women in this country should be seen in the context of a high rate of termination request amongst intravenous drug users, who contribute the largest proportion of women to the pool of HIV-positive individuals.[46]

Pregnancy as a risk to the HIV-positive woman

The consensus of opinion is that pregnancy will have no significant effect on the health of an HIV-positive mother. This assertion has been tested regarding infection in pregnancy,[47] complications during labour,[48] the clinical course of HIV infection[49] and by Berebbi et al,[50] who showed no variations in either parameters affecting immune function or evolution through the clinical stages of HIV disease. Data from the USA support the concept that in HIV-seropositive pregnant women without AIDS, pregnancy does little to accelerate clinical disease.[51] These reports are at odds with data from France where an adverse effect on both clinical and immunological parameters was seen in term pregnancies.[52] A report from Canada indicates that some of the measures of immune function are depressed in pregnancy and do not return to normal levels in the postpartum period in HIV-positive women.[53] It may be that pregnancy only has a deleterious effect in women who have laboratory or clinical evidence of immune compromise. Minkoff et al[54] reported five serious infections in 16 American women pregnant with CD4 counts less than 300/ml, but none in 40 women with counts in excess of 300.

HIV infection as a risk to pregnancy

HIV seropositivity seems to have little bearing on the immediate outcome of pregnancy in the developed world. The Edinburgh group found no association between HIV infection and problems in labour or any increase in the perinatal mortality rate.[48] Babies born to seropositive mothers were slightly smaller than those born to the HIV-negative control group. These results are substantiated by data gathered in France[55] and the USA.[56] It is of note that the majority of patients studied were intravenous drug users and any problems in pregnancy were common to both the HIV-positive and -negative drug users. In Africa there is evidence that HIV sero-positivity does have an adverse effect on pregnancy outcome. In Rwanda birth weights are marginally lower in HIV-seropositive women compared to seronegative controls, but the relative risk of bearing a baby of less than 1500 g in weight is 2.5 times that of the control group.[57] Although the perinatal death rate was 6% in both HIV-negative and HIV-positive women, infant mortality in those with low birth weight must be substantially higher. In Kinshasa HIV seropositivity was the strongest predictor of low birth rate compared to other sexually transmitted diseases.[58] The Nairobi group have shown a prematurity rate of 23% — double that seen among seronegative women.[59,60]

Predictors of HIV infection in the newborn

There is no consistent evidence that any of the markers of HIV infection in mothers are predictive of vertical transmission risk, especially if the mother is asymptomatic. Muggiasca et al[61] suggest that babies born to symp-tomatic HIV-positive drug users are more at risk of vertical transmission than pregnancies arising in asymptomatic individuals. The Edinburgh group add pregnancy within 12 months of seroconversion in the mother to factors which may influence vertical transmission rates.[62] Seroconversion during the index pregnancy apparently also confers added risk.[63] A study of pregnancy in HIV-positive women identified 100% vertical transmission rates in 17 women with AIDS-defining disease (CDC classification group 4) or who were P24 antigen-positive, but a vertical transmission rate of only 12% in 56 women in CDC groups 2 and 3 and 16% in those who were p24 antigen-negative. Data from Kinshasa relating to the offspring of 146 seropositive women found a strong relationship between maternal T4 lymphocyte count and the risk of vertical transmission.[64] A maternal count of above 30% of normal was associated with HIV carriage in 19% of babies (a figure close to that seen in the western world) but as the count fell to below 10% of normal the vertical transmission rate rose to 60%. These observations are supported by Ryder et al who found that perinatal infection was 33% amongst women with T4 lymphocyte counts less than 400/ml but zero amongst those with more favourable counts.[42] The balance of the evidence seems to be that pregnancy in recently infected women or women with advanced disease is more likely to lead to an infected child.

HETEROSEXUAL SPREAD OF HIV

During the early years of the HIV epidemic the question of heterosexual spread in general and heterosexually infected women in particular attracted little attention. Towards the end of the 1980s the obstetric and gynae-cological community awoke to the implications of extensive spread of HIV in the female population. Central to this question of spread amongst women is the efficiency with which heterosexual intercourse passes the infection, and the efficiency with which simple measures can contain it in well-defined risk groups.

Preliminary results of the European Collaborative Study of Heterosexual Transmission, which followed 206 monogamous couples, discordant for HIV infection, suggest that 50% of couples do not use barrier contra-ception despite understanding the implications of their actions. Sero-conversion rates were equal between the sexes and about 10% over 14 months, all conversions occurring amongst couples not using rigorous 'safe sex'. The risk of men contracting the infection from their seropositive female partners is estimated at 0.1% per episode of unprotected intercourse, and 0.2% for male-to-female transmission.[65]

That sexual intercourse can be a very efficient way of promoting spread of the infection is well-illustrated by recent figures from Thailand of a 4.8% per person-month seroconversion rate in brothel workers.[66] The influence of intravenous drug use in such studies is not known. In Zambia a 3% annual seroconversion rate is seen, the risk rising by a factor of 4 if the woman's husband is infected and by 12 if genital ulcerative disease is present.[67] In the west, where the majority of women gain infection through drug use, intercourse with a drug user or intercourse with a national of a pattern II country, counselling needs to emphasize strongly condom use.

It seems logical that women should suffer a greater seroconversion risk than men. Intercourse can cause trauma to the vagina and intravaginal ejaculation represents a high-dose inoculum of virus if the partner is seropositve. ABO blood group secretor-positive women may be more at risk of infection from heterosexual intercourse than secretor-negative women.[68] Other potent co-factors in the risk of transmission are the HIV status of the index case and the presence of genital ulcerative disease, and whether the male is circumcized. Hira et al[69] found seroconcordance of 70% in the spouses of men and women with either AIDS or AIDS-related complex in Zambia. Unprotected sexual intercourse is the rule in these communities and in initially discordant couples seroconversion occurred at an annual rate of 21% — a rate similar to that seen in the spouses of bisexual men in the west.[70]

Cameron et al[71] have shown that amongst men presenting to a sexually transmitted disease clinic in Nairobi after exposure to an HIV-seropositive prostitute, the risk of infection after a single act of intercourse was 2.5% and rises if the man is uncircumcized or there is coincident genitourinary disease. Although high rates of seroconversion are also seen in the west, especially in the spouses of men and women with high-risk behaviour who do not use condoms,[72] the transmission risk in heterosexual liaisons in Africa appears by far to outstrip the risk observed in the developed world. Rehmet et al[73] from Germany observed only one seroconversion in 40 discordant couples and Marinacci et al estimated an annual seroconversion rate of 5% amongst 88 discordant couples.[74] Musicco et al give a figure of 3.5% annually. All seroconversions took place in couples not using 'safe sex', the conscientious use of condoms for protection.[75]

The most powerful protection against HIV and sexually transmitted disease is probably the condom, although vigorous treatment of sexually transmitted disease has been advocated to reduce transmission rates.[76] Intervention with intensive education and promotion of condom use amongst 430 HIV-negative women in Kinshasa (14% of whom sero-converted during the 2 years of follow-up) allowed the intial seroconversion rate to fall from 18 to 2% annually.[77]

The condom offers both protection and contraception, and consistent use avoids the possibility that intercourse during menstruation increases the risk of female-to-male transmission of HIV. Theoretically low-grade endometritis brought about by the intrauterine contraceptive device, and oral contraceptive pill-induced cervicitis may also represent portals of transmission. With such uncertainties the condom must remain the contraceptive of choice in all at-risk populations.

RISKS TO HEALTH CARE WORKERS

Obstetricians are often in situations where their patients bleed un-expectedly and heavily and there is little time to don protective wear and certainly no time to establish HIV serostatus. Emergency procedures are commonplace and needlestick injury at caesarean section exceeds 50%.[78] Gynaecologists are exposed to the same injury risk as surgeons and in addition work in poorly exposed fields in the deep pelvis and upper vagina where accidental injury is all too easy. They should therefore be especially concerned over the question of occupational exposure to HIV.

Although well-informed of the risks, health care workers often do not observe necessary precautions.[79] They report good compliance with precautions but in reality their practice falls short of standard.[80] In the USA 22 health care workers without other risks have seroconverted after documented occupational exposure to HIV, nurses being most frequently affected. Eighty per cent of exposures were percutaneous and 18% muco-cutaneous. The source of risk was a known patient with AIDS in 75% of cases. These are, however, small numbers compared to the mortality and morbidity associated with occupational hepatitis B infection.[81]

Although the number of occupational exposures to HIV is unsatis-factorily high, seroconversion following challenge is low. In Italy[82] 1340 exposures have resulted in 2 seroconversions (0.14%) and in Canada[83] 0.31% of 1449 exposures resulted in seroconversion within 6 months. Zidovudine within a couple of hours of exposure as prophylaxis has been suggested. It is well-tolerated but its efficacy is unproven.[84]

In the UK the Royal College of Obstetricians and Gynaecologists has published a set of management recommendations for HIV-seropositive women undergoing gynaecological surgery, or under antenatal, intrapartum and postpartum care. The report recommends selective rather than elective screening and outlines guidelines for the management for all women, HIV-seropositive women and 'high-risk' patients. Minimum standards (for all labours) include the use of eye protection, overshoes, full-length, full-sleeved gowns with plastic aprons and surgical gloves. Any operative procedure (including perineal repair) requires masking and boots. Mouth-operated suction devices and fetal blood sampling tubes should be abandoned.

Such recommendations are clearly sensible but will require a marked change in approach to labour care, which for many years has encouraged a less 'medical' approach to maternity.

CONCLUSIONS

Obstetricians and gynaecologists treat patients who are young, fertile and sexually active. It is from amongst such groups, whatever other risk factors they have or risk behaviour they practise , that the bulk of women infected with HIV are found. We should therefore be aware of the extent and implications of HIV infections. This article has reviewed the scale of the female HIV epidemic in both the developed and developing world and the gynaecological, obstetric and perinatal complications that accompany a disease that in the space of a few years has become the major health issue of our time.

REFERENCES

1. Nahamas A, Weiss J, Yao X et al. Evidence for human infection with HTLVIII/LAV like virus in Central Africa, 1959. Lancet 1986; 1: 1279–1280
2. Piot P, Plummer F, Mhalu F, Lamboray J, Chin J, Mann J. AIDS: an international perspective. Science 1988; 239: 573–579
3. Barbacci M, Repke J, Chaisson R. Routine perinatal screening for HIV infection. Lancet 1991; 337: 709–711
4. Hom D, Guay L, Mmiro F, Ndugwa C, Goldfarb J, Olnese K. HIV-1 seroprevalence rates in women attending a prenatal clinic in Kampala, Uganda. 7th International Conference on AIDS, Florence, Italy, 1991; Abstract WC3262
5. Kengeya-Kayonda J, Kamalu A, Nunn A, Mudler D. Intervillage variations in HIV seroprevalence in a rural Ugandan community. 7th International Conference on AIDS, Florence, Italy, 1991; Abstract MC40
6. Mbugua G, Muthami L, Kimata M, Maina J, Ooga S, Waiyaki P. Rising trend of HIV infection among antenatal mothers in a Kenyan rural area. 7th International Conference on AIDS, Florence, Italy, 1991; Abstract WC3283

7. Ndinya-Achola J, Patta P, Embree J, Kreiss J, Maitha G, Plummer F. Increasing seroprevalence of HIV-1 in pregnant women in Nairobi. 7th International Conference on AIDS, Florence, Italy, 1991; Abstract WC3264

8. Doorly R, Kadio A, Brattergaardd K, Gnaaere E, Coulibaly I, DeCock K. Trends in HIV-1 and IV-2 infections in Abijan, Cote d'Ivoire, 1987–90. 7th International Conference on AIDS, Florence, Italy, 1991; Abstract MC42

9. Harries AD. Tuberculosis and human imunodeficiency virus infection in developing countries. Lancet 1990: 335: 387–389

10. Mokwa K, Batter V, Behets F et al. Prevalence of sexually transmitted disease (STD) in childbearing women in Kinshasa, Zaire, associated with HIV infection. 7th International Conference on AIDS, Florence, Italy, 1991; Abstract WC3251

11. Kreiss J, Koech D, Plummer F et al. AIDS virus infection in Nairobi prostitutes: spread of the epidemic to East Africa. N Engl J Med 1986; 314: 414–418

12. Carswell J. Lloyd G, Howells J. Prevalence of HIV-1 in East African lorry drivers. AIDS 1989; 3: 759–761

13. Berkley S, Naamara W, Okware S et al. AIDS and HIV infection in Uganda — are more women infected than men? AIDS 1990; 4: 1237–1242

14. Chin J. Plenary session, 7th International Conference on AIDS, Florence, Italy, 1991

15. Chin J. Current and future dimensions of the HIV/AIDS pandemic in women and children. Lancet 1991; 336: 221–224

16. Communicable Diseases Surveillance Centre (1991). AIDS and HIV-1 antibody reports — United Kingdom 1; 15: 67–68

17. Clarke S , McGarrigle C , Karunaratne M, Porter K, Evans B. Increasing HIV-1 infection in women in England and Wales and Northern Ireland. 7th International Conference on AIDS, Florence, Italy, 1991; Abstract WC3120

18. Forest B. Women, HIV and mucosal immunity. Lancet 1991; 337: 835–836

19. Peckham C, Tedder R, Briggs M et al. Prevalence of maternal HIV infection based on unlinked anonymous testing of newborn babies. Lancet 1990; 335: 516–519

20. Tappin D, Girdwood R, Follett E, Kennedy R, Brown A, Cockburn F. Prevalence of maternal HIV infection in Scotland based on unlinked anonymous testing of newborn babies. Lancet 1991; 337: 1565–1567

21. Banatvala J, Chrystie I, Palmer S, Sumner D, Kennedy J, Kenney A. HIV screening in pregnancy. Lancet 1991; 337: 1218

22. Warne P, Ehrhardt A, Schechter D, Williams D, Gorman J. Menstrual abnormalities in HIV+ and HIV– women with a history of intravenous drug use. 7th International Conference on AIDS, Florence, Italy, 1991; Abstract MC3113

23. Bradbeer C. Is infection with HIV a risk factor for cervical intraepithelial neoplasia? Lancet 1987; II: 1277–1278

24. Fahs M, Mandelblatt J, Garibaldi K, Senie R, Peterson H. The association between human immunodeficiency virus infection and cervical neoplasm. Implications for the clinical care of women at risk for both conditions. 7th International Conference on AIDS, Florence, Italy, 1991; Abstract WC3136

25. Vermund S, Kelley K, Klein R et al. High risk of human papilloma virus infection and cervical squamous intraepithelial lesions amongst women with symptomatic human immunodeficiency virus. Am J Obstet Gynecol 1991; 165: 392–400

26. Maiman M, Tarricone N, Vieira J, Suarez J, Serur E, Boyce J. Colposcopic evaluation of human immunodeficiency Virus seropositive women. Obstet Gynecol 1991; 78: 84–88

27. Schafer A, Friedman W, Mielke M, Schwartlander B, Koch M. The increased frequency of cervical dysplasia-neoplasia in women infected with the human immunodeficiency virus is related to the degree of immunosuppression. Am J Obstet Gynecol 1991; 164: 593–599

28. Feingold A, Vermund S, Burk R et al. Cervical cytological abnormalities and papilloma virus in women infected with human immunodeficiency virus. J AIDS 1990; 3: 896–903

29. Chiphangwi J, Dallabetta G, Motti P et al. Cervical squamous intraepithelial lesions and HIV-1 infections in Malawian women. 7th International Conference on AIDS, Florence, Italy, 1991; Abstract MC98

30. Alloub M, Barr B, McLaren K, Smith I, Bunny M, Smart G. Human papilloma virus and cervical intraepithelial neoplasia in women with renal allografts. Br Med J 1989; 298: 153–155

31. Conti M, Agarossi A, Muggiasca L, Casolati E, Ravasi L. Risk of genital HPV and CIN in HIV positive women. 7th International Conference on AIDS, Florence, Italy, 1991; Abstract MB2408

32. Agarossi A, Casolati E, Muggiasca L, Ravasi L, Brambilla T, Conti M. Natural history of cervical HPV and CIN in HIV positive women. 7th International Conference on AIDS, Florence, Italy, 1991; Abstract MB2425

33. Maiman M. Prevalence of human immunodeficiency virus in a colposcopic clinic. JAMA 1988; 260: 2214

34. Recchia O, Massi M, Graziani C et al. Seroepidemiological study of the association between HIV and *Chlamydia trachomatis infection*. 7th International Conference on AIDS, Florence, Italy, 1991; Abstract WC3099

35. Naiyer I, Carpenter C, Mayer K, Fisher A, Stein M, Danforth S. Hierarchical pattern of mucosal candidal infections in HIV seropositive women. Am J Med 1990; 89: 142–146

36. Anderson J, Horn J, Atkinson J, Smith M, Chaisson R. Gynaecological infection in women with HIV infection. 6th International Conference on AIDS, 1990; Abstract 2052

37. Sunderland A, Moroso G, Merthaud M et al. Influence of HIV infection on pregnancy decisions. 4th International Conference on AIDS, Stockholm, Sweden, 1988; Abstract 6607

38. European Collaborative Study. Children born to women with HIV-1 infection: natural history and risk of transmission. Lancet 1991; 337: 253–260

39. Hira S K, Kamanga J, Bhat G J et al. Perinatal transmission of HIV-1 in Zambia. Br Med J 1989; 299: 1250–1252

40. Prazuck T, Heybrick B, Yameogo J et al. Mother to child transmission of HIV viruses in South-West Burkino-Faso. Intermediate results. 7th International Conference on AIDS, Florence, Italy, 1991; Abstract MC3089

41. Mworzi E, Najjemba R, Niguli S, Ndugwa C, Katasha P. Five year follow up of HIV infected mothers and their children. 7th International Conference on AIDS, Florence, Italy, 1991; Abstract WB2011

42. Ryder R, Wato P, Hassiq E et al. Perinatal transmission of human immunodeficiency virus type 1 to infants of seropositive women in Zaire. N Engl J Med 1989; 320: 1637–1642

43. Kreiss J, Datta P, Willerford D et al. Vertical transmission of HIV in Nairobi: correlations with maternal viral burden. 7th International Conference on AIDS, Florence, Italy, 1991; Abstract MC3062

44. Nicholl A, Killewo J, Mgone C. HIV and infant feeding practices: epidemiological implications for sub-Saharan African countries. AIDS 1990; 4: 661–665

45. Selwyn P, Carter R, Schoenbaum E, Robertson V, Klein R, Rogers M. Knowledge of HIV antibody status and decisions to continue or terminate pregnancy among intravenous drug users. JAMA 1989; 261: 3567–3571

46. Johnstone F, Brettle R, MacCullum L, Mok J, Peutherer J, Burns S. Women's knowledge of their HIV antibody status; its effect on their decision whether to continue the pregnancy. Br Med J 1990; 33: 23–28

47. MacCullum L, Johnstone F, Brettle R et al. Population based, controlled study; effect of HIV infection on infectious complications during pregnancy. 7th International Conference on AIDS, Florence, Italy, 1991; Abstract WC3238

48. Johnstone F, MacCullum L, Brettle R. Population based, controlled study: effects of HIV infection on pregnancy. 7th International Conference on AIDS, Florence, Italy, 1991; Abstract WC3239

49. Mazzarello G, Canesa A, Melica F, Carrega G, Tarragna A. Influence of pregnancy on HIV disease progression. 7th International Conference on AIDS, Florence, Italy, 1991; Abstract WC3235

50. Berrebi A, Chraibi J, Kobuch W, Puel J, Grandjean H, Fournie A. Influence of pregnancy on HIV disease. 7th International Conference on AIDS, Florence, Italy, 1991; Abstract WB2046

51. Selwyn P, Schoenbaum E, Davenney K et al. Retrospective study of human immunodeficiency virus infection and pregnancy outcome in intravenous drug users. JAMA 1989; 261: 1289–1294

52. Delfraissey J, Pons J, Serini D et al. Does pregnancy influence disease progression in HIV? 5th International Conference on AIDS, 1989; Abstract MBP34

53. LaPointe N, Boucher M, Samson J, Charest J. Significant markers in the modulation of immunity during pregnancy and post-partum in a paired HIV positive and negative population. 7th International Conference on AIDS, Florence, Italy, 1991; Abstract WB2054

54. Minkoff H, Willoughby A, Mendez H et al. Serious infections during pregnancy among women in advanced human immunodeficiency virus infection. Am J Obstet Gynecol 1990; 162: 30–34

55. Berrebi A, Lahlou M, Puel J, Kobuch W, Fournie A. Effects of HIV infection on pregnancy. 7th International Conference on AIDS, Florence, Italy, 1991; Abstract WB2042

56. Minkoff H, Henderson C, Mendez H et al. Pregnancy outcomes amongst mothers infected with human immunodeficiency virus and uninfected control subjects. Am J Obstet Gynecol 1990; 163: 1598–1604

57. Bulterys M, Chao A, Kurawige B et al. Maternal HIV infection and intrauterine growth. A prospective cohort study in Butare, Rwanda. 7th International Conference on AIDS, Florence, Italy, 1991; Abstract WC3234

58. Kamenga M, Manzila T, Behets F et al. Maternal HIV infection and other sexually transmitted diseases and low birth weight in Zairan children. 7th International Conference on AIDS, Florence, Italy, 1991; Abstract WC3244

59. Temmerman M, Hawala D, Ndinya-Achola J, Plummer F, Piot P. Maternal HIV infection and low CD4/CD8 ratio as risk factor for prematurity and stillbirth. 7th International Conference on AIDS, Florence, Italy, 1991; Abstract MC93

60. Braddick M , Kreiss J, Embree J et al. Impact of maternal HIV infection on obstetric and early neonatal outcome. AIDS 1990; 4: 1001–1005

61. Muggiasca L, Agarossi A, Casolati E et al. Pregnancy, maternal stage and vertical transmission of HIV infection. 7th International Conference on AIDS, Florence, Italy, 1991; Abstract WB2000

62. Hague R, Mok J, MacCullum L, Mok J, Burns S, Yap P. Do maternal factors influence the risk of vertical transmission of HIV? 7th International Conference on AIDS, Florence, Italy, 1991; Abstract WC3237

63. d'Arminio M, Ravizza M, Muggiasca M et al. HIV infected women; possible predictors of vertical transmission. 7th International Conference on AIDS, Florence, Italy, 1991; Abstract WC49.

64. St Louis M, Kabagabo U, Brown C et al. Maternal factors associated with perinatal HIV transmission. 7th International Conference on AIDS, Florence, Italy, 1991; Abstract MC3027

65. DeVincenzi I, Ancelle-Park R. Heterosexual transmission of HIV: follow-up of a European cohort of couples. 7th International Conference on Aids, Florence, Italy, 1991; Abstract MC3028

66. Sawanpanyalert P, Ungchusak K, Thanprasertsuk S, Akarasewi P. Seroconversion rate and risk factors for HIV-1 infection among low class female sex workers in Chiang Mai, Thailand. A multi cross-sectional study. 7th International Conference on AIDS, Florence, Italy, 1991; Abstract WC3097

67. Hira S, Mangola V, Mwale C et al. Apparent vertical transmission of human immunodeficiency virus type-1 by breast feeding in Zambia. J Paediatr 1990; 117: 421–424

68. Blackwell C, James V, Davidson S et al. Secretor status and heterosexual transmission of HIV. Br Med J 1991; 303: 825–826

69. Hira S, Nkowane B, Kamanga J et al. Epidemiology of human immunodeficiency virus in families in Lusaka, Zambia. J AIDS 1990; 3: 83–86

70. Padian N, Marquis L, Francis D et al. Male to female transmission of HIV. JAMA 1987; 258: 788–790

71. Cameron D, Simonsen J, D'Costa L et al. Female to male transmission of human immunodeficiency virus type-1: risk factors for seroconversion in men. Lancet 1989; 2: 403–407

72. Fischl M, Dickinson G, Scott G. Evaluation of heterosexual partners children and household contacts of adults with AIDS. JAMA 1987; 257: 640–644

73. Rehmet S, Staszewski S, Helm E, Doerr H, Stille W. Cofactors of HIV transmission in heterosexual couples. 7th International Conference on AIDS, Florence, Italy, 1991; Abstract WC3132

74. Marinacci G, Costigliola P, Ricchi E, Chiodo F. Risk factors in heterosexual transmission of HIV. 7th International Conference on AIDS, Florence, Italy, 1991; Abstract WC3111
75. Musicco M, Saracco A, Nicolosi A et al. 7th International Conference on AIDS, Florence, Italy, 1991; Abstract MC4
76. Mertens T, Hayes R, Smith P. Epidemiological methods to study the interaction between HIV infection and other sexually transmitted diseases. AIDS 1990; 4: 57–65
77. Mulivanda T, Manoka AT, Nzila N et al. The impact of STD control and condom promotion on the incidence of HIV in Kinshasa prostitutes. 7th International Conference on AIDS, Florence, Italy, 1991; Abstract MC2
78. Smith J, Grant J. The incidence of glove puncture during Caesarean section. J Obstet Gynecol 1990; 10: 317–318
79. Gerschon R, Curbow B, Vlahoo D, Celentano D, Saah A. Low compliance with universal precautions among hospital employees despite high perceived risk. 7th International Conference on AIDS, Florence, Italy, 1991; Abstract WD4187
80. Henry K, Collier P, O'Boyle-Williams C, Campbell S. Observed and self reported compliance with universal precautions among emergency department personnel at two suburban community hospitals. 7th International Conference on AIDS, Florence, Italy, 1991; Abstract MD58
81. Smith J, Kitchen V. Reducing the risk of infection for obstetricians. Br J Obstet Gynaecol 1991; 98: 124–126
82. Ippolito G, Puro V. Efficiency of HIV transmission after at risk exposures in health care settings. The Italian multicentric study. 7th International Conference on AIDS, Florence, Italy, 1991; Abstract MD6
83. Tokars J, Marcus R, Culver D, McKibben P, Bell D. Zidovudine use after occupational exposure to HIV infected blood. 7th International Conference on AIDS, Florence, Italy, 1991; Abstract WD4184
84. Papillon M, Houle L, Lebel F. Zidovudine prophylaxis for health care workers following occupational exposure. 7th International Conference on AIDS, Florence, Italy, 1991; Abstract WD4182
85. Privertera G, Pocchiari M, De Donno A et al. Prevalence of HTLV-I/II and HIV infection in pregnant women and blood donors of 2 geographically defined Italian populations. 7th International Conference on AIDS, Florence, Italy, 1991; Abstract MC3230
86. Lo P, Benedetto A, Giannini V et al. Prevalence of HBV, HCV and HIV infection among women of reproductive age. 7th International Conference on AIDS, Florence, Italy, 1991; Abstract WC3272
87. Emanuelli F, Ermiglia M, Gabutti G et al. Human immunodeficiency virus among women attending obstetric and gynecology departments in Liguna Italy. 7th International Conference on AIDS, Florence, Italy, 1991; Abstract WC3275
88. Couturier E, Larsen C, Brossard Y, Henrion R, Brunet J. HIV-1 and HIV-2 seroprevalence in childbearing women at outcome of pregnancy in Paris area, France. 7th International Conference on AIDS, Florence, Italy, 1991; Abstract WC3246
89. Hoff R, Berardi V, Weiblen B, Mahoney-Traut L, Mitchell M, Grady G. Seroprevalence of human immunodeficiency virus among childbearing women. N Engl J Med 1988; 318: 525–530
90. Gwinn M, Pappaioanou M, George J. Prevalence of HIV infection in childbearing women in the US. JAMA 1991; 265: 1704–1708

14. Update on intrauterine devices

J. Newton

From the first intrauterine device (IUD) for contraception in 1909 came the original development of the Graefenberg ring in 1930[1] and the Ota ring in 1934.[2] Then in 1962 Jack Lippes introduced the now famous 'double S'-shaped Lippes loop of Silastic; this was widely used in national family planning programmes until the 1970s.

However, the next significant development was the introduction of copper-releasing devices pioneered by Zipper and others in 1969,[3] and the population council.[4] These two groups introduced the Copper 7 and the Copper T (Table 14.1). Various alterations in the shape of the IUD were tried in an effort to reduce the expulsion rate, e.g. Multiload,[5] and Copper Fix.[6] Copper surface area on the IUD was also increased to increase the length of action. Those devices with more than 300 mm² of copper (either as copper wire — Multiload 375 — or copper sleeves and wire — Cu

Table 14.1 IUD characteristics

| Device | Plastic frame | Copper | | |
		Thickness of copper (mm)	Surface area (mm²)	Type
Copper 7	Polypropylene + barium sulphate	(0.2)ª0.25	200	Wire
Copper T				
200	Polyethylene + barium sulphate	(0.2)0.25	200	Wire
300		0.25	300	Wire
380A	Polyethylene + barium sulphate	0.25	380	Wire plus collars
220C		0.25	220	7 collars
Multiload ML Cu250	Polyethylene	0.30	250	Wire
Nova T	Polyethylene + barium sulphate	0.30	200	Wire with 0.1 mm silver core
Multiload M1 Cu375	Polyethylene	0.40	375	Wire
Levonova	Polyethylene + barium sulphate	NR	NR	Releases levonorgestrel 20 µg from Silastic collar

NR = Not relevant.

Table 14.2 Grouping of devices by failure (pregnancy) rate

	Device	Pregnancy rates per 100 women years of use
Group I	Lippes loop Copper 7 Copper T 200	Significantly greater than 2.0
Group II	Nova T, Novagard Multiload ML Cu 250 Copper T 220C	Less than 2.0 but not less than 1.0
Group III	Copper T 380T Copper T 380 Slimline Multiload ML Cu 375 Levonova (levonorgestrel 20 µg/day)	Significantly less than 1, most less than 0.5

Reproduced with permission from WHO (1987).[7]

T380A or S) have been found to have a significantly lower pregnancy rate than earlier IUDs (Table 14.2).

In 1970 Scommegna et al[8] pioneered the hormone-releasing IUD which was shown to be effective at preventing pregnancy. From this the progesterone-releasing device was developed but this was only effective for 12 months. Over the last 10 years the development of a levonorgestrel-releasing device at 20 µg/day, Levonova,[9] has revolutionized the concept of long-term intrauterine contraception with a significantly better protection against pregnancy than any other device except the Copper T 380 series. However, the Levonova has other significant health benefits and no increase in risk.

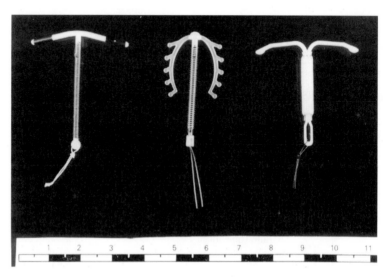

Fig. 14.1 Third generation IUDs; left to right, Copper T Cu 380, Multiload ML Cu 375 and the Levonova 20 µg/day.

TIMING OF INSERTION

Intermenstrual

The usual time for insertion of an IUD is at the time of a period or within the first 5–7 days. At this time the patient can be presumed not to be pregnant, and insertion is easier as the cervical canal is open during menstruation. Great care should be taken to insert an IUD under aseptic conditions. If there is a suspicion of vaginitis or cervicitis these should be treated and the IUD inserted later.

After a spontaneous miscarriage and after termination of pregnancy

There is now ample evidence that IUDs can be inserted immediately after a spontaneous miscarriage or immediately after termination.[10,11] There is no increase in side-effects, perforation of the uterus or infection. Only if the pregnancy has proceeded into the second trimester will there be a slightly increased risk of expulsion but this has to be balanced against the risk of a further unplanned pregnancy.

Post-delivery

Similar evidence now confirms that early puerperal insertion of IUDs, i.e. before 4 weeks, is safe and effective with no increase in side-effects.[12] IUDs can also be inserted after caesarean section without risk of perforation.[13] Care must be taken to sound the uterus to determine the direction of the cavity prior to insertion.

Post placental delivery

Insertion of standard IUDs immediately following delivery of the placenta has been tried[14] but a higher expulsion was found in the World Health Organization (WHO) study.[10,11] However, if a long inserter tube is used fundal placement can be achieved without risk of perforation or expulsion of the IUD. This may be a technique needed in certain family-planning programmes. Attempts to reduce the expulsion with an anchoring suture have been tried with mixed success.

CLINICAL EFFICACY AND DATA ANALYSIS

The usual way to express the performance of IUDs is to use cumulative life table analysis. (For a description of methods see Newton.[15]) The method to be recommended is that used by WHO (see Farley [16]) which uses a statistical package developed by WHO and is the Chiang model of cumulative discontinuation rates coupled with log rank statistical analysis,

Table 14.3 Pregnancy rates from clinical studies

Type of device	Number of studies	Pearl index ± s.e.		Number of woman-years		References[7]
		First year	First 2 years	First year	First 2 years	
Plastic						
Lippes loop D	4	2.8 ± 0.4	2.4 ± 0.3	2178	2787	17–20
Medicated						
Copper-bearing						
Copper 7	5	2.9 ± 0.3	2.7 ± 0.2	3077	5043	17, 19–28
T Cu-200	5	2.5 ± 0.2	3.0 ± 0.2	4592	6045	18, 21, 24, 25
T Cu-220C	10	0.9 ± 0.1	0.9 ± 0.1	6247	14184	17, 19, 20, 22–24, 29
T Cu-380A or Ag	5	0.5 ± 0.1	0.4 ± 0.1	5013	7289	23, 24, 26–28, 29
Nova T	3	1.2 ± 0.3	1.3 ± 0.2	1124	3671	25, 30–32
ML Cu-250	2	1.7 ± 0.7	1.2 ± 0.2	356	2568	22–28, 30–33
ML Cu-375	2	0.6 ± 0.2	0.5 ± 0.3	989	653	26, 27, 31, 32
Progesterone-releasing						
IPCS (25 mg)	2	1.6 ± 0.3	1.7 ± 0.2	2030	3300	34
Levonorgestrel-releasing						
Levonorgestrel (2 µg/day)	1	2.3 ± 0.5	2.1 ± 0.4	1030	1422	30
Levonorgestrel (20 µg/day)	1	0.2 ± 0.1	0.1 ± 0.1	968	1584	28, 35

which can be done on a daily basis. This method also allows stratification of the data by important variables, e.g. age and parity.

The reasons for discontinuation of an IUD are pregnancy (intrauterine or ectopic), removals for bleeding and/or pain, other medical reasons, confirmed pelvic inflammatory disease and expulsion of the IUD. Non-medical reasons (i.e. non-IUD-related) are no further need, planned pregnancy and sterilization. It is also important to know the lost-to-follow-up rate, which should be less than 10%.

IUDs can be divided into three groups according to the pregnancy rate — their clinical efficacy. Table 14.2 shows the allocation of devices to these groups. If one is only concerned about achieving the lowest pregnancy rates possible, then group III devices should be chosen in preference to others i.e. Copper T 380A or S, Multiload 375 or Levonova (levonorgestrel 20 μg/day). Group II devices are also effective (Multiload 250 and Nova T or Novogard), but their length of action is shorter than group III devices, except for the Copper T 220C which is not available in the UK. Groups III and II are to be preferred to those in Group I and the non-medicated devices.

Table 14.3 gives the pregnancy rates and length of action of these devices, together with the references for the clinical studies. All quoted are large multicentre studies which therefore avoid most biases associated with either single-centre or small studies (less than 500 patients per device).

MEDICAL REMOVALS

Still the most common reason for removal of an IUD is unacceptable blood loss, which may be either a longer but lighter period or a heavier period. Most studies have shown an increase in mean menstrual blood loss with IUDs of about 20–30%. It is lower with copper-releasing devices. The Levonova on the other hand significantly reduces menstrual blood loss, but in the first few months this is at the expense of an increase in inter-menstrual spotting. This however is tolerated by most patients. The range of discontinuation rates seen with group II and III devices is shown in Table 14.4. Pain may be associated with bleeding but is not an indication of infection, but rather of uterine cramping. This disappears when the IUD is removed but most cases respond to simple analgesics.

EXPULSION

With the smaller copper devices expulsion was found (Table 14.4). However these results have improved with the change in IUD design and are now at acceptable rates. The key to low expulsion rates is correct fundal placement of the device, by following the insertion instructions carefully. IUD insertion is easier for those who regularly insert IUDs and should not be carried out by those who only occasionally are called upon to insert an

Table 14.4 Discontinuation rates in selected clinic studies: medical reason for removal

Type of device	Expulsion	Removals for bleeding pain	Other medical reason
LL Loop D[4]	14.6	31.8	None at 5 years
ML Cu 250[2]	3.1	17.6	4.3 at 3 years
T Cu 220C[2]	4.5	17.3	4.2
T Cu 220C[1]	9.3	17.0	2.4 at 5 years
T Cu 380A[1]	8.2	18.5	2.9 at 5 years
T Cu 220C[3]	7.5	15.7	3.2 at 5 years
Nova T[3]	6.2	15.7	3.8
Levonova[5]	6.4	3.4	4.6 at 5 years (includes removals for amenorrhoea)

(1), (2) & (3) WHO[5]
(4) Tietze & Lewitt[18]
(5) Luukkainen 1991[36]

IUD. In this situation referral of the patient to an appropriate centre is essential. IUDs are now capable of being used without change for more than 5 years and therefore correct fitting is essential. Expulsion is less in multigravid than in nulliparous women and it is less in older women (over 30 years) than younger women.

ECTOPIC PREGNANCY

There has been an increase in ectopic rates in developed countries since the 1960s, which parallels exactly the rapid increase in sexually transmitted diseases. IUDs do not themselves cause ectopic pregnancy. Earlier copper-releasing devices were associated with a greater decrease in intrauterine pregnancy rate relative to tubal pregnancy, hence there was an apparent increase in ectopic pregnancy. However with the development of fundal copper in group III devices there was a reduction in this apparent effect on tubal pregnancy. Similarly, with the Levonova (levonorgestrel 20 µg/day) the ectopic mg rates are less than the background rates for tubal pregnancy, i.e. they are protective.

The importance of early diagnosis, using beta human chorionic gonadotrophin and ultrasound with laparoscopy if necessary, cannot be overstressed and routine investigations of patients should occur if an ectopic pregnancy is suspected. Careful selection of patients with avoidance of risk factors for ectopic pregnancies–previous ectopic, pelvic inflammatory and sexually transmitted disease will reduce the risk still further (see WHO[7] for a review).

PELVIC INFLAMMATORY DISEASE

The diagnosis of pelvic inflammatory disease is often difficult and still is usually based on series of signs and symptoms. Laparoscopy is needed to verify the diagnosis and should be used. It is routinely used in some Scandinavian countries and some centres in the UK. If one relies solely on the presence of abdominal pain, motion tenderness of the uterus and a purulent vaginal discharge, then there is only a 50% probability of being right. If one adds to that a pyrexia of 38°C or more and palpable adnexal swelling then the probability increases to 80%, and laparoscopy will allow an accurate diagnosis. As the majority of pelvic inflammatory diseases are sexually transmitted, especially in young women, and are often poly-bacterial, appropriate two-drug regimes of broad-spectrum antibiotics are needed. An example would be Flagyl plus ampicillin as a loading dose followed by 14 days of Flagyl plus doxycycline.

Earlier epidemiological studies overestimated the frequency of IUD-related infection (see WHO[7] for review). Studies since 1980 clearly indi-cated that the risk of pelvic inflammatory disease in a stable monogamous relationship was not higher than the background rate of pelvic inflam-matory disease. This has been confirmed by the work of Cramer[37] and Darling:[38] both these studies show the relative risk rates of pelvic inflam-matory disease to be lower with copper-releasing IUDs than with non-medicated devices, and to be no higher than background rates in the community. The Levonova device, releasing levonorgestrel, has a protective effect against the development of pelvic inflammatory disease and in this respect acts like oral contraception in decreasing the rate of infection (see Table 14.5 for rates). A recent review by Struthers[39] has shown an overall rate of 1.46 per 100 women-years of use for copper IUDs; in this large population study some 46% were nulliparous. Case selections and the avoidance of risk factors are important and data from the WHO multicentre studies show a very low rate of removals for pelvic inflammatory disease during long-term use of IUDs.[40]

CURRENT DEVELOPMENTS

Design changes in the IUD frame continue in an attempt to reduce the incidence of expulsion and the rate of removal for bleeding, e.g. the Cu

Table 14.5 Pelvic inflammatory disease rates

Authors	Rate	Device	Women	Database
Struthers (1991)[39]	1.49/100 women-years	Cu7	25 674	45 930 women-years
WHO (1990)[40]				
Study 1	0.27/100 women-months	T220C	1032	25 832 women-months
	0.33/100 women-months	ML250	1011	25 247 women-months
Study 2	0.11/100 women-months	T220C	1396	66 343 women-months
	0.05/100 women-months	T380A	1396	67 885 women-months
Study 3	0.08/100 women-months	T220C	1881	52 417 women-months
	0.11/100 women-months	Nova T	1847	51 322 women-months

Table 14.6   Levonova device multicentre study[41]

	At 3 years	At 5 years
Pregnancy	0.3	0.3
Bleeding	11.1	11.3
Amenorrhoea	4.6	4.6
'Hormonal'	8.2	9.0
Pelvic inflammatory disease	0.5	0.5
Number of insertions	937	1821

Safe. A different approach has been used in the Cu Fix[6] which is a non-adsorbable suture thread on which are six copper sleeves or collars; the upper and lower ones are crimped on to the thread to stop the collars slipping off. At the top of the thread is a knotted loop which is driven by the introducer stilette 1 cm into the myometrium. This increases retention and appears in the preliminary studies to reduce removals for bleeding and pain. Removal is easy by gentle traction on the thread.

The Levonova (levonorgestrel 20 µg/day) device is the most promising development of recent years. The hormone released affects all layers of the endometrium, unlike the earlier progesterone device.[9] Pregnancy and removal rates are low and ectopic rates are below the background rates, as is the rate for pelvic inflammatory disease (Table 14.6). This device lasts at least 5 years, if not 8 years. Menstrual blood loss is significantly reduced by at least 40–50% and therefore in areas where anaemia is endemic, it will be prevented. It also is very effective for the treatment of heavy periods, reducing menstrual blood loss from 250 to 10 ml within 3 months.[42] Its health benefits are considerable.

RISK-BENEFIT ANALYSIS

All drugs and devices, including contraceptive methods, are associated with a certain risk. The ratio of risk to benefit will vary from country to country and in developing countries the high maternal mortality and morbidity rates associated with pregnancy have to be assessed together with the much lower risk of contraceptive methods. The incidence of sexually transmitted disease and associated disease has to be balanced against providing essential contraception. For oral contraception there are the full-documented risks of cardiovascular disease, cerebral haemorrhage and benign liver tumours. While barrier methods may, if properly used, reduce infection they have higher failure rates and thus are related to the complication and risk of unwanted pregnancy.

The use of IUDs provides long-term effective contraception and with group III devices offers an alternative to sterilization. When compared with other reversible methods of contraception, women using an IUD have the lowest mortality resulting from deaths attributable to the method

Table 14.7 Death rates per 100 000 per annum in women using various methods of contraception

Method	Age (years)					
	15–19	20–24	25–29	30–34	35–39	40–44
None	5.6	6.1	7.4	13.9	20.8	22.6
Oral contraceptives						
Non-smokers	1.3	1.4	1.4	2.2	4.5	7.1
Smokers	1.5	1.6	1.6	10.6	13.4	58.9
IUDs	0.9	1.0	1.2	1.4	2.0	1.9
Barrier methods	1.1	1.6	2.0	3.6	5.0	4.2

Modified from Tietze (1978).[43]

(Table 14.7) It is also worth noting the increase in mortality rates with age of those who use no method of contraception (Table 14.7). The special risks discussed previously, e.g. removals for bleeding, pelvic inflammatory disease and uterine perforations, are much lower than first thought and can be significantly reduced by proper case selection and the use of an appropriate group III device.

SELECTION OF PATIENTS

It is essential to take a full history, including a sexual history of the patient and partner(s), and complete a full examination prior to the insertion of an IUD. Adequate verbal and written explanation needs to be given to prospective IUD users and suitable leaflets are produced by the Family Planning Association and others. If there is any suggestion of local infection then appropriate tests and treatment need to be completed before the IUD is fitted.

Absolute contraindications for insertion of an IUD include malignant disease of the cervix or uterus, undiagnosed vaginal bleeding, suspected pregnancy, and acute pelvic inflammatory disease, or sexually transmitted disease during past 12 months.[7]

Relative contraindications include nulliparity, previous ectopic pregnancy, anaemia or menorrhagia (except for the Levonova IUD), history of pelvic inflammatory disease since last pregnancy, current or recurrent lower genital tract infection, multiple sexual partners, rheumatic heart disease, immunosuppressive therapy and Wilson's disease (copper IUDs only).

It is important that the final informed choice is that of the patient; the professionals involved will need to advise of risks and benefits.

THE FUTURE

IUDs, especially the last generation of copper-releasing devices and the Levonova (levonorgestrel-releasing IUD), offer a highly acceptable and very effective method of contraception. IUDs are suitable for spacing or as a long-term (more than 5 years) method of reversible contraception. These devices described have significant health benefits with low risk and are found to have high continuation rates in clinical practice. They are a very important method of contraception that should be available to every family planning programme. It is clear that development will continue, making devices even more acceptable and effective.

REFERENCES

1. Graefenberg E. An intrauterine contraceptive method. In: Sanga M, Stone H M, eds. The practice of contraception. Proceedings of the 7th International Birth Control Conference. Baltimore: Williams & Wilkins, 1930: pp 33–47
2. Ota T A. A study on birth control with an intrauterine instrument. Jp J Obstet Gynaecol 1934; 17: 210–214
3. Zipper J, Tatum H J, Pasteur L et al. Contraception through the use of intrauterine metals. Am J Obstet Gynecol 1969; 105 (8): 1274–1278
4. Sivan I. A comparison of the Copper T 200 and the Lippes loop in four countries. Stud Fam Plann 1976; 15: 115–123
5. WHO task force on IUDs. Safety and efficacy of T Cu 220C Multiload 250 and Alza T IPCS 52. Clin Reprod Fertil 1983; 2: 113–128
6. Wildemeersch D, Van der Pas H, Thiery M et al. The Copper Fix: a new concept in IUD technology. Adv Contracept 1988; 4: 197–205
7. WHO. Mechanism of action, safety and efficacy of intrauterine devices (report of a WHO scientific group). Technical report series 753. Geneva: WHO, 1987
8. Scommegna A, Pandya G N, Christ M et al. Intrauterine administration of progesterone by a slow release device. Fertil Steril 1970; 21: 201–210
9. Luukkainen T, Nilsson C G, Lahteenmaki P L et al. Five years experience with a levonorgestrel releasing IUD. Contraception 1986; 33: 139–148
10. WHO task force in IUDs. Clinical trial of 3 IUDs inserted following termination of pregnancy. Stud Fam Plann 1983; 14: 109–114
11. WHO task force in IUDs. Clinical trial of 3 IUDs following spontaneous miscarriage. Stud Fam Plann 1983; 14: 109–114
12. Mishell D R, Roy S. Copper IUD rates following insertion at 4 to 8 weeks after delivery. Am J Obstet Gynecol 1982; 143: 29–35
13. Parikh V, Ghandi A S. Safety of copper T after caesarean section. J Indian Med Assoc 1989; 87: 113–115
14. Thiery M, Laufe L, Paveurijck W et al. Immediate post placental IUD insertion. Contraception 1983; 22: 299–313
15. Newton J. POP and contraception. In: Philipp E, Setchell M, eds. Scientific foundations of obstetrics and gynaecology 4E. Chicago, IL: Year Book Publishers, 1991: pp 691–708
16. Farley T M N. Life table methods for contraceptive research. Stat Med 1986; 5: 475–489
17. WHO. A randomized multicentre comparative trial of the Lippes Loop D. TCu220C and Copper 7. Contraception 1982; 26: 1–22
18. Tietze C, Lewitt S. Comparison of the Copper-T and Loop D: a research report. Stud Fam Plann 1972; 3: 277–278
19. WHO task force on intrauterine devices for fertility regulation. IUD insertion following termination of pregnancy: a clinical trial of the TCu 220C, Lippes Loop D and Copper 7. Stud Fam Plann 1983; 14: 99–108
20. WHO task force on intrauterine devices for fertility regulation. IUD insertion following spontaneous abortion. A clinical trial of the TCu220C, Lippes Loop D, and Copper 7. Stud Fam Plann 1983; 14: 109–114
21. Jain A K. Comparative performance of three types of IUDs in the United States. In: Hefnawi E F, Segal, S J, eds. Analysis of intrauterine contraception. Amsterdam, North-Holland/American Elsevier, 1975: pp 3–16

22. Hutapea H, McCarthy T, Goh T H et al. The acceptability of the Copper 7, Multiload 250 and Copper T 220 C intrauterine devices. Contracept Delivery Systems 1984; 5: 11–16
23. Sung S, Quian L J, Liu X. Comparative clinical experience with 3 IUDs, TCu 380 Ag, TCu 220 C and Mahua ring in Tianjin, People's Republic of China. Contraception 1984; 29: 229–239
24. Sivin I, Stern J. Long-acting, more effective Copper T IUDs: a summary of US experience, 1970–1975. Stud Fam Plann 1979; 10: 263–281
25. Luukkainen T, Allonen H, Nielsen N C et al. Five years experience of intrauterine contraception with the Nova-T and the Copper T 200. Am J Obstet Gynecol 1983; 147: 885–892
26. Cole L P, Aranda C, Potts D M et al. Comparative copper IUD trials. In: Zatuchni G I, Goldsmith A, Sciarra J J, eds. Intrauterine contraception: advances and future prospects. Philadelphia: Harper & Row, 1985: pp 95–100
27. Cole L P, Potts D M, Aranda C et al. An evaluation of the TCu 380 Ag and the Multiload Cu 375. Fertil Steril 1985; 43: 214–217
28. Sivin I, Stern J, Diaz J et al. Two years of intrauterine contraception with Copper or with levonorgestrel: a randomized comparison of the TCu 380 Ag and Levonorgestrel 20 mcg/day devices. Contraception 1987; 35: 245–255
29. Sung S, Quian L J, Liu X et al. Two-year comparative clinical experience with three IUDs in China. In: Zatuchni G I, Goldsmith A, Sciarra J J, eds. Intrauterine contraception: advances and future prospects. Philadelphia: Harper & Row, 1985: pp 109–114
30. WHO task force on intrauterine devices for fertility regulation: microdose intrauterine levonorgestrel for contraception. World Health Organization Annual Report, 1990
31. Hirvonen E, Kaivola S. Fincoid-350 IUD. In: Zatuchni G I, Goldsmith A, Sciarra J J, eds. Intrauterine contraception: advances and future prospects. Philadelphia: Harper & Row, 1985: pp 251–262
32. Saure A, Hirvonen E, Kivijarvi A et al. Comparative performance of Fincoid, Nova-T and ML 375 IUDs. In: Zatuchni G I, Goldsmith A, Sciarra J J, eds. Intrauterine contraception: advances and future prospects. Philadelphia: Harper & Row, 1985: pp 104–108
33. WHO special programme of research, development and research training in human reproduction. Intrauterine devices. 12th annual report. Geneva: World Health Organization, 1983: pp 40–45
34. WHO task force on intrauterine devices for fertility regulation. The Alza T IPCS52, a longer acting progesterone IUD: safety and efficacy compared to the TCu 220C and multiload 250 in two randomised multi-centre trials. Clin Repro Fertil 1983; 2: 113–128
35. Sivin I, Alvarez F, Diaz J et al. Intrauterine contraception with copper and with levonorgestrel: a randomized study of the TCu 380 Ag and levonorgestrel 20 mscg/day devices. Contraception 1984; 30: 443–456
36. Luukkainen T. Presentation at FIGO — 13th world congress of obstetrics and gynecology, Singapore, September 1991
37. Cramer D W, Schiff I, Schoenbaum S C et al. Tubal infertility and the IUD. N Engl J Med 1985; 312: 937–941
38. Darling J R, Weiss N S, Metch B J et al. Primary tubal infertility in relation to the use of an IUD. N Engl J Med 1985; 312: 937–941
39. Struthers B. PID with copper IUDs. Adv Contracept 1991; 7: 211–230
40. WHO comparative trials of Tcu 380A Multiload 750, T220C & Nova T. Contraception 1990; 142: 141–158
41. Luukkainen T. Presentation at SAC meeting, Singapore, 1990
42. Anderson J, Rybo G. Levonorgestrel releasing IUD in the treatment of menorrhagia. Br J Obstet Gynaecol 1990; 97: 690–694
43. Tietze C. What price fertility control? Contemp Obstet Gynaecol 1978; 1: 32–36

15. Antiprogesterones

R.C. Henshaw   A.A. Templeton

PROGESTERONE IN REPRODUCTIVE MEDICINE

A brief review of the central and indispensable role progesterone plays in reproductive medicine is required to interpret the effects of an antiprogesterone fully. In the follicular phase of the cycle there is some evidence that progesterone plays a role in initiating and defining the nature of the mid-cycle luteinizing hormone (LH) surge.[1,2] After ovulation the ovarian follicle becomes the corpus luteum (CL), which secretes increasing amounts of progesterone. In the uterus the luteal phase of the menstrual cycle is initially characterized by an increase in endometrial glycogen production and storage, vascular activity and secretory response, preparing the endometrium for implantation of the conceptus. If fertilization does not occur, then the activity of the CL starts to decline after about 12 days, and a fall in progesterone results in shedding of all but the basal layer of the endometrium.

If fertilization does occur, implantation begins about 6 days later. Trophoblastic tissue secretes human chorionic gonadotrophin (hCG) and other proteins, which signal the CL to continue secreting progesterone; this is indispensable for the support of the developing embryo.[3] Luteoplacental shift occurs around 8 weeks of amenorrhoea, when the placenta becomes mature enough to secrete adequate levels of progesterone. In later pregnancy placentally derived progesterone suppresses uterine reaction to endogenous and exogenous prostaglandins, making the uterus a quiescent organ. The clinical effects of an antiprogesterone therefore extend throughout the menstrual cycle and pregnancy, and reflect the precise time of administration. Progesterone receptors are present in high concentrations in other tissues, especially the breast and meninges. Tumours of these organs have long been known to be hormone-dependent, being more common in women as well as waxing and waning during pregnancy. Any organ containing progesterone receptors has the potential for clinical manipulation by an antiprogesterone.

INTRODUCTION TO ANTIPROGESTERONES

Antagonists are now available against all three classes of reproductive steroid hormones. Antioestrogens such as clomiphene citrate and tamoxifen are widely used in ovulation induction and in the management of breast cancer. Antiandrogens such as cyproterone acetate are used in the management of male hypersexuality and female hirsuitism. Mifepristone (RU486, Roussel-Uclaf, Paris) is the first antiprogesterone to become available for routine clinical use in the UK, having been granted a product licence in July 1991.

The direct antagonism of progesterone has been achieved and tested clinically in two alternative ways (the neutralization of circulating progesterone remains an experimental concept). Compounds such as mifepristone block the action of progesterone at the receptor level. Although other receptor level antiprogesterones do exist (e.g. onapristone, ZK 98299, Schering AG, Berlin), the overwhelming majority of clinical studies of this class of drug have been confined, as will this review be, to mifepristone. A number of drugs (e.g. epostane, trilostane, Sterling Winthrop, UK) have been developed to inhibit the 3 beta-hydroxysteroid dehydrogenase enzyme system, which during progesterone biosynthesis converts the precursor pregnenolone into progesterone. However, the development of these drugs as antiprogesterones was halted for commercial reasons in the 1980s (although trilostane has a product licence for its antiglucocorticoid activity), and has been overshadowed by the introduction of mifepristone.

This review will therefore only consider the progesterone receptor-blocking agent mifepristone. Readers wishing to explore the actions of enzyme-inhibiting drugs and antiprogesterones in lower mammals and non-human primates are referred to Van Look & Bygdeman.[4]

STRUCTURE AND MODE OF ACTION

Mifepristone, a 19 nor-steroid, is a derivative of the synthetic progestin norethindrone, and possesses a dimethylaminophenyl side chain at position 11; this hydrophobic moiety appears to be essential for antiprogestogenic activity (Fig. 15.1).

Steroid hormones, unlike polypeptide hormones, enter their target cells and bind to receptors in the cell nucleus. The activated receptor undergoes a conformational change, allowing it to bind to the regulating gene DNA; transcription of DNA into messenger RNA and eventually protein production ensues.

Progesterone binds to its receptor with high affinity and normally, when progesterone is absent, the receptor remains in a non-DNA binding conformation. The arrival of progesterone prompts gene transcription as described above, possibly by displacing the heat shock protein which caps the DNA binding area of the receptor. Mifepristone, acting as a competitive receptor antagonist with a three to five times greater receptor affinity than progesterone, is thought to stabilize the receptor in a non-DNA binding conformation, thus preventing gene transcription.[5]

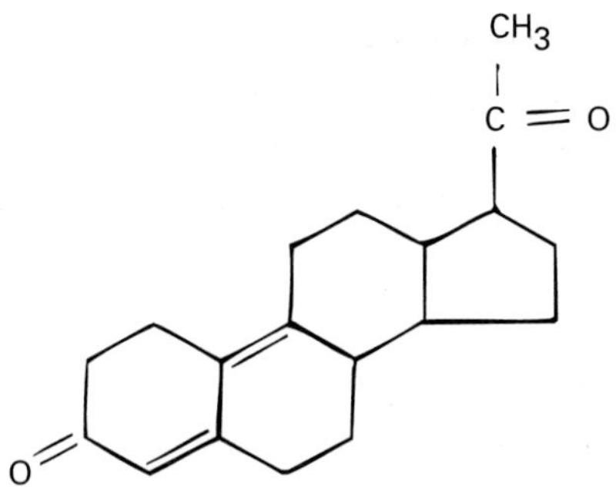

Progesterone

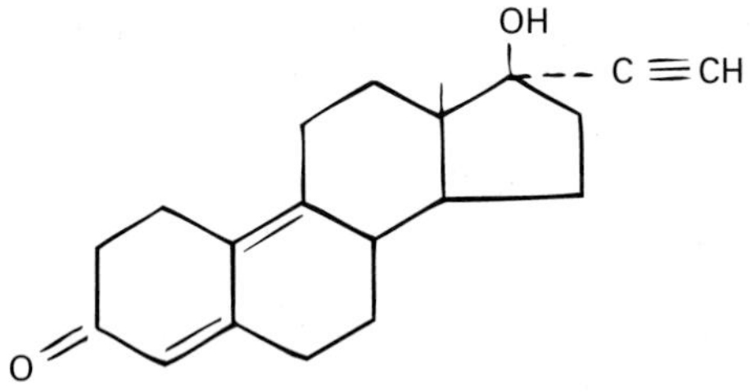

Norethindrone

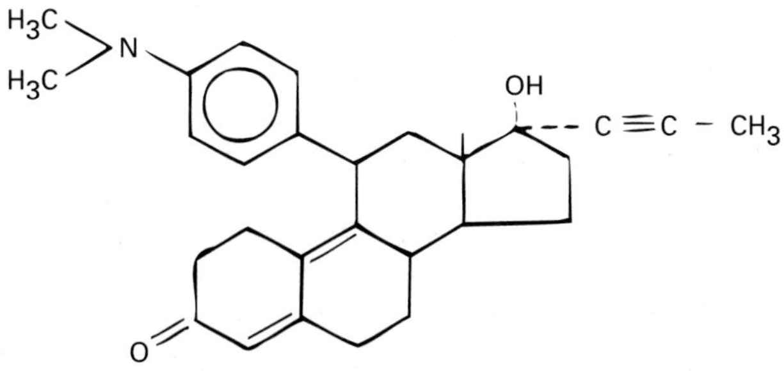

Mifepristone

Fig. 15.1 Chemical structures.

None of the antiprogesterones is a pure progesterone receptor antagonist. Mifepristone also acts as a competitive antagonist at the glucocorticoid receptor, binding up to four times more strongly than dexamethasone.[6] However this does not result in any clinically important glucocorticoid deficiency when the drug is used in effective antiprogestogenic doses in humans. Affinity of mifepristone for androgen receptors is low, and it has virtually no antioestrogenic or antimineralocorticoid effects.[5] In certain non-physiological experimental situations the drug may behave as a partial progesterone agonist.[7]

PHARMACOKINETICS

The bioavailabilty of mifepristone is approximately 60% of the administered dose, with 85% of the drug being absorbed after oral administration and peak serum levels occurring 1–2 hours later.[6]

The drug does not conform to standard linear pharmacokinetic models. Concentrations remain stable for 12 hours, then start to decline with a half-life of approximately 24 hours in both pregnant and non-pregnant women.[8] Some 95% of circulating mifepristone is bound to alpha$_1$ acid glycoprotein and, to a lesser extent, albumin. The major route of excretion is via bile and faeces, and the compound and its metabolites may undergo recirculation via the enterohepatic system. Both these factors contribute to the relatively long half-life of the drug.[9] The major metabolites of mifepristone are the demethylated and hydroxylated forms of the drug. These compounds are not thought to have any significant antiprogestogenic effects in humans.[10]

EFFECT ON THE NORMAL MENSTRUAL CYCLE

Mifepristone administered in the first 3 days of the follicular phase at effective dose levels seems to have no effect on the integrity of the menstrual cycle; the length of the follicular phase, the LH surge and the luteal phase length remain the same in treated and control cycles.[11] This is not the case when the drug is administered either throughout or later in the follicular phase, when inhibition of folliculogenesis and ovulation occurs; there is a reduction in LH and follicle-stimulating hormone (FSH) levels, with prolongation of follicular phase duration and collapse of the dominant follicle.[12,13] Whether this effect is primarily due to inhibition of pituitary gonadotrophin secretion, as some animal studies have demonstrated, or by a direct effect at ovarian level, is at present uncertain.[14] It appears important to give mifepristone in the mid to late follicular phase if ovulation is to be delayed; administering the drug in the immediate preovulatory period fails to prevent the LH surge.[13]

Luteal phase administration of the drug as a single dose within 2 days of the LH surge has been shown not to affect luteal phase duration, gonadotrophin secretion or CL function, but biopsy did show endometrial development to be retarded.[15]

Mifepristone administered sequentially during the first half of the luteal phase in normally cycling women affects the regulation of temperature, thirst and mood, suggesting a direct effect at the hypothalamus.[16] Further studies of mifepristone administration during the middle of the luteal phase confirm that the drug has a direct but independent inhibitory effect on pituitary gonadotrophin secretion, with reduction in the amplitude and frequency of the LH pulses.[17–19]

Endometrial shedding, which again occurs independently of the hypothalamic and pituitary inhibition caused by mifepristone, is reported in 40–100% of study subjects. This results from direct inhibition of the endometrial progesterone receptor, leading to decreased glandular secretory activity and accelerated degenerative changes which usually occur within 48–72 hours of drug administration.[16–20]

Luteolysis also occurs during these events. Although most of the data suggests that is in response to decreased gonadotrophin secretion, there is some evidence that mifepristone has a direct effect on ovarian CL function.[21]

There appear to be two distinct populations in response to mifepristone administration at this phase of the cycle, which are not related to drug dose or serum levels. In one group, comprising around 30% of subjects, CL function and gonadotrophin secretion are inhibited, complete luteolysis occurs and a single episode of uterine bleeding follows. In a second group, some inhibition of gonadotrophin secretion and CL function occurs, but this is short-lived and incomplete; the luteolytic process is then reversed, the luteal phase continues and a second episode of vaginal bleeding occurs at the end of the cycle.[19,20]

Late luteal phase administration of the drug causes uterine bleeding which is indistinguishable from normal menstrual bleeding. Menstrual cycle events in treatment and post-treatment cycles do not seem to be significantly affected when the drug is administered at the time of the natural progesterone withdrawal.[18,22] Prolactin levels seem to be increased in a mifepristone dose-dependent way during luteal phase administration of the drug.[19]

MENSTRUAL CYCLE EFFECTS: CLINICAL IMPLICATIONS

Drugs which inhibit folliculogenesis and ovulation may be used as a contraceptive or in the management of endometriosis. Mifepristone seems to be an effective contraceptive in monkeys.[23] However human data are limited; in one small study 25 mg was administered on days 1–14 of the cycle, followed by norethisterone 5 mg on days 15–24. Although some biochemical and ultrasonograpic evidence of follicle growth and ovulation was seen in the second half of the regime, by the third treatment cycle no ovulation occurred. Control of uterine bleeding was good, and mifepristone dose levels used were not associated with the side-effects typical of steroids used in oral contraceptives.[24] A small study, examining the effect of daily administration of mifepristone on women with endometriosis, resulted in acyclic ovarian function and an improvement in symptoms, but not laparoscopically assessed disease.[25]

The endometrial desynchronization, shedding and luteolysis caused by luteal phase administration of the drug may indicate a role as a post-ovulatory contraceptive agent. When given in the immediate postovulatory period mifepristone appears to be highly effective; 379 women who attended for emergency contraception within 72 hours of unprotected intercourse were randomly allocated to receive either mifepristone 600 mg as a single dose or the commonly used high-dose oestrogen (Yuzpe) regime. There were no pregnancies (and fewer side-effects) in the mifepristone group compared to a 1.1% pregnancy rate in the oestrogen-treated group.[26]

The boundary between contraception and abortion becomes somewhat blurred in the field of late luteal phase postovulatory contraception, and the introduction of terms such as contragestion and interception were coined in an attempt to defuse the abortion debate.[27] Unprotected mid-cycle intercourse in normal women results in a chance of conception varying from 7 to 35%;[28,29] the utilization of highly sensitive assays allows their detection within the late luteal phase prior to the first missed menstrual period. It is quite clear that a high proportion (25%) of these conceptions will fail to progress spontaneously.[30] Mifepristone administered in the late luteal phase will increase the number of conceptions that do not progress to 80–90%; an ongoing pregnancy rate of 10–20% is consistently reported, despite the induction of menses in virtually all women.[29-32]

The reasons for this relatively high failure rate are not clear; Li et al[33] postulated that although the drug induces uterine bleeding, this may not be associated with shedding of the functional layer of the endometrium, allowing a proportion of the pregnancies to persist. It is probable that combining the drug with a prostaglandin, or a gonadotrophin hormone-releasing antagonist to improve luteolytic properties, will reduce the failure rate in this situation.[34,35]

At present therefore it is not possible to use mifepristone alone during the late luteal phase as a regular 'once-a-month' postovulatory agent. However, one of the limiting features of currently used emergency contraception is the need to deliver treatment within a relatively short time-frame following unprotected mid-cycle intercourse (3 days if the Yuzpe regime is used, 5 days for insertion of an intrauterine device).[34] Using mifepristone in the late luteal phase extends this time-frame up to 14 days in regularly cycling women; however such treatment raises considerable medicolegal and ethical questions.[36]

EFFECTS IN PREGNANCY

Clinical evidence that mifepristone was able to procure abortion in early

Table 15.1   Mifepristone alone: studies with 50 or more subjects

Study	Number of women in trial	Duration of amenorrhoea (days)	Total mifepristone dose (mg)	Mifepristone administration regime	Efficacy (%)
Couzinet et al (1986)[37]	100	Within 10 days of missed menses	400–800 mg	Over 2–4 days	85%
Maria et al (1988)[38]	150	42	600 mg	Single dose	87%
Carol & Klinger (1989)[39]	50	42	600 mg	Single dose	80%
Ylikorkala et al (1989)[40]	50	42	600 mg	Single dose	72%
Somell & Olund (1990)[41]	70	42	600 mg	Single dose	80%
Birgerson & Olind (1988)[42]	153	49	140–700 mg	Over 7 days	64–73%
Maria et al (1988)[43]	205	49	200 or 600 mg	Single dose	63–84%
Shu-rong (1989)[44]	299	49	600 mg	Single dose	64%
Sitruk-Ware et al (1990)[45]	124	49	350–1000 mg	Single dose over 7 days	50–86%

human pregnancy was first provided in 1982, and a compendium of clinical trials involving 50 or more women exposed to mifepristone alone is shown in Table 15.1. To summarize these findings, mifepristone used alone at up to 7 weeks' amenorrhoea results in complete abortion in around 60–85% of cases, incomplete abortion in 10–30% and ongoing pregnancy in 5–10% of cases.

The low efficacy of the regimes employed and the infrequent but important complication of severe uterine haemorrhage in a proportion of the women with incomplete abortion were clearly unsatisfactory features that prevented the drug being employed in routine clinical practice. Subsequently efforts were made to improve the efficacy of the regime by altering dose schedules, including both the actual daily dose of the drug and the number of days for which it was administered. Reported regimes varied widely, ranging from 20 mg for 7 days up to 400 mg administered for 4 days.[4]

In an attempt to identify women who would fail to respond to the drug, Grimes et al[46,47] analysed clinical features in a large number of women undergoing abortion utilizing mifepristone alone. They concluded that the important arbiters of efficacy were the regime used (a single dose of 600 mg seems to be most effective), body mass (obesity increases failure rates) and serum beta hCG immediately prior to treatment (higher values were associated with higher failure rates). The diameter of the gestational sac and the duration of amenorrhoea were not statistically significant in predicting failure. Other authors who have reviewed the literature[4] contradict these findings, and suggest that the sole arbiter of success is the duration of amenorrhoea, with efficacy decreasing as gestational age advances.

The mechanism by which mifepristone terminates early pregnancy is not clear, although it is probably initiated by progesterone receptor antagonism of decidual glandular cells, resulting in changes in prostaglandin metabolism. Decidual prostaglandin synthesis increases and prostaglandin catabolism decreases,[48] leading to decidual necrosis with bleeding and detachment of the embryo. This embryonic detachment in turn leads to a fall in trophoblastic beta-hCG production and subsequent diminished progesterone production from the CL. There is also some evidence that mifepristone directly inhibits trophoblastic beta-hCG and placental progesterone production.[49] The net effect of these changes, once initiated, is a persistent decrease in progesterone levels, leading to increasing endogenous prostaglandin activity.

The increase in endogenous prostaglandin activity affects the cervix and myometrium. Coordinated uterine contractions commence within 24 hours of mifepristone administration. Cervical changes, which are similar to those observed after prostaglandin administration,[50] include dissolution of collagen fibres, an accumulation of mast cells and vascular proliferation. These morphological changes result in a decrease in cervical rigidity (see below), allowing easier expulsion of the conceptus as uterine contractility increases.

A further effect of mifepristone is a marked increase in myometrial sensitivity to orally, vaginally or intramuscularly administered prostaglandin E_1 (gemeprost, misopristol) and E_2 (sulprostone, meteneprost) analogues, but not to natural prostaglandin E_2 or oxytocin.[51,52] This is the explanation for the increased efficacy of combined mifepristone/prostaglandin regimes, first reported in 1985[4]; many large-scale trials have confirmed these findings. Studies including 100 or more women are shown in Table 15.2.

In summary, mifepristone followed 36 or more hours later by the administration of a vaginal, intramuscular or oral prostaglandin analogue is associated with a success rate (complete abortion without the need for subsequent surgical uterine evacuation) of around 95%, an incomplete abortion rate of around 4% and a less than 1% rate of missed abortion/viable pregnancy. Efficacy seems to be clearly linked to gestational age; the failure rate is increased in pregnancies of higher gestational age. Body mass seems not to be an important factor.[60]

This combined mifepristone/prostaglandin administration has become known as medical abortion,[65] and in the UK the currently recommended regime (for use up to 63 days' amenorrhoea) is mifepristone 600 mg followed 36–48 hours later by gemeprost 1 mg vaginal pessary.

SEQUELAE OF MEDICAL ABORTION

The main short-term sequelae of medical abortion are pain, bleeding and gastrointestinal disturbance. Women's self-reported experience of pain and bleeding at different times during the procedure are shown in Table 15.3.

Table 15.2 Mifepristone and prostaglandin: studies with 100 or more subjects

Study	Number of women in trial	Duration of amenorrhoea	Mifepristone dose	Mifepristone administration	Prostaglandin regime	Efficacy (%)
Rodger & Baird (1987)[53]	100	56	400–600 mg	Single dose	Gemeprost 0.5–1 mg	95
Dubois et al (1988)[54]	106	49	600 mg	Single dose	Gemeprost 1 mg	100
WHO (1989)[55]	251	49	50 mg bd	Over 3–4 days	Sulprostone 0.25 mg	89
Maria & Stampf (1989)[56]	338	49	600 mg	Single dose	Sulprostone 0.25 mg or Meteneprost 10 mg	96
Swahn & Bygdeman (1989)[57]	116	49	50–100 mg	Over 3–6 days	Sulprostone 0.25 mg	91–95
Rodger et al (1989)[58]	121	56	600 mg	Single dose	Gemeprost 0.5–1 mg	99
Rodger & Baird (1989)[59]	222	63	400–600 mg	Single dose	Gemeprost 0.5–1 mg	98
Shu-rong (1989)[44]	422	49	600 mg	Single dose	Chinese domestic vaginal prostaglandin analogue 1 mg	94
UK Multicentre Trial (1990)[60]	588	63	600 mg	Single dose	Gemeprost 1 mg	94
Silvestre et al (1990)[61]	2115	49	600 mg	Single dose	0.25–0.5 mg Sulprostone or gemeprost 1 mg	96
Hill et al (1990)[62]	100	63	600 mg	Single dose	Gemeprost 1 mg	95
WHO (1991)[63]	385	49	25 mg × 5 doses or 600 mg	12-hour increments	Gemeprost 1 mg	93
Aubery & Baulieu (1991)[64]	100	49	600 mg	Single dose	Misoprostol 400 µg	95

Prostaglandin administered at least 36 hours after mifepristone in single dose studies

Table 15.3   Self-reported pain and bleeding in medical abortion[60]

	Percentage reporting symptoms to be moderate or less	
	Pain	Bleeding
24–48 hours post mifepristone	97	90
4 hours post prostaglandin	89	91
2 days post prostaglandin	94	83
9 days post prostaglandin	100	99.6

Intensity of pain can also be assessed by analgesia requirements, although there is remarkably little consistency between individual units and groups of women. In some studies only 6% of women used narcotic analgesia,[63] varying to as high as 37% in primigravid UK women.[60] There is a similar discrepancy in non-narcotic analgesia requirements, varying from 9 to 30%.

There is a good deal more consistency in haemoglobin change; in the UK Multicentre Trial[60] only 0.9% of women experienced a fall in haemoglobin of more than 20 g/l when assessed before and 1 week following the procedure. A similar assessment suggests an average fall in haemoglobin of 7.8 (±7.4) g/l;[57] it seems that the typical change in haemoglobin is insignificant. This is supported by a study showing an average measured blood loss of 72 ml (range 72–398 ml) following medical abortion at up to 56 days' amenorrhoea.[59] Post abortal bleeding persists on average for around 10–12 days, and menses resume between 5–6 weeks later. However, a small proportion of women require blood transfusion following the procedure; reported rates vary from 1 in 2000 cases to 0.85%.[60,61]

Gastrointestinal sequelae such as vomiting or diarrhoea seem to be related to the administered prostaglandin. These symptoms occur in 25 and 13% of women respectively following 1 mg gemeprost. Other minor sequelae such as headache, malaise and faintness have been reported in a small proportion (5%) of cases. The literature suggests that smaller doses of both mifepristone and prostaglandin analogues may retain high efficacy, with the advantage of less procedure-related pain and gastrointestinal side-effects; multicentre trials are underway to confirm this hypothesis.

The frequency of unpleasant sequelae following any procedure will affect the acceptability and hence uptake by the population as a whole. In France, where over 100 000 women have undergone medical abortion, some 20% of eligible women opt for this method.[65] Limited acceptability studies have been performed; one suggested that 88% of women found the procedure acceptable.[62] Urquhart & Templeton[66] found that in a small number of women who had undergone both medical and surgical abortion, 77% preferred the medical approach. These findings are supported by trials assessing the acceptability of other methods of medical abortion;[67] women seem to value the lack of surgical intervention and avoidance of general anaesthesia highly.

MEDICAL ABORTION: IMPLICATIONS FOR REPRODUCTIVE HEALTH

Prior to the introduction of mifepristone in the UK, 99% of first trimester pregnancy terminations were performed by vacuum aspiration.[68] Over half of these were treated as day-cases, and general anaesthesia was used in over 96% of cases.[69] In developed countries where abortion is legal, this procedure is extremely safe and effective. Maternal mortality occurs in less than 1 in 100 000 cases.[70] Other serious complications occur in less than 1% of cases, and minor complications, including psychological disturbances, in less than 10% of cases.[69] The procedure seems to have no effect on subsequent fertility or pregnancy outcome,[71,72] and leads to complete abortion in 95–98% of cases.[73]

In developed nations medical abortion must be assessed against this background. Although efficacy rates appear to be very similar, it must be stressed that a large-scale comparison of medical and surgical abortion, using standard techniques and similar outcome measures, remains to be reported. Comparisons have to be made on the basis of literature reports, with all the inaccuracies inherent in using different investigators and a variety of end-points to measure the incidence of complications.

Rare events such as maternal death seem to be of the same order in both medical and surgical abortion; one death has occurred amongst the 100 000 women who have been exposed to the drug. This single death (which was probably more related to the type of prostaglandin used than mifepristone) prompted a revision of clinical guidelines to exclude women who are over the age of 35 years or more than light smokers. Two women died following surgical abortion in the UK in 1985–1987.[70] The death of one of the women following surgical abortion occurred in almost identical clinical circumstances as the death of the woman following medical abortion; it is probable that severe coronary artery disease represents an increased risk for sudden death, no matter which procedure is undertaken.

The serious complication rate of medical abortion, when assessed by parameters such as the need for blood transfusion, is not dissimilar to that associated with surgical abortion (0.85 and 0.5% respectively).[60,69] Evidence of infection appears to be as infrequent following medical abortion as surgical abortion (1–2 and 2–5% respectively),[55,62,69] although these figures must be interpreted cautiously. Medical abortion, by its very nature, liberates 95% of women from the rare but serious complications of surgical abortion, such as genital trauma and anaesthetic mishaps. There does not seem to be any increased risk of psychological complications when the procedures are compared.[66] There are not yet any data on fertility following medical abortion, although it is hard to formulate a mechanism by which this method could exert an effect. Neither are there any data on subsequent pregnancy outcome.

A large-scale pragmatic randomized controlled trial comparing outcomes following medical and surgical abortion has recently been completed in our unit. Interim analysis supports the view that there is no difference in medical or psychological outcomes between either method of abortion.

Although legal surgical abortion is extremely safe in developed nations, the same is not true in developing countries. Worldwide some 40 million abortions are performed each year, many in non-medical circumstances, resulting in around 200 000 maternal deaths, and a huge amount of morbidity. Ninety-nine per cent of this burden falls on developing countries.[74a] Reasons include shortages of adequately trained personnel and surgical facilities, as well as recourse to highly dangerous methods of abortion in countries where the procedure is illegal. The need for a safe non-invasive method of medical abortion was expressed by WHO in 1978,[74b] and the mifepristone/prostaglandin combination goes a long way towards fulfilling this concept; the potential for improving maternal reproductive health on a global scale is considerable.[75]

Medical abortion, as well as providing an alternative for those women who wish to avoid surgery,[76] has a number of other advantages. The drug is licensed for use at up to 9 weeks' gestation; this prompts earlier referral, and reduces the morbidity associated with increasing gestation.[73] Nearly 20% of women return with another unplanned pregnancy,[77] due to a widespread failure to deliver adequate post abortal contraceptive advice. The mandatory follow-up visit provides an excellent opportunity for reinforcing contraceptive counselling.

MEDICAL ABORTION: IMPLICATIONS FOR ABORTION SERVICES

There have been suggestions that the introduction of mifepristone may have major implications for women's access to abortion services. Whilst mifepristone has renewed debate about the provision of services, factors other than medical technology are of more importance.

In nearly all countries of the world access to abortion is controlled by the process of law.[78] Ten per cent of countries ban abortion completely, 24% of countries allow abortion if the mother's life is at risk, and on eugenic, genetic or juridical grounds. A further 25% of countries allow socio-economic reasons to be taken into account when determining whether an abortion should be granted. Finally 40% of countries allow abortion at the request of the individual in the first trimester.[79] It is not realistic to suggest that the development of mifepristone will lead to a major change in cultural and religious objections to abortion in those states where it remains illegal. Access to abortion services is not therefore likely to be affected; indeed Roussel-Uclaf have established that the drug will only be introduced into countries where abortion is legal, widely accepted and where adequate control can be maintained upon distribution.

In France, where early abortion is available on request, mifepristone provides a useful alternative method which is utilized by about one-fifth of eligible women,[65] with advantages that will tend to decrease morbidity in the long term.

In the UK, where abortion is not available on request, there are vast discrepancies affecting the standards of abortion provision available within the National Health Service (NHS). The reasons for this are complex and interrelated, but two of the most important are the level of resource allocation and consultant gynaecologists' attitude to abortion;[80,81] many districts in the NHS are either unable or unwilling to provide a good quality of service.

At present in England and Wales only about 20% of NHS abortions are performed prior to 9 weeks' gestation, the upper limit for utilizing medical abortion, despite the fact that 79% of women approach a doctor prior to 8 weeks' gestation.[80,82] Until this number is increased, it is apparent that medical abortion is going to have only minor impact. In Scotland, where nearly 95% of abortions are performed within the NHS, centralized referral services allow nearly three times as many abortions to be performed prior to 9 weeks' gestation.[83] The implementation of such a referral mechanism, like all other aspects of abortion service provision, is dependent not on the invention of a new drug but upon the values, willingness and actions of health service managers and gynaecologists. Mifepristone has renewed the debate at a time of great change within the NHS; purchasing authorities have a golden opportunity to improve abortion services.

Medical abortion has important resource implications, and although its introduction is unlikely to lead to the high level of resource savings originally predicted,[65,84] there will be some scope for resource benefit. Operating theatre time that is currently utilized to perform surgical abortions will be released. Moreover the marginal cost of the procedure will tend to fall as, for example, less expensive prostaglandins become available.

SIDE-EFFECTS AND TERATOGENICITY

When taking into account factors such as the high incidence of nausea, vomiting and lower abdominal pain in early pregnancy, and the symptoms due to the abortion mifepristone causes, the incidence of true drug-related adverse events is uncommon; headache has been reported in 5%, gastrointestinal upset in 3.5%; there are rare reports of malaise, faintness and maculopapular rash. Overdosage of the drug may lead to signs of adrenal failure, although a massive ingestion would be required.[85]

Mifepristone is known to cross the placenta,[86] and concern has been expressed that the drug may have a teratogenic potential. This is difficult to assess in a drug which is used as an abortifacient; surgical uterine evacuation is recommended when the procedure fails and a viable intrauterine pregnancy persists. It is perhaps inevitable that some women will have a change of heart about the fate of their pregnancy after ingesting mifepristone but prior to prostaglandin administration. This has only happened in a handful of cases, and is testament to the quality of counselling available to women who opt for this method of abortion. Consequently data on infants exposed to mifepristone in utero are rare, but that which does exist suggests that mifepristone does not have a teratogenic potential in humans.[87,88] This is supported by animal work, although contradictory reports exist on the drug's teratogenic potential in rabbits.[89-91]

OTHER USES OF MIFEPRISTONE IN INDUCED ABORTION AND LATER PREGNANCY

In the first and early second trimesters the value of softening and dilating ('priming') the pregnant cervix prior to surgical vacuum aspiration/ evacuation is well-established, with a decrease in genital trauma and intra-operative blood loss.[92-94] Controlled randomized trials using an objective methodology all affirm that mifepristone is a highly effective priming agent (Table 15.4). Randomized trials using subjective methodology support these findings.[101-103] Mifepristone is as effective as the commonly used prostaglandin priming agent gemeprost, and has the advantage of a reduced rate of side-effects.[99] Further trials comparing the drug to priming agents such as laminaria are awaited. Mifepristone also exerts a significant dilating effect in the non-pregnant cervix, and may facilitate procedures such as colposcopy and the insertion of intrauterine devices[100] although uterine contractility is also increased.[104]

The increased myometrial sensitivity to administered prostaglandins persists into the second and third trimesters. Commonly used methods of second-trimester termination include the administration of extra-amniotic,

Table 15.4   Mifepristone in cervical priming: objective placebo-controlled randomized trials

Study	Number of women in trial	Mifepristone dose	Time mifepristone administered prior to surgery (hours)
Radestad et al (1988)[95]	43	100 mg	12 and 24
Urquhart & Templeton (1990)[96]	40	600 mg	48 Single dose
Radestad et al (1990)[97]	55	600 mg	36 or 48 Single dose
Cohn & Stewart (1991)[98]	80	600 mg	48 Single dose
Henshaw & Templeton (1991)[99]	90	200 mg	36 Single dose
Gupta & Johnson (1990)[100]	30	600 mg	42–53 Single dose

All studies show a significant (P < 0.05) reduction in the force required to dilate the cervix.

Table 15.5 Randomized trials of mifepristone prior to second-trimester prostaglandin termination

Study	Number of women in trial	Mifepristone dose*	Prostaglandin induction to abortion interval (hours)		
			Standard regime	Mifepristone + standard regime	Reduction in interval
Urquhart & Templeton (1990)[105]	70	600	11.6	6.4	45%
Rodger & Baird (1990)[106]	100	600	15.8	6.8	57%
Gottlieb & Bygdeman (1991)[107]	71	200	13.2	6.6	50%

* Given as a single dose 24–48 hours before prostaglandin induction.

intramuscular or vaginal prostaglandins. Randomized controlled trials have confirmed that pretreatment with mifepristone (200–600 mg administered as a single dose 24–48 hours earlier) significantly augments the effect of prostaglandins in achieving uterine evacuation, reducing the induction-to-abortion time interval by 50% (Table 15.5). Consequently procedure-related side-effects and analgesia requirements are also significantly reduced. The drug remains effective in the presence of an abnormal or dead fetus, and is therefore of benefit in the management of missed abortion, intra-uterine fetal death and fetal malformations.[108–110] The efficacy of mifepristone persists into the third trimester, and it has been used to induce labour at term.[111]

Mifepristone has been used as a non-surgical method of managing ectopic pregnancy. However, only a small number of women have been treated, without reference to an expectant management control group. Further research is required to determine what role the drug may have in this condition.[112,113]

OTHER USES OF MIFEPRISTONE

Progesterone receptors are present in other tissues, such as the meninges and breast. Mifepristone has been used, with some clinical benefit, to treat neoplastic disease affecting these structures.[114,115] The drug also has some clinically useful antiglucocorticoid activity, explaining its use in the management of Cushing's syndrome.[116,117]

The role of the drug as a pre- and postovulatory contraceptive, and in endometriosis, has already been discussed. It may also have a role in premenstrual syndrome,[118] but a small placebo-controlled randomized trial has not supported this hypothesis.[119]

Mifepristone is equally useful in a non-clinical setting as an experimental tool, and has been used extensively to investigate the physiology of the menstrual cycle and early pregnancy, the actions of progesterone and

Table 15.6   Clinical roles of mifepristone

Follicular phase
   Contraceptive agent
   Endometriosis management
Luteal phase
   Post ovulatory contraceptive agent
First trimester
   Medical abortion
   Non-surgical evacuation of missed abortion
Second trimester
   Cervical priming agent
   Augmentation of second-trimester abortion
   Management of fetal anomalies and intrauterine fetal death
Third trimester
   Induction of labour at term
Endocrinology
   Cushing's syndrome
Oncology
   Breast and meningeal tumours
Research tool
   Especially in reproductive endocrinology, biology of steroid-dependent tumours, actions
   of steroid hormones

---

glucocortical steroids at the cellular level, the behaviour of breast and endometrial tumour cell lines and the actions of antineoplastic chemotherapeutic agents in vitro.[120] The actions and clinical roles of mifepristone are summarized in Table 15.6.

CONCLUSIONS

To view antiprogesterones simply as abortifacients of limited use is greatly to underestimate their potential. Clinical management in many areas of reproductive medicine, obstetrics, endocrinology and oncology will be enhanced. Their value as research tools is beyond doubt. As abortifacients in the first and second trimesters they will reduce morbidity, release resources and widen the choice available to women. In countries where abortion is legal, medical professionals who feel that abortion should be a punitive procedure, whether financially, mentally or physically, contravene the medical ethics of beneficence and non-maleficence.[84] Finally in developing nations they have a potential for providing a safe non-surgical method of abortion that will assist in relieving the hardship of maternal mortality.

REFERENCES

1. Messinis I E, Templeton A A. Effects of supraphysiological concentrations of progesterone on the characteristics of the oestradiol-induced gonadotrophin surge in women. J Reprod Fertil 1990; 88: 513–519
2. Permezel J M, Lenton E A, Roberts I, Cooke I D. Acute effects of progesterone and

the antiprogestin RU 486 on gonadotropin secretion in the follicular phase of the menstrual cycle. J Clin Endocrinol Metab 1989; 68: 960–965

3. Csapo A I, Pulkkinen M. Indispensability of the human corpus luteum in the maintenance of early pregnancy luteectomy evidence. Obstet Gynecol Surv 1989; 33: 69–81

4. Van Look P F A, Bygdeman M. Antiprogestational steroids: a new dimension in human fertility regulation. In: Milligan S R, ed. Oxford Reviews of Reproductive Biology, Vol II. Oxford: Oxford University Press. 1989, pp 1–60

5. Cameron I T, Healy D L. Anti-progesterones: background and clinical physiology. Bailliere's Clin Obstet Gynaecol 1988; 2: 597–607

6. Heikinheimo O, Kontula K, Croxatto H, Spitz I, Luukkainen T, Lahteenmaki P. Plasma concentrations and receptor binding of RU 486 and its metabolites in humans. J Steroid Biochem 1987; 26: 279–284

7. Gravanis A, Schaison G, George M et al. Endometrial and pituitary responses to the steroidal antiprogestin RU 486 in postmenopausal women. J Clin Endocrinol Metab 1985; 60: 156–163

8. Swahn M L, Wang G, Aedo A R, Cekan S Z, Bygdeman M. Plasma levels of antiprogestin RU 486 following oral administration to non-pregnant and early pregnant women. Contraception 1986; 34: 469–481

9. Liu J H, Garzo V G, Yen S S C. Pharmacodynamics of the antiprogesterone RU 486 in women after oral administration. Fertil Steril 1988; 50: 245–249

10. Heikinheimo O. Antiprogesterone steroid RU486. Pharmacokinetics and receptor binding in humans. Acta Obstet Gynecol Scand 1990; 69: 357–358

11. Stuenkel C A, Garzo V G, Morris S, Liu J H, Yen S S C. Effects of the antiprogesterone RU 486 in the early follicular phase of the menstrual cycle. Fertil Steril 1990; 53: 642–646

12. Luukkainen T, Heinkinheimo O, Haukkamaa M, Lahteenmaki P. Inhibition of folliculogenesis and ovulation by the antiprogesterone RU 486. Fertil Steril 1988; 49: 961–963

13. Liu J H, Garzo G, Morris S, Stuenkel C, Ulmann A, Yen S S C. Disruption of follicular maturation and delay of ovulation after administration of the antiprogesterone RU 486. J Clin Endocrinol Metab 1987; 65: 1135–1140

14. Shoupe D, Mishell D R, Page M A, Madkour H, Spitz I M, Lobo R A. Effects of the antiprogesterone RU 486 in normal women. Administration in the late follicular phase. Am J Obstet Gynecol 1987; 157: 1421–1426

15. Swahn M L, Bygdeman M, Cekan S, Xing S, Masironi B, Johannisson E. The effect of RU 486 administerd during the early luteal phase on bleeding pattern, hormonal parameters and endometrium. Hum Reprod 1990; 5: 402–408

16. Li T C, Dockery P, Thomas P, Rogers A W, Lenton E A, Cooke I D. The effects of progesterone receptor blockade in the luteal phase of normal fertile women. Fertil Steril 1988; 50: 732–742

17. Schaison G, George M, Le Strat N, Reinberg A, Baulieu E E. Effects of the antiprogesterone steroid RU 486 during midluteal phase in normal women. J Clin Endocrinol Metab 1985; 61: 484–489

18. Garzo V G, Liu J, Ulmann A, Baulieu E, Yen S S C. Effects of an antiprogesterone (RU 486) on the hypothalamic-hypophyseal-ovarian-endometrial axis during the luteal phase of the menstrual cycle. J Clin Endocrinol Metab 1988; 66: 508–517

19. Shoupe D, Mishell D R, Lahteenmaki P et al. Effects of the antiprogesterone RU 486 in normal women. Single dose administration in the midluteal phase. Am J Obstet Gynecol 1987; 157: 1415–1420

20. Swahn M L, Johannisson E, Daniore V, de la Torre B, Bygdeman M. The effect of RU 486 administered during the proliferative and secretory phase of the cycle on the bleeding pattern, hormonal parameters and the endometrium. Hum Reprod 1988; 3: 915–921

21. DiMattina M, Albertson B D, Tyson V, Loriaux D L, Falk R J. Effect of the antiprogestin RU 486 on human ovarian steroidogenesis. Fertil Steril 1987; 48: 229–233

22. Croxatto H B, Salvatierra A M, Romero C, Spitz I M. Late luteal phase administration of RU 486 for three successive cycles does not disrupt bleeding patterns or ovulation. J Clin Endocrinol Metab 1987, 65: 1272–1277

23. Nieman L K, Choate T M, Chrousos G P et al. The progesterone antagonist RU 486. A potential new contraceptive agent. N Engl J Med 1987; 316: 187–191
24. Kekkonen R, Alfthan H, Haukkamaa M, Heikinheimo O, Luukkainen T, Lahteenmaki P. Interference with ovulation by sequential treatment with the antiprogesterone RU 486 and synthetic progestin. Fertil Steril 1990; 53: 747–750
25. Kettel L M, Murphy A A, Mortola J F, Liu J H, Ulmann A, Yen S S C. Endocrine responses to long-term administration of the antiprogesterone RU 486 in patients with pelvic endometriosis. Fertil Steril 1991; 56: 402–407
26. Glasier A, Thong K J, Dewar M, Mackie M, Baird D T. Postcoital contraception with mifepristone. Lancet 1991; 337: 1414–1415
27. Baulieu E-E. Contragestion with RU 486: a new approach to postovulatory fertility control. Acta Obstet Gynecol Scand 149 (suppl): 5–8
28. Dixon G W, Schlesselman J J, Ory H W, Blye R P. Ethinyl estradiol and conjugated estrogens as postcoital contraceptives. JAMA 1980; 244: 1336–1339
29. Dubois C, Ulmann A, Baulieu E E. Contragestion with late luteal administration of RU 486 (mifepristone). Fertil Steril 1988; 50: 593–596
30. Lahteenmaki P, Rapeli T, Kaariainen M, Alfthan H, Ylikorkala O. Late postcoital treatment against pregnancy with antiprogesterone RU 486. Fertil Steril 1988; 50: 36–38
31. Couzinet B, Le Strat N, Silvestre L, Schaison G. Late luteal administration of the antiprogesterone RU 486 in normal women: effects on the menstrual cycle events and fertility control in a long-term study. Fertil Steril 1990; 54: 1039–1044
32. Van Santen M R, Haspels A A. Interception III: Postcoital luteal contragestion by an antiprogestin (mifepristone RU 486) in 62 women. Contraception 1987; 35: 423–431
33. Li T C, Lenton E A, Dockery P, Rogers A W, Cooke I D. Why does RU 486 fail to prevent implantation despite success in inducing menstruation? Contraception 1988; 38: 401–406
34. Glasier A, Baird D T. Post-ovulatory contraception. Bailliere's Clin Obstet Gynaecol 1990; 4: 283–291
35. Roseff S J, Kettel L M, Rivier J, Burger H G, Baulieu E, Yen S S C. Accelerated dissolution of luteal-endometrial integrity by the administration of antagonists of gonadotropin-releasing hormone and progesterone to late-luteal phase women. Fertil Steril 1990; 54: 805–810
36. Editorial. Mifepristone — contragestive agent or medical abortifacient? Lancet 1987; ii: 1308–1310
37. Couzinet B, Le Strat N, Ulmann A, Baulieu E E, Schaison G. Termination of early pregnancy by the progesterone antagonist RU 486 (mifepristone). N Engl J Med 1986; 315: 1565–1570
38. Maria B, Stampf F, Goepp A, Ulmann A. Termination of early pregnancy by a single dose of mifepristone (RU 486), a progesterone antagonist. Eur J Obstet Gynecol Reprod Biol 1988; 28: 249–255
39. Carol W, Klinger G. Experience with the antigestagen mifepristone (RU 486) in the interruption of early pregnancy. Zentralbl Gynakol 1989; 111: 1325–1328
40. Ylikorkala O, Alfthan H, Kaariainen M, Rapeli T, Lahteenmaki P. Outpatient therapeutic abortion with mifepristone. Obstet Gynecol 1989; 74: 653–657
41. Somell C, Olund A. Induction of abortion in early pregnancy with mifepristone Gynecol Obstet Invest 1990; 29: 13–15
42. Birgerson L, Olind V. The antiprogestational agent RU 486 as an abortifacient in early human pregnancy: a comparison of three dose regimens. Contraception 1988; 38: 391–400
43. Maria B, Chaneac M, Stampf F, Ulmann A. Early pregnancy interruption using an antiprogesterone steroid: mifepristone (RU 486). J Gynecol Obstet Biol Reprod 1988; 17: 1089–1094
44. Shu-rong Z. RU 486 (mifepristone): clinical trials in China. Acta Obstet Gynecol Scand 149 (suppl): 19–23
45. Sitruk-Ware R, Thalabard J C, De Plunkett T L et al. The use of the antiprogestin RU 486 (mifepristone) as an abortifacient in early pregnancy — clinical and pathological findings; predictive factors for efficacy. Contraception 1990; 41: 221–243
46. Grimes D A, Mishell D R, Shoupe D, Lacarra M. Early abortion with a single dose of the antiprogestin RU 486. Am J Obstet Gynecol 1988; 158: 1307–1312

47. Grimes D A, Bernstein L, Lacarra M, Shoupe D, Mishell D R. Predictors of failed attempted abortion with the antiprogestin mifepristone (RU 486). Am J Obstet Gynecol 1990; 162: 910–917

48. Norman J E, Wu W X, Kelly R W, Glasier A F, McNeilly A S, Baird D T. Effects of mifepristone in vivo on decidual prostaglandin synthesis and metabolism. Contraception 1991; 44: 89–98

49. Das C, Catt K J. Antifertility actions of the progesterone antagonist RU 486 include direct inhibition of placental hormone secretion. Lancet 1987; ii: 599–601

50. Di Lieto A, Catalano D, Campanile M et al. The morphological characteristics and ultrastructural aspects of cervical ripening induced by sulprostone. Acta Eur Fertil 1988; 19: 33–36

51. Swahn M L, Bygdeman M. The effect of the antiprogestin RU 486 on uterine contractility and sensitivity to prostaglandin and oxytocin. Br J Obstet Gynaecol 1988; 95: 126–134

52. Swahn M L, Ugocsai G, Bygdeman M, Kovacs L, Belsey E M, Van Look P F A. Effect of oral prostaglandin E_2 on uterine contractility and outcome of treatment in women receiving RU 486 (mifepristone) for termination of early pregnancy. Hum Reprod 1989; 4: 21–28

53. Rodger M W, Baird D T. Induction of therapeutic abortion in early pregnancy with mifepristone in combination with prostaglandin pessary. Lancet 1987; ii: 1415–1418

54. Dubois C, Ulmann A, Aubeny E et al. Abortion induced by RU 486: importance of its combination with a prostaglandin derivative. CR Acad Sci 1988; 306: 57–61

55. World Health Organization. Termination of early human pregnancy with RU 486 (mifepristone) and the prostaglandin analogue sulprostone: a multicentre, randomised comparison between two treatment regimens. Hum Reprod 1989; 4: 718–725

56. Maria B, Stampf F. Termination of early pregnancy using mifepristone in combination with prostaglandin analogs. Acta Obstet Gynecol Scand 1989; 149 (suppl): 31–32

57. Swahn M, Bygdeman M. Termination of early pregnancy with RU 486 (mifepristone) in combination with a prostaglandin analogue (sulprostone). Acta Obstet Gynecol Scand 1989; 68: 293–300

58. Rodger M W, Logan A F, Baird D T. Induction of early abortion with mifepristone (RU 486) and two different doses of prostaglandin pessary (gemeprost). Contraception 1989; 39: 497–502

59. Rodger M W, Baird D T. Blood loss following induction of early abortion using mifepristone (RU 486) and a prostaglandin analogue (gemeprost). Contraception 1989; 40: 439–447

60.. UK Multicentre Trial. The efficacy and tolerance of mifepristone and prostaglandin in first trimester termination of pregnancy. Br J Obstet Gynaecol 1990; 97: 480–486

61. Silvestre L, Dubois C, Renault M, Rezvani Y, Baulieu E E, Ulmann A. Voluntary interruption of pregnancy with mifepristone (RU 486) and a prostaglandin analogue. N Engl J Med 1990; 322: 645–648

62. Hill N C W, Ferguson J, MacKenzie I Z. The efficacy of oral mifepristone (RU 38,486) with a prostaglandin E_1 analog vaginal pessary for the termination of early pregnancy: complications and patient acceptability. Am J Obstet Gynecol 1990; 162: 414–417

63. World Health Organization. Pregnancy termination with mifepristone and gemeprost: a multicenter comparison between repeated doses and a single dose of mifepristone. Fertil Steril 1991; 56: 32–40

64. Aubeny E, Baulieu E E. Contragestive activity of RU 486 and oral active prostaglandin combination. CR Acad Sci 1991; 312: 539–545

65. Heard M, Guillebaud J. Medical abortion. Br Med J 1992; 304: 195–196

66. Urquhart D R, Templeton A A. Psychiatric morbidity and acceptability following medical and surgical methods of induced abortion. Br J Obstet Gynaecol 1991; 98: 396–399

67. Rosen A S. Acceptability of abortion methods. Bailliere's Clin Obstet Gynaecol 1990; 4: 375–390

68. Botting B. Trends in Abortion. Popul Trends 1991; 64: 19–29

69. Joint Study of the Royal College of General Practitioners and the Royal College of Obstetricians and Gynaecologists. Induced abortion operations and their early sequelae. J R Coll Gen Pract 1985; 35: 175–180

70. Report on confidential enquiries into maternal deaths in the UK 1985–1987. London: HMSO, 1991
71. Obel E B. Fertility following legally induced abortion. Acta Obstet Gynecol Scand 1979; 58: 539–542
72. Frank P I, McNamee R, Hannaford P C, Kay C R, Hirsch S. The effect of induced abortion on subsequent pregnancy outcome. Br J Obstet Gynaecol 1991; 98: 1015–1024
73. Castadot R G. Pregnancy termination: techniques, risks, and complications and their management. Fertil Steril 1986; 45: 5–17
74a. Mahler H. The safe motherhood initiative: a call to action. Lancet 1987; i: 668–670
74b. WHO. Induced abortion. Technical Report Series, No. 623. Geneva: WHO, 1978
75. Kovacs L. Future direction of abortion technology. Bailliere's Clin Obstet Gynaecol 1990; 4: 407–414
76. Editorial. Mifepristone: widening the choice for women. Lancet 1989; Lancet ii: 1112–1113
77. Hull M G R, Gordon C, Beard R W. The organisation and results of a pregnancy termination service in a National Health Service hospital. J Obstet Gynaecol Br Commonwlth 1974; 81: 577–587
78. Cook R J. Antiprogestin drugs: medical and legal issues. Fam Plann Perspect 1989; 21: 267–272
79. Loraine J A. Abortion: world perspectives in the mid-1980s. Fam Pract 1986; 3: 266–271
80. Munday D, Francome C, Savage W. Twenty one years of legal abortion. Br Med J 1989; 298: 1231–1234
81. Savage W, Francome C. Gynaecologists' attitudes to abortion. Lancet 1989; ii: 1323–1324
82. Editorial. The Abortion Act twenty years on. Lancet 1987; i: 91–92
83. Glasier A, Thong J K. The establishment of a centralised referral service leads to earlier abortion. Health Bull 1991; 49: 254–259
84. Editorial. Reproductive health and mifepristone. Lancet 1990s 336: 1480–1481
85. Laue L, Lotze M T, Chrousos G P, Barnes K, Loriaux D L, Fleisher T A. Effect of chronic treatment with the glucocorticoid antagonist RU 486 in man: toxicity, immunological and hormonal aspects. J Clin Endocrinol Metab 1990; 71: 1474–1480
86. Frydman R, Taylor S, Ulmann A. Transplacental passage of mifepristone. Lancet 1985; 2: 1252.
87. Lim B H, Lees D A R, Bjornsson S et al. Normal development after exposure to mifepristone in early pregnancy. Lancet 1990; 336: 257–258
88. Pons J C, Imbert M C, Elefant E, Roux C, Herschkorn P, Papiernik E. Development after exposure to mifepristone in early pregnancy. Lancet 1991; 338: 763
89. Wolf J P, Chillik C F, Dubois C, Ulmann A, Raulieu E E, Hodgen E B. Tolerence of perinidatory primate embryos to RU 486 exposure in vitro and in vivo. Contraception 1990; 41: 85–92
90. Hardy R P, New D A T. Effects of the anti-progestin RU 38486 on rat embryos growing in culture. Food Chem Toxicol 1991; 29: 361–362
91. Jost A. Animal reproduction — new data on the hormonal requirement of the pregnant rabbit; partial pregnancies and fetal anomalies resulting from treatment with a hormonal antagonist given at a sub-abortive dosage. CR Acad Sci 1986; 303: 281–284
92. Schulz K F, Grimes D A, Cates W. Measures to prevent cervical injury during suction curettage abortion. Lancet 1983; i: 1182–1185
93. Grimes D A, Schultz K F, Cates W. Prevention of uterine perforation during curettage abortion. JAMA 1984; 251: 2108–2111
94. MacKenzie I Z, Fry A. Prostaglandin E$_2$ pessaries to facilitate first trimester aspiration termination. Br J Obstet Gynaecol 1981; 88: 1033–1037
95. Radestad A, Christensen N J, Stromberg L. Induced cervical ripening with mifepristone in first trimester abortion. A double blind randomised biomechanical study. Contraception 38: 301–312
96. Urquhart D R, Templeton A A. Mifepristone (RU 486) for cervical priming prior to surgically induced abortion in the late first trimester. Contraception 1990; 42: 191–199
97. Radestad A, Bygdeman M, Green K. Induced cervical ripening with mifepristone (RU

486) and bioconversion of arachidonic acid in human pregnant uterine cervix in the first trimester. A double blind, randomised, biomechanical and biochemical study. Contraception 1990; 41: 283–292

98. Cohn M, Stewart P. Pretreatment of the primigravid uterine cervix with mifepristone 30h prior to termination of pregnancy: a double blind study. Br J Obstet Gynaecol 1991; 98: 778–782

99. Henshaw R C, Templeton A A. Pre-operative cervical preparation before first trimester vacuum aspiration: a randomised controlled comparison between gemeprost and mifepristone (RU 486). Br J Obstet Gynaecol 1991; 98: 1025–1030

100. Gupta J K, Johnson N. Effect of mifepristone on dilatation of the pregnant and non-pregnant cervix. Lancet 1990; 335: 1238–1240

101. Durlot F, Dubois C, Brunerie J, Frydman R. Efficacy of progesterone antagonist RU 486 (mifepristone) for pre-operative cervical dilatation during first trimester abortion. Hum Reprod 1988; 3: 583–584

102. World Health Organization. The use of mifepristone (RU 486) for cervical preparation in first trimester pregnancy termination by vacuum aspiration. Br J Obstet Gynaecol 1990; 97: 260–266

103. Lefebvre Y, Proulx L, Elie R, Poulin O, Lanza E. The effects of RU-38486 on cervical ripening. Am J Obstet Gynecol 1990; 162: 61–65

104. Gemzell K, Swahn M L, Bygdeman M. Regulation of non-pregnant human uterine contractility. Effect of antihormones. Contraception 1990; 42: 323–335

105. Urquhart D R, Templeton A A. The use of mifepristone prior to prostaglandin-induced mid-trimester abortion. Hum Reprod 1990; 5: 883–886

106. Rodger M W, Baird D T. Pretreatment with mifepristone (RU 486) reduces interval between prostaglandin administration and expulsion in second trimester abortion. Br J Obstet Gynaecol 1990; 97: 41–45

107. Gottlieb C, Bygdeman M. The use of antiprogestin (RU 486) for termination of second trimester pregnancy. Acta Obstet Gynecol Scand 1991; 70: 199–203

108. Asch R H, Weckstein L N, Ralmaceda J P, Rojas F, Spitz IM, Tadir Y. Non-surgical expulsion of non-viable early pregnancy: a new application of RU 486. Hum Reprod 1990; 5: 481–483

109. Cabrol D, Dubois C, Cronje H et al. Induction of labor with mifepristone (RU 486) in intrauterine fetal death. Am J Obstet Gynecol 1990; 163: 540–542

110. Frydman R, Fernandez H, Pons J C, Ulmann A. Mifepristone (RU486) and therapeutic late pregnancy termination: a double-blind study of two different doses. Hum Reprod 1988; 3: 803–806

111. Frydman R, Baton C, Lelaidier C, Vial M, Bourget P H, Fernandez H. Mifepristone for induction of labour. Lancet 1991; 337: 488–489

112. Pansky M, Golan A, Bukovski I, Caspi E. Nonsurgical management of tubal pregnancy. Am J Obstet Gynecol 1991; 164: 888–895

113. Avrech O M, Golan A, Weinraub Z, Bukovsky I, Caspi E. Mifepristone (RU 486) alone or in combination with a prostaglandin analologue for termination of early pregnancy: a review. Fertil Steril 1991; 56: 385–393

114. Grunberg S M, Weiss M H, Spitz I M et al. Treatment of unresectable meningiomas with the antiprogesterone agent mifepristone. J Neurosurg 1991; 74: 861–866

115. Klijn J G, de Jong F H, Bakker G H, Lamberts S W, Rodenburg C J, Alexieva-Figusch J. Antiprogestins, a new form of endocrine therapy for human breast cancer. Cancer Res 1989; 49: 2851–2856

116. Nieman L K, Chrousos G P, Kellner C et al. Successful treatment of Cushing's syndrome with the glucocorticoid antagonist RU 486. J Clin Endocrinol Metab 1985; 61: 536–540

117. Van der Lely A J, Foeken K, Van der Mast R C, Lamberts S W. Rapid reversal of acute psychosis in the Cushing syndrome with the cortisol receptor antagonist mifepristone (RU 486). Ann Intern Med 1991; 114: 143–144

118. Halbreich U. Treatment of premenstrual syndromes with progesterone antagonists (e.g., RU 486): political and methodological issues. Psychiatry 1990; 53: 407–409

119. Schmidt P J, Nieman L K, Grover G N, Muller K L, Merriman G R, Rubinow D R. Lack of effect of induced menses on symptoms in women with premenstrual syndrome. N Engl J Med 1991; 324: 1174–1179

120. Crowley W F. Progesterone antagonism. N Engl J Med 1986; 315: 1607–1608

16. Primary amenorrhoea

D. K. Edmonds

Menstruation is the end-point of a cascade of events which begin in the hypothalamus and end at the uterus. The mechanism is the fundamental basis of reproduction and menstruation represents failure to achieve such reproductive success in the time-frame of the menstrual cycle. Amenorrhoea will ensue if any part of the cascade either fails to function endocrinologically or if there is developmental deficiency. Thus, management of patients with primary amenorrhoea demands a knowledge of the embryology of female development and an understanding of the endocrinology of puberty and assessment of the patient in her entirety.

DEFINITION

Whilst most gynaecologists are familiar with the concept of primary amenorrhoea, it is misleading to consider menstruation in this isolated way. Like the other changes associated with puberty, there is a range of ages between which menstruation may occur and be classified as normal. Thus, a child who has normal sexual development at age 15 and has failed to menstruate is probably normal, whereas the equivalently aged child with no secondary sexual characteristics is more likely to require investigation. Therefore, the previously held belief that investigation of primary amenorrhoea be commenced if menstruation had not occurred by age 16 must be abolished. As a general rule therefore, failure of the development of any secondary sexual characteristic by age 14 should be investigated and failure of menstruation by age 16 in the presence of normal secondary sexual characteristics should arouse concern. However, any child brought by her mother at any age because of concern about development must be treated seriously and investigated appropriately. As can be seen, it is not possible to define primary amenorrhoea in a clinically useful way, as it simply means no onset of menses; a better term for the condition would be delayed puberty as this encompasses all the problems we shall encounter.

NORMAL PUBERTY

Puberty is the time when one becomes functionally able to procreate; this includes physical and psychological development. The most important aspect of the changes is the variation in time that these changes take. There are five classical changes that occur which we call the secondary sexual characteristics — breast, pubic hair and axillary hair development, the growth spurt and the onset of menstruation (and subsequent establishment of ovulation).

1. Breast growth is divided into five stages,[1] and the age of onset begins around 9 years, full development taking 5 years. It is unusual for no breast tissue to develop by 13 years of age.

2. Pubic hair growth occurs almost in parallel with breast development and has five stages also.

3. Axillary hair is described in only three stages, and this development tends to occur later, around age 13.

4. The growth spurt is an interesting phenomenon. The rate of growth is constant from age 2 to the onset of puberty, with a growth rate of around 6 cm/year; at the time of accelerated growth, this reaches 11 cm/year (known as peak height velocity). Most girls will reach their maximum height between their 10th and 14th birthdays, with peak height velocity being around 12.14 years.[2]

5. Menstruation occurs in 95% of UK girls by age 13 years, although delay in the remainder may reach 16 or 17 years. Many factors influence the age of menarche, including nutritional status, genetic factors and racial elements.[3]

All the physical changes of puberty occur as a result of endocrine maturation. During childhood, gonadotrophin levels are very low and as puberty approaches, there is a gradual increase in the pulse frequency of luteinizing hormone-releasing hormone (LHRH) released from the hypothalamus, and a resultant increase in the selection of follicle-stimulating hormone (FSH). This tends to begin at night initially and as the pulse frequency and amplitude increase, so the pulses of FSH begin to occur in daytime.[4] This maturation of the hypothalamus is associated with increased growth hormone secretion and hence the growth spurt.

The ovarian response to the increase of FSH is an increase in oestradiol 17β and the initiation of breast growth. Ultrasound studies[5] suggest that follicular growth may begin at age 8.5 years, giving a multicystic appearance to the ovary, although development of a dominant follicle does not occur until some years later. The secretion of androgen (primarily DHEA and DHEAS) begins to rise at age 6 (adrenarche) and continues to rise until age 12 and seems to be the prime instigator of pubic and axillary hair growth.

EMBRYOLOGY

Sexual differentiation occurs as a result of a number of maxims.

1. Two X chromosomes are necessary for normal ovarian development.

2. Absence of a gonad results in a female phenotype.

3. H-Y antigen and testis-determining factor control the evolution of the gonad to become a testis in the presence of an X and Y chromosome.

4. Sertoli cells produce müllerian inhibitor and this leads to disappearance of the müllerian duct.

5. Fetal testosterone induces wolffian duct development.

6. Masculinization of the cloaca can only occur if testosterone is bound to a receptor and converted to dihydrotestosterone (via 5α-reductase).

7. Absence of 5α-reductase will fail to allow masculinization of the cloaca but wolffian development will be normal.

8. Exogenous androgen exposure during cloacal development in the female will masculinize the cloaca but has no effect on müllerian structures.

The ovary and the müllerian ducts develop separately. The cephalic end of the müllerian duct develops into the fallopian tube and the caudal end becomes the uterus following fusion with its counterpart. Subsequently, the cervix develops from the condensed lower aspect of the fused müllerian bulbs and this leads to the appearance of the vaginal plate. A cord of dense tissue now exists between the cervix and the cloaca and this eventually canalizes and the vagina is formed. Any error in development of the gonad or müllerian ducts will therefore lead to amenorrhoea when functional demands are made on the organs involved with reproduction.

AETIOLOGY OF PRIMARY AMENORRHOEA

In trying to classify these disorders, the presence or absence of secondary sexual characteristics allows the integration of endocrine and anatomical problems in most circumstances. Under some circumstances, development may be heterosexual and in these patients, height is normal (Table 16.1).

Secondary sexual characteristics normal

Imperforate hymen

This typically presents in 14–16-year-old girls who complain of intermittent abdominal pain which is often cyclical. The pain is due to dysmenorrhoea associated with the accumulation of menstrual blood and, as the vagina is a very distensible organ, large quantities of blood can collect before any presenting symptoms occur. The situation is known as a haematocolpos; blood collects in the uterus much more rarely, but if it does, it is known as a haematometra. Occasionally, the size of the mass may lead to difficulty with micturition and defecation. Examination may reveal an abdominal swelling and observation of the introitus will reveal a tense, bulging, bluish membrane which is the hymen.

Table 16.1 Classification of primary amenorrhoea

Secondary sexual characteristics normal
Imperforate hymen
Transverse vaginal septum
Absent vagina and functioning uterus
Absent vagina and non-functioning uterus
XY female — androgen insensitivity
Resistant ovary syndrome
Constitutional delay

Secondary sexual characteristics absent
Normal stature
  Hypogonadotrophic hypogonadism
    Congenital
      Isolated gonodotrophin-releasing hormone deficiency
      Olfactogenital syndrome
    Acquired
      Weight loss/anorexia
      Excessive exercise
      Hyperprolactinaemia
  Hypergonadotrophic hypogonadism
    Gonadal agenesis
      XX agenesis
      XX agenesis
    Gonadal dysgenesis
      Turner's mosaic
      Other X deletions or mosaics
      XY enzymatic failure
      Ovarian failure
      Galactosaemia
Short stature
  Hypogonadotrophic hypogonadism
    Congenital
      Hydrocephalus
    Acquired
      Trauma
      Empty sella syndrome
      Tumours
  Hypergonadotrophic hypogonadism
    Turner's syndrome
    Other X deletions or mosaics

Heterosexual development
Congenital adrenal hyperplasia
Androgen-secreting tumour
5α-reductase deficiency
Partial androgen receptor deficiency
True hermaphrodite
Absent müllerian inhibitor

Transverse vaginal septum

These are much more complicated cases which present in a very similar
manner to the imperforate hymen. Again there is cyclical abdominal pain
and examination will reveal an abdominal mass which can be surprisingly

large. However, inspection of the introitus may reveal a bulging membrane but it will *not* be blue in colour and the hymenal remnants are often seen separately. As the transverse vaginal septum may be at three levels — lower third, middle third or upper third — there may be no introital swelling and vaginal or rectal examination may discover a mass. As the management requires a very different approach to the imperforate hymen, careful assessment of the introitus is essential.

Absent vagina and functioning uterus

This is a rare phenomenon, and may be associated with an absent cervix. The presenting symptom is again cyclical abdominal pain but there is no pelvic mass to be found — solely a haematometra.

Absent vagina and non-functioning uterus

This is the second most common way for primary amenorrhoea to present, superseded only by Turner's syndrome. Secondary sexual development is normal, as would be expected, as ovarian function is normal. However, examination of the genital area discloses normal female external genitalia but a blind-ending vaginal dimple which is usually not more than 1.5 cm deep. This is known as the Mayer–Rokitansky–Kuster–Hauser syndrome or, for short, the Rokitansky syndrome. It is important to remember that 40% of these patients have renal anomalies, 15% being major, e.g. absent kidney. There are also recognizable skeletal abnormalities associated with this syndrome.[6]

XY female — androgen insensitivity

There are a number of ways in which an individual may have an XY karyotype and a female phenotype. These are:

1. Failure of testicular development.
2. Enzymatic failure of the testis to produce androgens.
3. Androgen receptor absence or failure.

In androgen insensitivity, there is thought to be a structural abnormality with the androgen receptor which prevents the masculinizing effect of testosterone during development and subsequently. The patients are phenotypically female with good breast development which occurs because of peripheral conversion of androgen to oestrogen and subsequent stimulation of breast growth. Pubic hair is scanty, the vulva is normal, the vagina is short, and the uterus and tubes are absent. The testes are found in the lower abdomen but occasionally they are found in hernial sacs in childhood, which alerts the physician to the diagnosis[7].

Resistant ovary syndrome

This is a very rare condition as a cause of primary amenorrhoea but is described. In this syndrome, there is elevated levels of gonadotrophins in the presence of apparently normal ovarian tissue. It is believed that these women have absence of FSH receptors in the ovarian follicles and therefore are unable to respond to FSH.

Constitutional delay

Here, all the normal sexual characteristics exist and there is no anatomical anomaly. Endocrine investigations are normal and it is thought that there is a delay in hypothalamic maturation of the pulsatile frequency/amplitude release of gonadotrophin-releasing hormone (GnRH).

Secondary sexual characteristics absent

Isolated GnRH deficiency/olfactogenital syndrome

In this condition, the hypothalamus lacks the ability to produce GnRH and therefore there is a hypogonadotrophic state. The pituitary is normal and stimulation with GnRH leads to normal release of gonadotrophins. If the patient also suffers with anosmia it is known as the olfactogenital syndrome or Kallmann's syndrome. It is presumably a gene deletion as it may occur either sporadically or in families.

Weight loss/anorexia

The association of weight loss and secondary amenorrhoea is more common than in primary amenorrhoea but it is being increasingly identified as an aetiology. The condition of anorexia nervosa is now recognized as a disease of children and adults and requires equal attention to therapy in the young. There is usually normal growth and secondary sexual characteristics and so the fault lies in the pulsatile release of gonadotrophins, because of the effect of low body mass on the secretion of GnRH.

Excessive exercise

This has been increasingly recognized as a problem initially in girls who are ballet dancers. The constant desire for a very thin body in order to succeed in their vocation means that dieting is essential. These girls fail to menstruate and may develop frank anorexia nervosa. Other athletes undertake excessive training and their body mass remains normal or sometimes is actually elevated. However their percentage body fat is much reduced and as a result there is suppression of GnRH release and therefore failure to establish menstruation.

Hyperprolactinaemia

Although this is more commonly seen as a cause of secondary amenorrhoea, it is recognized in primary amenorrhoea also. There may be a
recognizable prolactinoma in the pituitary but often no apparent lesion is
seen.

Gonadal agenesis

In this situation, there is failure of development of the gonad. They may
be 46,XY or 45,X/46,XY when the absence of testicular-determining
factor (TDF) or its receptor is postulated as the cause of failure of
differentiation of the gonad, but in the 46,XX — pure gonadal agenesis —
this explanation is not valid. This condition is an autosomal recessive
disorder and therefore other genes than those located on the X chromosome must be involved in ovarian development. The location of these
mutant genes remains unclear. In all of these patients, their genotype does
not affect their phenotype, all of them being female since no androgens
cause masculinization, and absence of müllerian inhibitor means the development of the normal müllerian structures, i.e. uterus, tubes and vagina.
As there is no hypothalamo-pituitary disorder, height is normal.

Ovarian failure

These unfortunate girls have ovarian failure as a result of chemotherapy or
radiotherapy for childhood malignancy.

Galactosaemia

This disorder is an inborn error of galactose metabolism due to the
deficiency of galactose-1-phosphate uridyl transferase. The relationship
with hypergonadotrophic hypogonadism is documented; the aetiology
however remains obscure.

Gonadal dysgenesis

The gonad is said to be dysgenetic if it is imperfectly formed and this
encompasses a spectrum of conditions which vary with the degree of
gonadal differentiation.

    The commonest condition is a single X chromosome, 45,X, known as
Turner's syndrome. The missing chromosome may be either an X or a Y.
However, there are many circumstances where cases of gonadal dysgenesis
are associated with a mosaic karyotype. Here two cell lines coexist within
one individual, the most common being 45,X/46,XX or 45,X/46,XY.
Other chromosomal anomalies associated with gonadal dysgenesis are

those with structural abnormalities, known as deletions. The deletion may be of the long arm of the X chromosome (46,XXq-) or the short arm (46,XXp-), and the loss of genetic material affects the individual.

In Turner's syndrome, the ovarian development is normal until 20 weeks and oocytes are found in the ovaries until this stage. Thereafter, there is failure of the oocyte to undergo further maturation, which requires the influence of both X chromosomes and the oocytes begin to undergo a process of atresia which probably continues beyond birth and up until puberty in limited individuals. The ovary in most individuals at this stage consists solely of stroma and therefore is unable to produce oestrogen. There is normal female organ development as the absence of a Y chromosome means the presence of a uterus, tubes and a vagina. The loss of the X chromosome is associated with short stature as the determining genes for height are lost, most Turner's girls being of similar stature.

In mosaicism, the proportion of each cell line determines the manifestation of the condition. Thus, the higher the percentage of 45,X cells, the more likely the features of Turner's syndrome. The presence of some normal 46,XX cells means that there is the possibility of ovarian differentiation and the associated development of secondary sexual characteristics. Some 10–15% of girls exhibit some oestrogenic activity and a few have conceived.

Deletion of genetic material and its impact is much more variable in its clinical presentation. The loss of a short or long arm of a chromosome may be partial or complete and the genetic material lost determines the impact on the patient. For example, the deletion of the X chromosome may or may not be associated with amenorrhoea (Table 16.2).

In chromosomally normal males embryonic development may result in enzymatic failure such that androgen production is inhibited. In these circumstances a non-functional testis exists and failure of masculinization leads to normal female development of the external genitalia. However these enzymatic failures result in a hypergonadotrophic state with elevated levels of FSH. Testosterone levels are very low, if not absent, and the intra-abdominal position of the gonads carries the incumbent risk of malignant transformation and therefore the gonads should be removed.

The second group of disorders are associated with short stature.

Hydrocephalus. In this group of patients, who often have hydrocephalus from birth, it is presumed that damage to the hypothalamus leads to the resultant amenorrhoea.

Table 16.2 Deletion of genetic material and its impact on amenorrhoea

Abnormality	Percentage with amenorrhoea
Deletion of short arm of X chromosome	35%
Deletion of long arm of X chromosome	15%

Trauma. As in hydrocephalus, trauma resulting in severe head injuries followed by primary amenorrhoea is again presumably due to hypothalamic damage.

The empty cellar syndrome. In this disorder there is an absence of sufficient pituitary tissue to allow GnRH to influence FSH production. These patients are therefore hypogonadotrophic but the problem lies at the level of the pituitary rather than the hypothalamus. Computed tomographic scanning of the pituitary fossa will identify this syndrome.

Tumours. Intracranial neoplasms must always be considered in patients with primary amenorrhoea. Pituitary tumours must be especially considered and pituitary adenomas may be found producing hyperprolactinaemia. Other tumours such as craniopharyngioma may also be present and may, through their extension by growth, interfere with the portal circulation from the hypothalamus to the pituitary gland, as well as acting primarily through destruction of the pituitary gland itself.

Hypergonadotrophic hypogonadism. The commonest situation of the short-statured person with primary amenorrhoea is Turner's syndrome. This chromosomal abnormality is typically 45,XO with deletion of one of the sex chromosomes. It is uncertain as to the numbers of cases of 46,XX and 46,XY genotypes in which a sex chromosome is lost, although it has been suggested that in as many as 20-30% of cases genetic material arising from the Y chromosome can be found translocated to other chromosomes in Turner's girls. Not all cases of Turner's syndrome are 46,XO and a substantial number of them will have a mosaic appearance with 45,XO, 46,XX or 45,XO/46,XY. The Turner's syndrome is characterized by short stature and sexual infantilism and there may be webbing of the neck, wide-spaced nipples, pectus cavum, shortening of the fourth metacarpal and sometimes congenital heart disease. The gonadal development that occurs in Turner's syndrome is characterized by normal ovarian development until around 20 weeks of gestation when failure of the primordial follicle to develop a granulosa cell layer leads to atresia and by the time of birth there are almost no oocytes remaining. Occasionally however oocytes do remain and pure Turner's girls have been known to have a few periods at puberty and undergo some secondary sexual development. There have in fact been cases of pregnancy in pure Turner's girls, which must be explained by the retention of a few oocytes which last until puberty.

The majority however have stromal tissue only remaining in the ovary and therefore no possibility of folliculogenesis. FSH levels rise during puberty in response to ovarian failure and remain elevated.

Heterosexual development

Congenital adrenal hyperplasia

This is the most common condition presenting at birth which exhibits heterosexual features but it can also present initially at puberty with clitoral enlargement. It is an autosomal recessive disorder which leads to an enzyme deficiency in the synthesis of cortisol, the most common being 21 hydroxylase deficiency. The genome includes two genes for 21 hydroxylase alternating with genes for complement factors C4a and C4b; they are located on the short arm of chromosome 6. Abnormal mutations of the active gene leads to 21 hydroxylase deficiency and the failure to produce cortisol in normal quantities leads to elevation of adrenocorticotrophic hormone and increased production of cortisol precursors which are converted via 17 α-hydroxyprogesterone to androgens.[8,9] This elevated level of circulating androgens leads to variable degrees of masculinization and thus ambiguity of the genitalia at birth. The vagina is always present and internal genitalia are normal but the external genitalia vary from thin fused labia to severe stenosis of the lower two-thirds of the vagina, with an associated urogenital sinus.

At puberty clitoral enlargement may be the first sign of elevated levels of androgen and should alert the clinician to the hyperandrogenic state which may be adrenal in origin.

Failure of steroid control during childhood and puberty will inhibit normal puberty and delay the onset of menstruation. Evidence exists to suggest that the average age of menarche in congenital adrenal hyperplasia is around 15 years, but this would seem to be totally dependent on steroid control.[10,11]

Androgen-secreting tumours

These are extremely rare but may occur on infrequent occasions and may be tumours arising in the adrenal cortex or the ovary. The most common would be Cushing's syndrome of the adrenal and hilar cell tumours of the ovary, but the most florid forms of polycystic ovarian syndrome may also delay the onset of puberty if androgen production is sufficiently elevated.

5α-reductase deficiency

In patients with 5α-reductase deficiency the ambiguity of their genitalia is associated with the findings of a male karyotype, normal levels of 17 hydroxyprogesterone and complete absence of the uterus and fallopian tubes. If left untreated the steroidogenically competent testes will produce normal amounts of testosterone at puberty, causing rapid virilization in a child who has been brought up as a female, as the external genitalia have a female appearance. Thus a child with primary amenorrhoea and virilization must be thought to have 5α-reductase deficiency if this has not been diagnosed previously. Testosterone levels are in the normal male range.

True hermaphrodites

The majority of true hermaphrodites are 46,XX and are reared as apparent males because at birth they are found to have some degree of masculinization. However, ambiguous genitalia may lead to investigation of the situation, which may reveal the presence of both testicular and ovarian tissue. More commonly they present with menstruation or bleeding at puberty in association with male external genitalia and in these circumstances difficulty may exist in deciding the continued sex of rearing. It is much better to determine the gonadal sex and gonadal structure as early as possible so that the sex of rearing will not be discrepant at puberty.

EVALUATION AND MANAGEMENT

In assessing a teenager with primary amenorrhoea it is important to remember that the most common aetiology is constitutional delay in the onset of puberty. However as the differential diagnosis of primary amenorrhoea can be extensive it is important that the child is appropriately investigated before the diagnosis of constitutional delay is made. Whenever a child presents with her parents and concern is expressed about her wellbeing it is important fully to record history and examination and then to institute the appropriate diagnostic investigations. Physical examination is extremely important to identify the presence or absence of secondary sexual characteristics and these must be classified according to the staging system of Tanner. It is important to realize that normal breast tissue indicates either normal ovarian production of oestrogen or peripheral conversion of androgen to oestrogen. It is unlikely that full breast development will occur from peripheral conversion, thus the presence of secondary sexual characteristics is extremely important in evaluating the patient for investigation. The second important recording is that of the patient's height as the combination of secondary sexual characteristics and height will lead the clinician along the most appropriate investigative pathway (Fig. 16.1).

Normal secondary sexual characteristics

The presence of normal secondary sexual characteristics on physical examination should alert the clinician to the possibility of outflow tract obstruction. The presence of an imperforate hymen may be visible at the introitus but it is inappropriate to perform pelvic examinations on the teenager. The clinician should arrange for a pelvic ultrasound to assess pelvic anatomy. The absence of a uterus indicates the necessity to perform a karyotype and if that karyotype is 46,XX then the Mayer–Rokitansky–Kuster–Hauser syndrome is the most likely diagnosis. If the chromosome is 46,XY then the patient is an XY female. The presence of a uterus on ultrasound scan may well be seen in association with a haematometra or

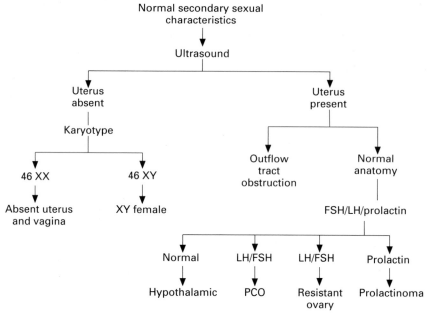

Fig. 16.1 Investigative pathway for a patient with normal secondary sexual characteristics. FSH = Follicle-secreting hormone; LH = luteinizing hormone; PCO = polycystic ovary.

haematocolpos and appropriate reconstructive surgery should be recommended. The presence of a normal pelvic anatomy indicates a necessity to perform FSH, LH and prolactin levels. Normal levels of gonadotrophins would indicate a hypothalamic cause for the amenorrhoea — so-called constitutional delay. Elevation of the LH:FSH ratio indicates the presence of polycystic ovaries which again will have been seen on ultrasound. An elevated level of FSH and LH indicates the development of the resistant ovary syndrome, while elevation of the prolactin level indicates a prolactinoma.

Management

Patients with an absent uterus and vagina should be carefully counselled as to their anatomical problem. It is important to be extremely sensitive in discussing the situation of sexual activity in the future, and their infertility. At the appropriate time of development and interest in sexual activity, a vagina may be created either non-surgically or surgically, depending on the circumstances.[6] Girls who are found to be XY females should be advised that they have abnormal gonads and that these gonads will need to be removed because of the 30% risk of malignancy. It is not felt appropriate to inform these girls of their karyotype as this may be extremely distressing to them. It is of no benefit to them as they are not fertile, although a careful explanation of the lack of development is extremely important in helping them to understand their problem.

Outflow tract obstructions may be at various levels. The imperforate hymen is simply treated with hymenectomy or a cruciate incision, allowing subsequent drainage of retained menses. However transverse vaginal septa are more difficult to deal with and require a careful reconstructive approach in order to obtain a functional vagina in the end. In rare circumstances, the vagina and the cervix may be absent but the incidence of this is extremely small. Surgical approaches to the management of outflow tract obstructions are varied and readers are referred to other texts for greater detail.[12]

In girls in whom constitutional delay is suggested, great reassurance may be given but it is important to ensure that the girl has an opportunity to return to her clinician at regular intervals for continued reassurance until menses commence. The diagnosis of polycystic ovarian syndrome as a cause of primary amenorrhoea is not common and the clinician can reassure the patient that spontaneous menses may occur but the necessity for the use of ovulation induction agents in the future may be mentioned, such that an understanding of the condition is complete. There is no contraindication to the use of the oral contraceptive pill in order to reassure the patient of her ability to menstruate if she so desires. The diagnosis of resistant ovary syndrome is somewhat more complex in differentiating it from premature ovarian failure and this really can only be done by direct ovarian biopsy in which the presence of oocytes confirms the diagnosis of the resistant ovary syndrome.

Finally the presence of an elevated prolactin level should provoke the clinician to perform a computed tomography scan of the pituitary fossa to determine the presence of a prolactinoma.

The absence of secondary sexual characteristics (Fig. 16.2)

In this set of circumstances it is extremely important for the clinician to record the patient's height. If the patient is of normal height for her age, then gonadotrophin measurement will reveal levels that are either low or high. Low levels of gonadotrophins confirm the diagnosis of hypogonadotrophic hypogonadism and elevated levels should provoke the necessity for karyotyping: the 46,XX patient will have premature ovarian failure, the resistant ovary syndrome or gonadal agenesis, while the 46,XY patient will have 46, XY agenesis or testicular enzymatic failure. In the patient who is short in stature measurement of gonadotrophins will indicate either low levels associated with an intracranial lesion, or high levels which again should be followed with a karyotype, almost certainly indicating Turner's syndrome or a variant of it.

Management

In hypogonadotrophic hypogonadism treatment should be directed

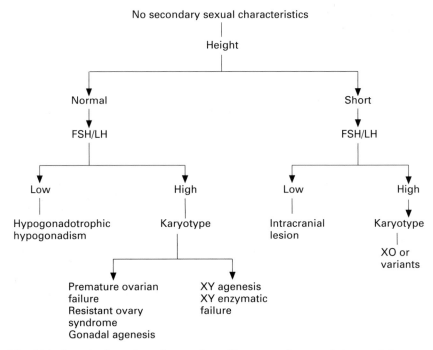

Fig. 16.2 Investigative pathway for a patient with no secondary sexual characteristics. FSH = Follicle-stimulating hormone; LH = luteinizing hormone.

towards any avoidable cause or in the isolated GNRH deficiency, hormone replacement therapy may be instituted in order to induce secondary sexual characteristic development. The patient should be informed that she will be fertile but that ovulation induction will be necessary in order to fulfil this wish. The use of hormone replacement therapy in these girls is controversial but it seems that the most prudent hormone replacement therapy regimes involve the commencement of very low doses of oral oestrogen which are gradually increased over a 2-year period to induce good secondary sexual characteristic growth. The introduction of progestogens should not be included until between 12 and 18 months after the beginning of oestrogen therapy. Patients in whom XY dysgenesis and XY enzymatic failure are suspected should have gonadectomies performed and those patients in whom intracranial lesions are suspect should be investigated appropriately.

Finally physicians must be aware of the fact that any chronic illness will delay the onset of puberty and whilst it is prudent to exclude other causes of primary amenorrhoea, the coexistence of chronic illness may be pertinent.

Absence of menstruation in a teenager is an extremely stressful problem psychologically, and the difficult psychological changes occurring in teenage years demand that the clinician handles the cases with great sensitivity.

Inappropriate consulting can do untold long-term harm and thus care in counselling is paramount in the management of these cases.

REFERENCES

1. Tanner J M. Growth at adolescence. Oxford: Blackwell Scientific Publications, 1962
2. Marshall W A, Tanner J M. Variation in the pattern of pubertal changes in girls. Arch Dis Child 1969; 44: 291
3. Marshall W A. Growth and secondary sexual characteristics and related abnormalities. Clin Obstet Gynecol 1974; 1: 593
4. Lee P A, Plotnick L P, Migeon C J et al. Integrated concentrations of follicle stimulating hormone and puberty. J Clin Endocrinol Metab 1978; 46: 488
5. Stanhope R, Adams J, Jacobs H S, Brook C G D. Ovarian ultrasound assessment in normal children and idiopathic precocious puberty. Arch Dis Child 1985; 60: 116
6. Edmonds D K. Congenital malformations of the vagina and their management. Semin Reprod Med 1988; 3: 91
7. Dewhurst C J, Spence J E H. The XY female. Br J Hosp Med 1977; 17: 498
8. White P C, Grossberger D, Onufer B J. Two genes encoding steroid 21-hydroxylase are located near the genes encoding the fourth component of complement in man. Proc Natl Acad Sci 1985; 82: 1089
9. Donohoue P A, Van Dop C, Jospe N et al. Congenital adrenal hyperplasia: molecular mechanisms resulting in 21 hydroxylase deficiency. Acta Endocrinol (suppl) 1986; 279: 315
10. Grant D, Muram D, Dewhurst C J. Menstrual and fertility patterns in patients with congenital adrenal hyperplasia. Pediatr Adol Gynecol 1983; 1: 97
11. Edmonds D K. Dewhurst's practical paediatric and adolescent gynaecology. London: Butterworths, 1989
12. Edmonds D K. Sexual developmental abnormalities and their reconstruction. In: Sanfillipo J, ed. Pediatric and adolescent gynecology. Philadelphia: W B Saunders, 1993 (in press)

17. Alternatives to surgery for stress incontinence

R. S. Rai   E. Versi

Urinary incontinence is defined by the International Continence Society as being a condition in which the involuntary loss of urine is a social or hygienic problem and is objectively demonstrated.[1] It has been variously reported as occurring in approximately 8.5% of women.[2-4] However, there is little doubt that this is a condition that is under-reported because of the degree of stigma that is attributed to it. This view is substantiated by several large-scale studies. Thomas et al[3] reported a postal questionnaire of 9323 women in which 28% were found to leak urine either frequently or occasionally; and Wolin[5] reported a series of 4211 American nursing students of whom 35% leaked urine occasionally. A MORI poll[6] has reported that between 3.5 and 10 million people in the UK suffer from urinary incontinence.

Genuine stress incontinence (GSI), the stress-induced involuntary loss of urine occurring in the absence of detrusor contraction, accounts for about 50% of all cases of incontinence.[7] Despite the reported success rates of up to 95%[8] for the Burch colposuspension, for various reasons surgery is not the first line of treatment indicated for all.

Stanton et al[9] have identified increasing age, previous incontinence surgery and the presence of detrusor instability as being indicators of adverse surgical outcome. More recent reports[10-12] have added the preoperative finding of a low maximum urethral closure pressure (MUCP) to this list. In addition, women who have not completed their child-bearing and the medically unfit are not ideal candidates for surgical treatment, nor are those in whom stress incontinence is only a slight or occasional problem.

A recent National Institutes of Health[13] conference has reiterated that urinary incontinence is not part of normal ageing and that every person with urinary incontinence has the right to evaluation and treatment. With our greater appreciation of the prevalence of this condition, the potential postoperative voiding complications of surgery[14] and the ever-increasing demands on limited health service resources, attention has once again fallen on the conservative methods of treatment of urinary incontinence. These have the advantages of having a reasonable success rate, being free of complications and do not preclude the surgical option at a later date if they prove to be unsuccessful.

In order to understand the rationale behind the various physio-therapeutic interventions that are employed, we shall briefly consider the functional anatomy of the urethra and its supports with relation to the maintenance of continence.

STRUCTURE IN RELATION TO FUNCTION

In the majority of young women continence is maintained at the bladder neck. However, with advancing age the bladder neck mechanisms tend to fail and so urethral sphincter mechanisms become more important.[15] The maintenance of urinary continence depends on the pressure at some point in the urethra exceeding the intravesical pressure at all times, even under stress.[16] The difference between the intravesical pressure and urethral pressure is known as the urethral closure pressure. The generation of this urethral pressure is achieved by two components, which may be divided into the intrinsic and extrinsic sphincter. The intrinsic sphincter comprises the smooth muscle of the urethral wall together with the submucosal collagen and elastin as well as the blood vessel tone.[17] These components act along the whole length of the urethra and contribute approximately two-thirds of the urethral closure pressure at rest.[17]

The extrinsic sphincter is composed of those structures influencing urethral pressure that lie outside the walls of the urethra. They comprise the striated urogenital sphincter muscle consisting of the urethral sphincter, compressor urethrae and the urethrovaginal sphincter.[18] It is this external sphincter that is the principal component of the distal sphincteric

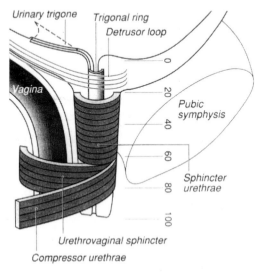

Fig. 17.1 Diagrammatic representation of the component parts of the urethral sphincter. The numbers indicate the distance from the bladder neck in terms of the percentage of the urethral length. Reproduced with permission from DeLancey (1990).[18]

mechanism (Fig. 17.1). At different points along the urethra external forces will vary and their contribution to the maintenance of continence will also vary.

In an attempt to relate structure with function, Delancey[19] correlated his anatomical findings, obtained from the dissection of 22 cadavers, with urethral pressure measurements obtained using urethral pressure profilometry.[20] It has been variously demonstrated that maximum urethral pressure at rest occurs between the 40th and 54th percentile of the total urethral length.[21,22] This region corresponds to the same area, demonstrated by Delancey,[19] as that surrounded by the striated urethral sphincter (Fig. 17.1). Constantinou & Govan[21] have shown that when a patient is asked to hold her urine, urethral pressure increases between the 15th and 85th centile and within this area there are two regions which show marked increases in pressure. One of these, occurring along the 50th to the 85th centile of the urethra, corresponds to the location of the compressor urethrae and urethrovaginal sphincter. The other area, located between the 15th and 20th centile, corresponds to the area of attachment of the urethra to the levator muscles via the arcus tendineus fasciae pelvis (ATFP), indicating an active role for the levator muscle group in the maintenance of continence. The ATFP is the condensation of the superior fascia of the levator muscle and the obturator internus fascia stretching from the lower border of the pubic symphysis to the ischial spine bilaterally. A separate group of connective tissue fibres, the precervical arc, runs in a transverse orientation between the two ATFPs in their anterior half and attaches to the anterior bladder neck. Posterior and lateral to the bladder neck the vaginal wall and its adventitia are attached to the levators, allowing it to control bladder neck position through these connections. As can be seen from Figure 17.2, when the levator muscle contracts it moves the urethra anteriorly, compressing the bladder neck against the precervical arc and favouring closure of the bladder neck.[23]

The levator muscle is well-suited to this role, as histochemical studies[24] have shown that it comprises a heterogeneous population of Type I and Type II cells. These are thought to correspond to slow and fast twitch fibres respectively. It can therefore not only maintain tone over a long period, but also has the ability to contract rapidly and therefore produce a strong occlusive force.

At times when intra-abdominal pressure rises the intravesical pressure also rises, as the bladder is an intra-abdominal organ. To maintain continence, the intraurethral pressure also has to increase. The three mechanisms whereby urethral pressure rises are voluntary striated muscle contraction, reflex striated muscle contraction and pressure transmission.

The part played by voluntary muscle contraction has already been discussed. As for reflex contraction, Constantinou & Govan[21] have shown that sudden increases in intra-abdominal pressure induce reflex contractility of the periurethral striated muscle. This reflex contraction occurs

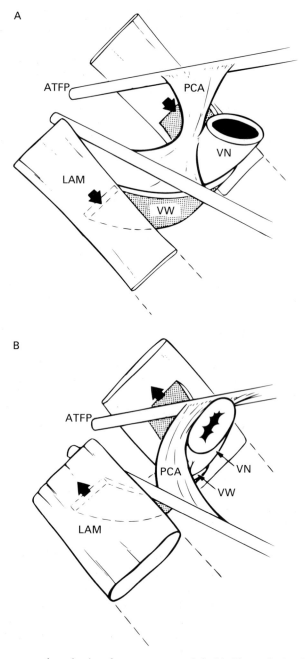

Fig. 17.2 Anatomy and mechanics of structures around the bladder neck. A = Relaxation; B = contraction. ATFP = Arcus tendineus fasciae pelvis; PCA = precervical arc; VN = vesical neck; LAM = medial levator ani muscle; VW = vaginal wall. Reproduced with permission from DeLancey (1988).[23]

before the effect of either pressure transmission or voluntary contraction. It is probably mediated via the fast twitch fibres of the levators and may be a learned reflex.

Transmission of the intra-abdominal pressure to the proximal urethra is thought to be important for the maintenance of continence.[11,25] The diagnostic potential of this has been questioned by us[26] as we were unable to differentiate between patients with an intact sphincter and those with GSI on the basis of pressure transmission. Defects in transmission most commonly occur due to defects in support of the urethra, causing it to become extra-abdominal either at rest or at times of exertion.

CONSERVATIVE TREATMENT OF GENUINE STRESS INCONTINENCE

All physiotherapeutic interventions employed in the treatment of GSI are aimed at improving function of the pelvic floor musculature.

In a postal questionnaire of all 192 English district health authorities, Mantle & Versi[27] obtained responses from 98.4% of them, making their report a fair representation of the current practice employed by physiotherapy departments in England. They found that pelvic floor exercises (PFE) and inferential treatment were the most favoured in terms of availability, efficacy, and preference. PFE were preferred by 178 (94%) and inferential therapy by 144 (76%). Forty per cent of respondents thought that a combination of these two modalities was more effective than either treatment alone.

PELVIC FLOOR EXERCISES

The rationale behind PFE is that repeated voluntary contractions of the pelvic floor muscles will lead to improved voluntary and reflex contractility of these muscles. How this is achieved may be elucidated from electrophysiological studies which have shown that repetitive activity of a muscle leads to increased motor unit recruitment and to axonal sprouting together with reinnervation of the muscle.[28]

Kegel[29] was among the first to postulate the use of conservative treatment in patients with GSI. In addition, he correctly identified that the most important factors influencing the successful training of such women involved them in correctly identifying the muscles of the pelvic floor, and the use of biofeedback. Using his perineometer (a pneumatic device placed in the vagina and connected to a manometer in order to give a visual feedback of muscle contraction), and a regimen of 300 contractions per day he reported a cure rate of 80% among 500 of his patients.

Since Kegel's report, his techniques of PFE have come into widespread clinical use and been further refined. Current practice in England, largely for historical reasons, involves the physiotherapist taking the primary role in the conservative management of patients with stress incontinence. However, more recently there has been an increasing interest amongst continence advisors. Mantle & Versi[27] reported that in teaching PFE almost all physiotherapy departments start by explaining the anatomy and nature of the condition. This took an average of 22 minutes. Instruction in pelvic floor contraction took on average 20 minutes to explain to a new patient. In the majority of cases women were encouraged to hold a contraction for 4 or 5 seconds if possible, and to perform four or five such contractions at each practice session. Fifty-nine per cent of respondents taught quicker, shorter contractions. This is important because the levator muscles are composed of both slow and fast twitch muscle fibres, which are thought to respond to different training regimens. Finally, it was the practice in the majority of clinics to advise patients to practise every hour. Given this rather demanding requirement, the authors[27] questioned compliance and emphasized the obvious necessity of motivation.

Results of PFE

It was not until this decade that objective results of treatment with PFE have been reported. Earlier reports tended to be subjective and grouped together patients who reported improvements as well as cure. In addition, the exact technique used and expertise of the educator were often not quoted. More recent reports tend to show a cure rate ranging from a low of 8%[30] to 27%.[31] However, the rates for those reporting a significant improvement are much more impressive, with most reports suggesting a figure of around 60% for those either cured or reporting a significant improvement in symptoms.[31,32]

Tapp et al[33] reported the results of a randomized study comparing the results of PFE with those of the Burch colposuspension. Three groups of women, who all had urodynamically proven GSI, were randomized to treatment which consisted of either PFE, PFE and faradism (PFE + F) or Burch colposuspension. At 6-month assessment 2 of 21 in the PFE group were cured, 7 of 21 were symptomatically improved, and 12 requested surgery. Of the PFE + F group 8 of 23 were symptomatically better and 13 requested surgery. Of those who had a colposuspension, 18 of 24 were objectively cured and 23 of 24 noted an improvement. These results suggest that faradism adds little to the effect of PFE and would indicate a disappointingly poor comparative performance of PFE as against surgery. However, it has been argued that this is not an entirely appropriate comparison. It is generally accepted that surgery offers a better cure rate than physiotherapy and this has certainly been demonstrated by this well-controlled study. However, in the clinical situation patient selection is critical for appropriate management. Thus patients who elect for PFE may regard a significant improvement in their symptomatology to be a satisfactory outcome, especially when this can be achieved without the potential perils of surgery.[14] On the other hand, only a cure could be deemed as being acceptable after major surgery. The drop-out rate in the PFE groups is not surprising in that some patients want a rapid resolution of their symptoms and so opt for surgery, thereby shifting the responsibility from themselves to the surgeon. This is another reason why selection is critical.

In 1991 Klarskov et al[34] reported the results of a long-term follow-up (median 6 years) of patients who had earlier been randomized to treatment with either PFE or surgery. At earlier follow-up (4 and 12 months) patients not satisfied were offered the alternative form of treatment. Forty-two per cent were satisfied following PFE and did not request surgery and 71% were satisfied after surgery. At late follow-up, the results were practically the same as at 1 year, indicating that the beneficial effects of PFE are continued for years after the end of a formal treatment programme. At long-term follow-up 59% were still using PFE at least once per week and 28% occasionally.

Factors affecting outcome of PFE

In view of the relatively low objective cure rates reported, and the time-consuming nature of PFE, Tapp et al[33] have attempted to identify those patients who might be cured by PFE. Good prognostic features were a shorter duration of symptoms, less severe symptoms (lower visual analogue score), and better urethral function (i.e. a longer functional urethral length and a maximum urethral pressure of greater than 9.4 cm of water). Mantle & Versi[27] reported that physiotherapists viewed positive motivation as the single most important prognostic feature. Other positive features were recent onset of symptoms, ability to contract the pelvic floor at the time of presentation and youth. On the negative side were listed previous surgery, concomitant prolapse and a chronic cough. What is urgently needed are large, possibly multicentre trials to examine formally these predictive variables with a view to developing a more rational patient selection policy.

BIOFEEDBACK

We have already alluded to the role of biofeedback, which represents a form of operant learning. Kegel[29], appreciated that the first step in muscle re-education was to establish awareness of the muscle. He used the perineometer, as described above, in order to provide his patient with continuous visual feedback of the pressures she was generating using her pelvic floor. However, because the top of the instrument was placed in the vagina above the level of the levators, he was in addition also recording intra-abdominal pressure. As the essence of pelvic floor training is to educate the patient to contract her pelvic floor without contracting her abdominal muscles, this is a serious flaw in the design of the perineometer. Recently,

Wilson et al[35] have investigated the reproducibility of perineometry measurements and found some inconsistencies and so have recommended that measurements be carried out with an empty bladder and the first recording of each visit be discarded.

The importance of biofeedback was reinforced by Burgio et al[36] who reported the results of a study comparing the effectiveness of simultaneous visual biofeedback with intermittent verbal feedback based on vaginal palpation. They found a significant 76% reduction in incontinence in the biofeedback group, which was also significantly greater than the 51% reduction seen in the verbal feedback group, thus emphasizing the importance of biofeedback. It is possible that the much lower success rates of recent studies as compared to Kegel's[29] are due to the non-use of biofeedback techniques.

VAGINAL CONES

Plevnik[37] introduced the use of weighted vaginal cones in order to improve the muscles of the pelvic floor. The cones (initially nine in a set, now five) are of similar shape and volume, but of increasing weight, ranging from 20 to 100 g (Fig. 17.3). They are placed in the vagina, with the rounded end uppermost, and held in position by the action of the levator muscles. The

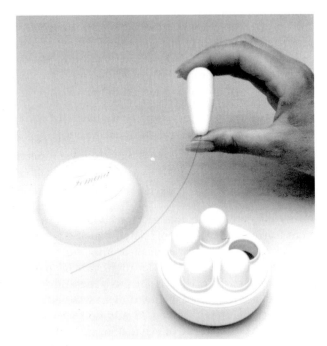

Fig. 17.3 A set of five vaginal cones. Reproduced with permission from Colgate Medical, Berkshire.

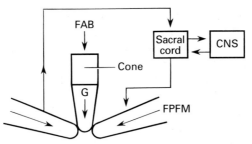

Fig. 17.4 Diagrammatic representation of forces on cones in situ. G = Weight of cone; FAB = force due to abdominal pressure; CNS = central nervous system; FPFM = force developed by pelvic floor muscles. Reproduced with permission from Peattie et al (1988).[38]

patient is given a complete set of cones and is instructed to retain the cone for 15 minutes twice per day. Once successful for two consecutive occasions, she moves up in weight to the next cone.

The tendency is for the cone to fall out, and this feeling of losing the cone is thought to provide a sensory feedback response that causes the pelvic floor to contract in order to retain the cone (Fig. 17.4). This was confirmed by Hesse et al[39] using electromyographical recordings of the pubococcigei muscles after a vaginal cone is inserted. Their recordings showed a waxing and waning pattern of electrical activity, probably reflecting repetitive contraction of these muscles in 'pushing up' the cone which tends to slip.

Mantle & Versi[27] reported that physiotherapists thought that it took an average of 15 minutes in order to teach a patient to use a cone, as opposed to an average of 42 minutes to teach pelvic floor anatomy and exercises. Current practice is that patients are reviewed after an average of 13 days and then reviewed five times. The mean time taken for these reviews was 19 minutes. However there has been no adequate evaluation of the follow-up required.

Patient acceptability of cones is good, but Wilson & Borland[40] reported that after 12 months only 6 of 14 women were still using them. The rest preferred to use PFE alone, primarily due to convenience. This might indicate that cones are useful for initiating pelvic floor contractions as the patient is initially made aware of her pelvic floor muscles. Subsequently they may not be necessary. For aesthetic reasons some women decline their use. They would not be suitable in those with vaginal stenosis, for example following previous surgery or secondary to postmenopausal vaginal atrophy, and in those women with a significant degree of vaginal wall prolapse.

As a way of providing biofeedback, cones are in some ways superior to the perineometer. The latter records rises in pressure due not only to contraction of the pelvic floor but also to contraction of the abdominal muscles, thereby giving the patient false information as to the effectiveness of her PFE. With vaginal cones, any increase in intra-abdominal pressure would tend to push the cone downwards, thus stimulating contraction of the pelvic floor muscles. The patient can therefore be sure that she is contracting the correct muscles, and at the same time the ability to hold cones of increasing weight provides a form of biofeedback. As mentioned earlier, this may be more important at the beginning of an exercise programme.

Results from cone use

Peattie et al[38] reported an objective improvement or cure rate, based on a standardized 1-hour pad test, of 70% in 30 premenopausal women after 1 month of treatment. However Versi & Mantle[41] have criticized this paper on the grounds that there was a 23% drop-out rate and the results may therefore merely represent a placebo effect. In addition, the validity and reproducibility of the 1-hour pad test that was used are open to question. Wilson & Borland[40] in a study of 34 women reported an objective improvement rate of 68% at 6 weeks. In addition, 47% thought that no treatment other than cones was required. At 12-month follow-up 41% still reported an improvement and were satisfied to continue with conservative treatment.

Two small randomized preliminary studies[42,43] have compared the results of vaginal cones against those of conventional PFE. Unfortunately the numbers were too small to make any valid statistical inference. However Haken et al[43] noted that difficulty in remembering the technique was a significant feature in those treated with PFE. Before a definitive conclusion can be reached as to the relative merits of cones as opposed to PFE, Larger-scale studies are needed, with standardization of techniques and treatment protocols.

ELECTRICAL STIMULATION

Mantle & Versi[27] reported that this was the second most common form of conservative treatment in England for patients with stress incontinence. Despite its widespread use the exact mechanism by which its effect is mediated is not clear.

One mode of action is that electrical stimulation may be a kind of muscle training, the pelvic floor muscles being activated by stimulation of the pudendal nerve, with an effect similar to that of PFE. This idea is supported by work on cats[44] which found that the urethral pressure increases with intravaginal electrical stimulation were attributable to direct stimulation of efferent motor axons. In addition, Ridge & Betz[45] have shown that electrical stimulation promotes the development of large motor units. Therefore, stimulation may improve the re-innervation of partly denervated pelvic floor muscles by enhancing the sprouting of surviving motor axons. An additional point is that there are somatic afferent nerves travelling with the pudendal nerve. These ascend via the dorsal columns to convey proprioception from the pelvic floor. Their stimulation may therefore be expected to restore cortical awareness of this muscle group.

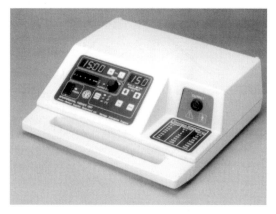

Fig. 17.5 EMS interferential therapy unit, manufactured by Electro-Medical Supplies, Wantage, Oxfordshire.

FARADISM

This technique uses low-frequency alternating-current treatment in various modulations in order to produce contraction of the pelvic floor muscles (Fig. 17.5). Two electrodes are needed: the current practice in England is to have an indifferent electrode over the lumbar or sacral region and either an active vaginal electrode or pad electrode over the perineum.[27] The current is provided by a small Faradic battery which produces surges of current lasting 2 seconds at a repetition frequency of 12 surges/minute. The major disadvantage of faradism is that one has to provide a large current in order to overcome skin resistance at the effective frequencies for muscle stimulation. This can be associated with pain. This problem has led to interest in other ways of delivering a stimulatory current to the pelvic floor muscles.

INFERENTIAL TREATMENT

This involves the delivery of two slightly different medium frequency currents of around 4000 Hz, from different directions, in order to overcome skin resistance. Where the currents cross, the difference between the original frequencies is known as the interference or beat frequency. It is this frequency that is the stimulatory frequency to the pelvic floor muscles (Fig. 17.6).

Crucial to the effectiveness of inferential treatment is the position of the electrodes, whether two or four electrodes should be used, and the interference frequencies used. Laycock & Green[46] have addressed these questions and suggest a two-electrode method, with one electrode placed centrally over the anus and the other on the anterior part of the perineum immediately inferior to the pubic symphysis. Using this method minimal patient discomfort is caused, application of the electrodes is easy and the

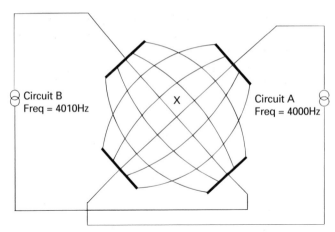

Fig. 17.6   Interferential effect in homogeneous medium, X (frequency = 10 Hz). Reproduced with permission from Laycock & Green (1988).[46]

current flows along the path of least resistance, avoiding bony tissue. In addition, they have demonstrated that using the bipolar method, which is in effect amplitude-modulated faradism, a greater current can be used than by employing the four-electrode technique.

As the levator muscles consist of both fast and slow twitch muscle fibres the stimulatory frequency should perhaps mimic these. Eccles et al[47] have shown that motor neurons innervating slow twitch muscles discharge at a frequency of 10–20 Hz and fast twitch muscle at a frequency of between 30 and 60 Hz. Laycock & Green[46] suggest that a frequency sweep of 10–50 Hz be used with a gradual rise and fall ensuring that a full range of frequencies is covered. However such theoretical considerations have not been tested and shown to influence outcome in a formal trial.

Results of electrical stimulation

Olah et al[48] using inferential therapy reported a subjective cure rate of 33% at 6-month follow-up of a group of patients, the majority of whom gave a history of incontinence of longer than 1 year, and a 40% cure rate of those who completed treatment. Seventy-three per cent of patients who completed treatment at 6-month follow-up showed an objective improvement on 1-hour pad testing. These results are broadly similar to those reported earlier by Wilson et al.[49] Indeed, the results of inferential treatment were deemed to be so impressive that Laycock[50] suggested that this should be a first-line treatment in the management of those patients with stress incontinence unable to cooperate in a course of PFE (e.g. the elderly). However, one study has indicated that adding inferential or faradic treatment to PFE confers no extra benefit.[49]

In a comparative study of inferential treatment and cones, Olah et al[48] reported no significant difference between the two groups in either cure rate or improvement at 6 months. They recommended the use of cones over inferential treatment as it required less supervision and the patient could carry out the treatment regimen at home.

Most of these studies are flawed by the lack of a control group. Studies with end-points which are purely subjective are particularly susceptible to a placebo effect.

OESTROGEN TREATMENT AND MEDICAL MANAGEMENT

It is well-recognized that the prevalence of incontinence increases with age.[51] Several authors[3,52,53] have demonstrated that at the time of the menopause stress incontinence is the most common symptom of urinary incontinence. In view of the oestrogen deficiency at this time, attention has been focused on the role of oestrogen replacement in the treatment of stress incontinence.

Credence for a role for oestrogen has been lent by the identification of high-affinity oestrogen receptors in the urethra, predominantly in the middle and distal one-third, and also in the bladder itself.[54] These findings are not surprising as both the lower urinary and genital tracts are derived embryologically from the urogenital sinus.

Urethral pressure profilometry has revealed that the vascular pulsations of the submucosal plexuses, which provide one-third of the intraurethral pressure,[55] decrease in size after the menopause, but this decrease can be reversed by oestrogen treatment.[56]

Similarly, it has been shown that skin collagen (which is probably similar to that forming the connective tissue layer of the urethral wall and plays a part in the generation of intraurethral pressure) has its decline after the menopause reversed by oestrogen replacement treatment.[57] Skin collagen has been shown to correlate with urethral pressures[58] and consequently it has been suggested that oestrogens may influence urethral pressure via this axis. Therefore, there are several sound reasons for believing that oestrogen replacement will be beneficial in the treatment of GSI.

Salmon et al[59] were the first to use oestrogens as a treatment for incontinence, but theirs and later studies were subjective in nature and uncontrolled. Evidence from more recent objective studies is confusing. Rud[55] using high doses of oral oestrogen reported small increases in total urethral pressure and urethral closure pressures after oestrogen treatment. Significantly, in those patients who reported an improvement in their symptomatology, Rud reported an increase in the transmission of rises in intra-abdominal pressure to the proximal urethra. This was a similar finding to that of Hilton & Stanton[60] and Bhatia et al[61] who used intra-vaginal oestrogen. The most likely explanation for this effect of increased transmission pressure is that it is mediated via an effect on the periurethral connective tissue elements. Certainly a moderate degree of prolapse is thought to improve following oestrogen replacement therapy.[62]

Unfortunately, the above studies were not placebo-controlled and also the results are at variance with those of Wilson et al,[31] who reported a double-blind placebo-controlled objective study of 36 postmenopausal women who received 3 months of cyclical treatment with oral oestrone. They found no significant difference in the urethral pressure profile variables or nappy test (Urilos) measurements between the two groups. Another placebo-controlled subjective study of 70-year-old women was unable to show any effect of oestriol treatment on women with stress incontinence.[63] The only placebo-controlled study to show that stress incontinence can be improved by oestrogen therapy was carried out by Walter et al[64] on a small number of patients. Nine out of 12 women preferred oestriol to placebo and there was a significant objective decrease in urine loss.

The most promising drug treatment for GSI is the combination of oestrogen with the alpha-adrenoceptor agonist phenylpropanolamine. The rationale behind this combination is that animal studies have shown oestrogens to increase two-or threefold the urethral adrenoceptor population. Controlled studies using phenylpropanolamine and oestrogens separately and in combination have shown a synergistic effect of the combination treatment.[65,66] The study by Kinn & Lindskog[66] reported a cure rate of 28% with 53% of patients reporting an improvement in their condition.These findings have been confirmed in an objective trial by Hilton et al.[67]

Due to the lack of large-scale controlled studies using objective measurements of lower urinary tract function it is difficult to draw a definitive conclusion on the role of oestrogen replacement in the treatment of GSI. Caution has to be exercised on the use of unopposed oestrogen in those women who have not had a hysterectomy due to the well-recognized potential complication of endometrial hyperplasia and malignancy.[68] The situation is further complicated by the fact that progesterone has been shown to increase incontinence,[69] though progesterone receptors have not been identified in the urethra. Benness et al[70] reported preliminary results of a study of postmenopausal women with incontinence, receiving a combined hormone replacement treatment regimen of Estraderm patches and Cyclogest pessaries. The studies (videocystourethography, urethral pressure profilometry, 40-minute pad testing) were performed in the two phases of hormone treatment and showed a significantly higher urine loss on pad-testing performed during the progestogen phase as compared to that recorded during the oestrogen-only phase. Indeed, in the only long-term reported series of oestrogen replacement treatment combined with norethisterone, Versi et al[62] reported no improvement in the symptoms of stress incontinence and no significant improvement in the urethral closure pressure after 1 year of treatment with 50 mg subcutaneous estradiol implant with 5 mg norethisterone for 7 days per month. Cyclical treatment with progestogens to oppose exogenous oestrogen may therefore negate any beneficial effect of the administered oestrogen.

Paraurethral implants

Paraurethral implants aim to cure stress incontinence by increasing urethral pressure through external compression of the urethra. To achieve this aim, a variety of substances have been injected in the past, but attention is now focused on the use of Teflon and glutaraldehyde cross-linked collagen. To date, the experience with Teflon is longer, but the use of this material is complicated by the findings of distant microembolization of Teflon and its associated inflammatory reaction, which is similar to that produced by asbestos.[71] The significance of these findings is debatable. On the other hand, collagen has the advantage of being easier to inject periurethrally (either paraurethrally using a spinal-type needle or transurethrally). In addition, there are no reports of microembolization of collagen.

Vesey et al[72] investigated the urodynamic effects of Teflon injection and demonstrated a reduction of 23% in mean urine flow rate, a 9% increase in functional length but only a 2% increase in maximum urethral closure pressure. Due to the relatively small numbers in this trial, none of the above changes reached statistical significance. This study does, however, suggest that the increased outflow resistance produced by Teflon injection is achieved by an increase in functional urethral length rather than by a rise in maximum urethral closure pressure.

Regrettably, most reports on the use of periurethral implants are subjective. In addition the range of reported cure rates vary from 20%[72] to 70%.[73] These variations can probably be explained to some extent by the degree of operator experience.

There is, however, general agreement that patients who would benefit most from this form of treatment are those who have undergone previous vaginal surgery, especially when the anterior vaginal wall is well-supported. This is perhaps due to the areas of fibrosis providing a firm base into which injection can be made. Also bladder neck surgery in this group has a lower success rate.

The advantages of this technique are that it is relatively straightforward, can be repeated as required, and in a certain group of women can be an effective form of treatment, especially when previous surgery has failed.

FUTURE RESEARCH

We have already highlighted the importance of selecting patients suitable for conservative treatment based on certain factors such as motivation and age. Only the small study by Tapp et al[33] has looked at the urodynamic parameters that influence the outcome of physiotherapeutic treatment. As large numbers are required to resolve this issue statistically, multicentre trials are needed in order to determine which factors in the history, clinical and urodynamic examination of the patient can be shown to influence the outcome of conservative treatment. In addition, parameters need to be identified that indicate which of the different treatment modalities discussed above is most likely to give a satisfactory outcome for a particular patient. When such studies come to fruition we will be in a position to identify those patients who are most likely to benefit from conservative management and thus increase the cost-effectiveness of this mode of treatment.

CONCLUSIONS

Since the introduction of the Burch colposuspension, an effective form of treatment for GSI has been available, and interest in non-operative treatment declined. However, recent reports over the last decade indicating that relatively good objective results could be obtained from the use of physiotherapy have reawakened interest in conservative treatment. Given our awareness that the prevalence of GSI is higher than previously thought, together with a greater appreciation of the potential of complications from surgery[8,14] attention has increasingly focused on the conservative management of this condition.

Whilst attempts have been made to identify those patients who might be cured by conservative treatment (e.g. the highly motivated, young and fit), it should be remembered that many would find a significant improvement to be an acceptable outcome. In addition failure does not preclude the surgical option of treatment at a later date, if that is what is requested. Nonetheless, a greater attention to the selection of patients would result in a more efficient use of resources.

The medical management of GSI is limited. Hormone replacement therapy does not result in adequate long-term improvement, though there may be a role for this form of treatment concomitantly with surgery or even conservative therapy. Oestrogens may improve the local tissues and so possibly improve the effect of surgery whilst physiotherapy may be more successful if the fascial muscle connections are strengthened. Therefore the role of oestrogens may be as a supplement[74] rather than as a primary therapeutic agent. The role of collagen implants needs to be evaluated further. The success rate is limited but this technique may have a place in certain circumstances: determination of these is to be awaited.

In terms of success rates, PFE are generally thought to be the most effective mode of conservative treatment.[27] There is little to choose between the use of vaginal cones and inferential treatment. The former may be preferred, in that it requires much less supervision and provides a form of biofeedback to the patient, encouraging her to persist with her treatment regimen. In addition, this is a form of treatment the patient may undertake in the privacy of her own home.

The most important aspect in the successful conservative treatment of GSI is that the patient understands that it involves a change in her pattern of life and represents a lifelong commitment. An understanding of this, together with enthusiasm and commitment from both the patient and her teachers, can lead to results that may obviate, in some, the necessity of surgery and its attendant risks.

REFERENCES

1. Abrams P, Blaivas J G, Stanton S L, Andersen J T. The standardiztion of terminology of lower urinary tract function. Br J Obstet Gynaecol 1990; 97 (suppl 6): 1–16
2. Fenely R C L, Shepard A M, Powell P H et al. Urinary incontinence: prevalence and needs. Br J Urol 1979; 51: 493–496
3. Thomas T M, Plymat K R, Blannin J, Meade T W. Prevalence of urinary incontinence. Br Med J 1980; 281: 1243–1245
4. Elving L B, Foldspang A, Lam G W, Mommsen S. Descriptive epidemiology of urinary incontinence in 3100 women age 30–59. Scand J Urol Nephrol 1989; 125 (suppl): 37–43
5. Wolin L H. Stress incontinence in young healthy nulliparous female subjects. J Urol 1969; 101: 545–549
6. Market and Opinion Research Institute. Survey of attitudes and prevalence of incontinence (for the British Association for continence care). MORI Health Research Unit, 1991
7. Yarnell J W, Voyle G J, Richards C J, Stephenson T P. The prevalence and severity of urinary incontinence in women. J Epidemiol Community Health 1981; 35: 71–74
8. Pow-Sang J M, Lockhart J L, Suarez A, Lansman H, Politano V A. Female urinary incontinence: preoperative selection, surgical complications and results. J Urol 1986; 136: 831–833
9. Stanton S L, Cardozo L, Williams J E, Ritchie D, Allan V. Clinical and urodynamic features of failed incontinence surgery in the female. Obstet Gynecol 1978; 51: 515–520
10. McGuire E J. Urodynamic findings in patients after failure of stress incontinence operations. Prog Clin Biol Res 1981; 78: 351–360
11. Hilton P, Stanton S L. A clinical and urodynamic evaluation of the Burch colposuspension for genuine stress incontinence. Br J Obstet Gynaecol 1983; 90: 934–939
12. Bowen L W, Sand P K, Ostergard D R et al. Unsuccessful Burch retropubic urethropexy: a case controlled urodynamic study. Am J Obstet Gynecol 1989; 160: 452–458
13. National Institutes of Health. Consensus Conference on Urinary Incontinence. Bethesda, Md: NIH. 1988
14. Stanton SL. Surgical management of urethral sphincter incompetence. Clin Obstet Gynecol 1990; 33: 346–357
15. Versi E, Cardozo L D, Studd J W, Brincat M, O'Dowd T M, Cooper D J. Internal urinary sphincter in maintenance of female continence. Br Med J 1986; 292: 166–167
16. Enhoring G. Simultaneous recording of the intravesical and intraurethral pressures. Acta Obstet Gynecol Scand 1961; 276 (suppl): 1
17. Rud T, Andersson K E, Asmussen M, Hunting A, Ulmsten U. Factors maintaining the urethral pressure in women. Invest Urol 1980; 17: 343–347
18. DeLancey J O L. Anatomy and physiology of urinary incontinence. Clin Obstet Gynecol 1990; 33: 298–307
19. DeLancey J O L. Correlative study of paraurethral anatomy. Obstet Gynecol 1986; 68: 91–97
20. Rai R S, Versi E. Urethral pressure profilometry. Int Urogynecol J 1991; 2: 222–227
21. Constantinou C E, Govan D E. Spatial distribution and timing of transmitted and reflexly generated urethral pressures in healthy women. J Urol 1982; 127: 964–969
22. Hilton P, Stanton S L. Urethral pressure measurement by microtransducer; the results in symptom free women and in those with genuine stress incontinence. Br J Obstet Gynaecol 1983; 90: 919–933

23. DeLancey J O L. Anatomy and mechanics of structures around the vesical neck: how vesical neck position might affect its closure. Neurourol Urodyn 1988; 7: 1–2

24. Gosling J A, Dixon J S, Critchley H O D, Thompson S A. A comparative study of the human external sphincter and periurethral levator ani muscles. Br J Urol 1981; 53: 35–41

25. Collins C D, Montgomery E, Williams J P et al. Treating incontinence electrically. Br Med J 1972; 3: 112–113

26. Versi E, Cardozo L, Cooper D J. Urethral pressures: analysis of transmission pressure ratios. Br J Urol 1991; 68: 266–270

27. Mantle J, Versi E. Physiotherapy for stress urinary incontinence: a national survey. Br Med J 1991; 302: 753–755

28. Fall M, Lindstrom S. Electrical stimulation: a physiologic approach to the treatment of urinary incontinence. Urol Clin North Am 1991; 18: 393–407

29. Kegel A H. Progressive resistance exercise in the functional restoration of the perineal muscles. Am J Obstet Gynecol 1948; 56: 238–248

30. Tapp A J S, Hills B, Cardozo L D. Randomized study comparing pelvic floor physiotherapy with the Burch colposuspension. Neurourol Urodyn 1989; 8: 356–357

31. Wilson P D, Faragher B, Butler B, Bulock D, Robinson E L, Brown A D G. Treatment with oral piperazine oestrone sulphate for genuine stress incontinence in postmenopausal women. Br J Obstet Gynaecol 1987; 94: 568–574

32. Henalla S M, Kirwan P, Castleden C M, Hutchins C J, Bresson A J. The effect of pelvic floor exercises in the treatment of genuine stress incontinence in women at two hospitals. Br J Obstet Gynaecol 1988; 95: 602–606

33. Tapp A J S, Cardozo L, Hills B, Barnick C. Who benefits from physiotherapy? Neurourol Urodyn 1988; 7: 259–261

34. Klarskov P, Nielsen K K, Kromann-Andersen B, Maegaard E. Long term results of pelvic floor training and surgery for female genuine stress incontinence. Int Urogynecol J 1991; 2: 132–135

35. Wilson P D, Herbison G P, Heer K. Reproducibility of perineometry measurements. Neurourol Urodyn 1991; 10: 399–400

36. Burgio K L, Robinson J C, Engel B T. The role of biofeedback in Kegel exercise training for stress urinary incontinence. Am J Obstet Gynecol 1986; 154: 58–64

37. Plevnik S. New methods for testing and strengthening the pelvic floor muscles. Neurourol Urodyn 1985; 4: 265–266

38. Peattie A B, Plevnik S, Stanton S L. Vaginal cones: a conservative method of treating genuine stress incontinence. Br J Obstet Gynaecol 1988; 95: 1049–1053

39. Hesse U, Vodusek D B, Deindl F M, Lukanovic A, Schubler B. Neurophysiological assessment of treatment with vaginal cones. Neurourol Urodyn 1991; 10: 394–395

40. Wilson P D, Borland M. A preliminary study of vaginal cones for the treatment of genuine stress incontinence. Proc Univ Otago Med Sch 1988; 66: 37

41. Versi E, Mantle J. Vaginal cones: a conservative method of treating stress incontinence. Br J Obstet Gynaecol 1989; 96: 752–753

42. Peattie A B, Plevnik S. Cones versus physiotherapy as conservative management of genuine stress incontinence. Neurourol Urodyn 1988; 7: 265–266

43. Haken J, Benness C, Cardozo L, Cutner A. A randomized trial of vaginal cones and pelvic floor exercises in the management of genuine stress incontinence. Neurourol Urodyn 1991; 10: 393–394

44. Fall M, Erlandson B E, Carlsson C A, Lindstrom S. The effect of intravaginal electrical stimulation on the feline urethra and urinary bladder: neuronal mechanisms. Scand J Urol Nephrol 1978; 44 (suppl): 19–30

45. Ridge R M A P, Betz W J. The effect of selective, chronic stimulation on motor unit size in developing rat muscle. J Neurosci 1984; 4: 2614–2620

46. Laycock J, Green R J G. Inferential therapy in the treatment of incontinence. Physiotherapy 1988; 74: 161–168

47. Eccles J C, Eccles R M, Lundberg A. The action potentials of the alpha motor neurones supplying fast and slow muscles. J Physiol 1958; 142: 275–291

48. Olah K S, Bridges N, Denning J, Farrar D J. The conservative management of patients with symptoms of stress incontinence: a randomized, prospective study comparing weighted vaginal cones and inferential therapy. Am J Obstet Gynecol 1990; 162: 87–92

49. Wilson P D, Al Sammari T, Deakin M, Kolbe E, Brown A D G. An objective assessment of physiotherapy for female genuine stress incontinence. Br J Obstet Gynaecol 1987; 94: 575–582
50. Laycock J. Inferential therapy in the treatment of genuine stress incontinence. Neurourol Urodyn 1988; 7: 268–269
51. Cardozo L, Versi E. Oestrogens and the lower urinary tract. In: Asch R, Studd J W W, eds. Progress in reproductive medicine, vol 1. Carnforth, Lancashire: Parthenon Publishing, 1992 (in press)
52. Hagstad A, Janson P O. The epidemiology of climacteric symptoms. Acta Obstet Gynecol Scand 1986; 134 (suppl): 59–65
53. Jolleys J V. Reported prevalence of urinary incontinence in women in general practice. Br Med J 1988; 296: 1300–1302
54. Isoif M D, Batra S, Ef A, Astedt B. Oestrogen receptors in the human female lower urinary tract. Am J Obstet Gynecol 1981; 141: 817–820
55. Rud T. The effects of oestrogens and gestogens on the urethral pressure profile in urinary incontinent and stress incontinent women. Acta Obstet Gynecol Scand 1980; 59: 265–270
56. Versi E, Tapp A, Cardozo L D, Montgomery J C. Urethral vascular pulsations and the menopause. Proc Int Menop Soc 1987; 5: 201
57. Brincat M, Versi E, O'Dowd T M et al. Skin collagen changes in postmenopausal women receiving oestradiol gel. Maturitas 1987; 9: 1–5
58. Versi E, Cardozo L D, Brincat M, Cooper D, Montgomery J, Studd J W W. Correlation of urethral physiology and skin collagen in postmenopausal women. Br J Obstet Gynaecol 1988; 95: 147–152
59. Salmon U L, Walter R I, Geist S H. The use of estrogens in the treatment of dysuria and incontinence in postmenopausal women. Am J Obstet Gynecol 1941; 42: 845–851
60. Hilton P, Stanton S L. The use of intravaginal estrogen cream in genuine stress incontinence. Br J Obstet Gynaecol 1983; 90: 940–944
61. Bhatia N N, Bergman A, Karam M M. Effects of estrogen on urethral function in women with urinary incontinence. Am J Obstet Gynecol 1989; 141: 176–181
62. Versi E, Cardozo L, Studd J. Long-term effect of estradiol implants on the female urinary tract during the climacteric. Int Urogynaecol J 1990; 1: 87–90
63. Samsioe G, Jansson I, Mellstrom D, Svandborg A. Occurrence, nature and treatment of urinary incontinence in a 70 year old female population. Maturitas 1985; 7: 335–342
64. Walter S, Kjaergaard B, Lose G et al. Stress urinary incontinence in postmenopausal women treated with oral estrogen (estriol) and alpha adrenoceptor-stimulating agent (phenylpropanolamine): a randomised double blind placebo controlled study. Int Urol J 1990; 12: 74–79
65. Beisland H O, Fossberg E, Moer A, Sander S. Urethral sphincter insufficiency in postmenopausal females: treatment with pheylpropanolamine and estriol separately and in combination. Urol Int 1984; 39: 211–216
66. Kinn A C, Lindskog M. Estrogens and phenylpropanolamine in combination for stress urinary incontinence in postmenopausal women. Urology 1988; 32: 273–280
67. Hilton P, Tweddell A L, Mayne C. Oral and intravaginal estrogens alone and in combination with alpha adrenergic stimulation in genuine stress incontinence. Int Urogynecol J 1990; 1: 80–86
68. Whitehead M I, McQueen J, Minardi J, Campbell S. Progestogen modification of oestrogen-induced endometrial proliferation in climacteric women. In: Cooke I D, ed. The role of oestrogen/progestogen in the management of the menopause. Lancaster: MTP Press, 1978: Chapter 10, pp 121–133
69. Caine M, Raz S. The role of female hormones in stress incontinence. Abstracts of the International Society of Urology, presented at the 16th Congress of Société Internationale d'Urologie, Amsterdam, 1973: p 30
70. Benness C, Ganger K, Cardozo L, Cutner A, Whitehead M. Do progestagens exacerbate urinary incontinence in women on HRT? Neurourol Urodyn 1991; 10: 316–317
71. Malizia A A, Reiman M M, Myers R P et al. Migration and granulation after peri-urethral injection of Polytef (Teflon). JAMA 1984; 251: 3277–3281
72. Vesey S G, Rivett A, O'Boyle P J. Teflon injection in female stress incontinence. Effect on urethral pressure profile and flow rate. Br J Urol 1988; 62: 39–41

73. Schulman C C, Simon J, Wespes E et al. Endoscopic injection of teflon for female urinary incontinence. Br Med J 1984; 288: 192
74. Fantl J A, Wyman J F, Anderson R L, Matt D W, Bump R C. Postmenopausal urinary incontinence: comparison between non-oestrogen supplement and oestrogen-supplemented women. Obstet Gynecol 1988; 71: 823–826

18. Vaginal hysterectomy

S. S. Sheth

The debate on whether the uterus should be removed vaginally or abdominally was sparked when Langenbeck first performed a vaginal hysterectomy in 1813.[1] Vaginal hysterectomy described in the days of Soranus of Ephesus (AD 120)[2a] was technically revived by Czerny[2b] in 1879 and credit for the modern operation is given to Koeberle.[3] In 1885 Jackson[4] suggested it should be abandoned, but Schauta,[5] treating carcinoma of the cervix, gave a boost to vaginal surgery in 1890. Before the turn of the century, brilliant French surgeons were most successful with the use of clamps and produced remarkable morcellation and hemisection techniques. They stressed the use of the vaginal approach for pelvic inflammatory disease. The famous French Surgeon Doyen[6] insisted in 1939 that no one could call himself a gynaecologist until he performed vaginal hysterectomy 'in private'. The Germans developed a methodical suture technique. From the UK, ardent promoters of this technique were Green-Armytage,[7] Palmer,[8] Howkins,[9] Stallworthy[10,11] and Watson.[12] Van Bastiaanse[13] from Amsterdam and Navratil[14] from Austria were eminent vaginal surgeons while Mitra[15,16] and Purandare[17] were advocates from the eastern world.

The superiority of hysterectomy by the vaginal route is not denied. In 1932 Babcock[18] felt vaginal hysterectomy was the operation of choice. Dicker and associates[19] documented that women who undergo vaginal hysterectomy experience significantly fewer complications than women who undergo abdominal hysterectomy. However, there is a vast difference between precept and practice.

Too often a hysterectomy which should be done vaginally is done abdominally merely because this has become a routine procedure in that particular clinic.[20] The ease and convenience by which hysterectomy can be performed through a wide open abdominal incision, along with a lackadaisical attitude to acquiring the necessary surgical expertise required for vaginal hysterectomy, have led to a large number of gynaecologists removing the uterus abdominally. This path of least resistance is justified by the mistaken belief that the vaginal route should be avoided in the absence of uterine descent or visible prolapse. In the last two decades, there has been a paucity of literature emphasizing the rightful place of vaginal hysterectomy.

CONTRAINDICATIONS

The universally accepted contraindications are a uterus of more than 12 weeks' size, absence of free mobility of uterus and the presence of adnexal pathology.

Many gynaecologists even at teaching institutes and in the affluent world perform an abdominal hysterectomy in total absence of any of the contraindications for the vaginal route on the flimsiest excuse.

Often, a gynaecologist who is not adept at vaginal hysterectomy will avoid it on one pretext or another.

1. 'There is an absence of uterine prolapse.'
2. 'The uterus is enlarged.'
3. 'A good look at the abdominal organs, particularly at the appendix, is essential'.
4. 'She is a nullipara.'
5. 'She needs ovarian removal.'
6. 'A decision will be taken after she has been examined under anaesthesia.'

Unfortunately, in nine out of 10 cases, an abdominal hysterectomy is a foregone conclusion and examination under anaesthesia is a mere formality.

It should be standard practice to teach that absence of prolapse is not a contraindication. Likewise, its presence is not essential to indicate the vaginal route. It is essential to emphasize that, in the absence of any contraindications, the preferred route for hysterectomy should be vaginal.

The contraindications to vaginal hysterectomy are only relative,[21] vary with the experience and skill of the surgeon,[22] or are to be evaluated as only relative and not absolute.[14] Weaver & Johnson[23] state that contraindications and operative difficulties are exaggerated. With a personal experience of having performed more than 3800 vaginal hysterectomies, the author strongly feels that only a genuine contraindication to vaginal hysterectomy should indicate an abdominal hysterectomy.

Points to remember are:

1. Uterine prolapse is not a prerequisite for vaginal hysterectomy.
2. As a rule, uterus without surrounding pathology descends (downward mobility) when traction is applied under anaesthesia.
3. Uterine descent becomes progressively easier as the uterosacral and Mackenrodt's ligaments are cut.
4. Nulliparity per se does not contraindicate a vaginal hysterectomy.
5. To have a look at the abdominal contents, particularly the appendix, the abdominal route should be used only if a surgical opinion so indicates.
6. The size of the uterus that can be removed vaginally increases with experience.

7. Should the need for oophorectomy arise, it should not pose a problem for an experienced vaginal surgeon.

ABSOLUTE CONTRAINDICATIONS

1. Uterus more than 12 weeks' size.
2. Restricted uterine mobility.
3. Limited vaginal space.
4. Adnexal pathology.
5. Vesicovaginal fistula repair.
6. Cervix flush with vagina.
7. Invasive cancer of the cervix.

INDICATIONS

These vary according to the experience of the operator and the traditions at various institutes. As Krige[22] has rightly noted, 'The surgeon's list of indications not only reveals his mental attitude towards the operation but also his confidence in or lack of operative ability and techniques'.

The majority of indications in the past 50 years have been related to pelvic relaxation and uterine bleeding.[24] Kovac[25] feels that vaginal hysterectomy is the technique of choice for the management of patients with non-malignant pelvic disease.

Ideally, the vaginal route should be the primary route when a hysterectomy is to be performed. Indeed, it is a gynaecological route, unlike the abdominal one, which is used by all and sundry — general surgeons, oncologists, urologists, biliary and plastic surgeons!

An indication for hysterectomy and absence of any contraindications to the vaginal route for hysterectomy are sufficient markers to perform vaginal hysterectomy.

The incidence of vaginal hysterectomy to abdominal hysterectomy varies from 1 : 4 or less. Ideally, this ratio should be reversed. Most series in the world literature mention uterine prolapse as the main indication for vaginal hysterectomy.

Repair was part of vaginal hysterectomy in 90% of Hawksworth & Roux's series of 1000 cases.[26] Centaro et al[27] had 52% with repair in a series of 1438 cases. There are no details of the repair. In Gray's 386 vaginal hysterectomies, 99% had repair.[47] Richter reported 3468 hysterectomies, of which 2611 (75%) were vaginal; 87.4% of these were with repair.[29]

In a series of 3800 hysterectomies, 3388 vaginal hysterectomies were done in the absence of prolapse (Table 18.1).

The indications discussed here include conditions where hysterectomy:

1. should be routinely by the vaginal route, e.g dysfunctional uterine bleeding and adenomyosis;

Table 18.1   Indications for vaginal hysterectomy in 3800 patients

	Indications	Associated conditions
Dysfunctional uterine bleeding } Adenomyosis	2415	
Enlarged uterus		2857
Fibroids	875*	
Nullipara		146
Severe mental handicap	60	
Previous abdominal surgery		558
Previous vaginal surgery		61
Cervical polyp/fibroid	24	
Carcinoma-in-situ of the cervix	10	
Endometrial cancer	4	
High-risk patients		54
Emergency conditions		8
Uterine prolapse	412	
Total	3800	

* Out of 875 with fibroids a total of 486 were menorrhagic due to fibroids while the remaining 389 could have been menorrhagic because of dysfunctional uterine bleeding and/or fibroids.

2. need not be by the abdominal route merely because of fibroids, nulliparity etc.;

3. by the vaginal route will make a difference to the patient, anaesthetist and surgeon, e.g. in high-risk cases.

Dysfunctional uterine bleeding

Dysfunctional uterine bleeding is exceedingly common and forms the commonest indication for hysterectomy if prolapse is excluded. Apart from correction of endometrial hyperplasia by progestogen,[31] an effective and safe long-term therapy for dysfunctional uterine bleeding has been disappointing. Noble[32] was of the opinion that hysterectomy has a worthwhile place in the treatment of menorrhagia. Studd[33] finds a paucity of literature concerning the role of hysterectomy in the treatment of menorrhagia. In dysfunctional uterine bleeding, there is an absence of adnexal pathology and a freely mobile normal-size uterus which make for an ideal indication for vaginal hysterectomy. An enlargement up to 10–12 weeks' size does not form a contraindication, nor does nulliparity. A multiparous state makes the operation easier.

From 687 vaginal hysterectomies reported by Sheth & Asher,[34] 41.9% were for dysfunctional uterine bleeding. Of 889 vaginal hysterectomies for benign disease,[14] 47.8% were for uterine bleeding. Dysfunctional uterine bleeding in women at or after menopause with or without relaxation is regarded as a universally acknowledged indication for vaginal hysterectomy.[7,26,27,35,36] Jeffcoate[37] has stated that hysterectomy can easily be carried out by the vaginal route and this involves little risk and upset.

In the last 25 years, 3800 vaginal hysterectomies have been done for various indications. In all, 2359 were for dysfunctional uterine bleeding or adenomyosis. In the absence of dysmenorrhoea, it is impossible to make a definite diagnosis of dysfunctional uterine bleeding or adenomyosis until the removed uterus is examined histopathologically

Adenomyosis

This is an ideal indication for vaginal hysterectomy, though the definitive diagnosis is made only after careful histopathological examination of the removed uterus. Menorrhagia with dysmenorrhoea does signify adenomyosis, but there is a large number of patients without dysmenorrhoea who are usually diagnosed clinically as having dysfunctional uterine bleeding and found later to have adenomyosis on histopathological examination.

A uterus with adenomyosis is likely to be enlarged but rarely more than 12 weeks' size. The enlargement is uniform, often soft to feel and may give the fallacious impression of a bulging soft myoma.

All adenomyotic uteri less than 12 weeks' size can be removed by the vaginal route. Out of 3800 vaginal hysterectomies, 2415 were diagnosed clinically as adenomyosis or dysfunctional uterine bleeding. As many as 1766 (73.1%) turned out to be adenomyosis on histopathological examination.

Fibroids and enlarged uterus

Fibroids that cause symptoms need to be operated upon. It is important to ascertain the cause of the symptoms as bleeding may be due to dysfunctional uterine bleeding or adenomyosis and the small fibroids may only be an incidental finding. Sonography fairly frequently reveals an insignificant myoma which can be ignored. The mere presence of a fibroid does not contraindicate the vaginal route.

Edwards & Beebe[36] advocated vaginal hysterectomy for myoma up to 14 weeks' size. Navratil[14] goes on to state: 'In general, it can be said that uteri enlarged to the size of a pregnancy of approximately 3–4 months do not represent a contraindication'. Of Navratil's vaginal hysterectomies for benign disease, 50.8% were for uterine fibroids. In the author's series of 3388 vaginal hysterectomies for conditions other than prolapse, 486 were for uterine fibroids. The size of a fibroid is not as important as the size to which the uterus is enlarged and how accessible the fibroid is. Kovac[25] performed intramyometrial coring in 76% of vaginal hysterectomies. He recommends coring for vaginal removal of many uteri for which abdominal hysterectomy has been a traditional choice. The present author feels that if at examination under anaesthesia, particularly on applying traction to the cervix, the fundus in an uterus of 12–14 weeks' size descends to disappear in the pelvis, the vaginal route should not pose a problem.

An anterior wall myoma may demand extra attention whilst opening the uterovesical pouch of the peritoneum. Careful inspection and feeling with the index and middle fingers on the uterine wall will differentiate between a bulge that is due to a myoma — firm and fixed — and that due to the bladder — soft, mobile and able to be rolled. A posterior wall myoma does not obstruct the opening of the posterior pouch, unlike the anterior wall one which can obstruct the opening of the anterior pouch.

Nulliparity

For many gynaecologists, nulliparity per se is a sufficient reason to avoid the vaginal route. As long as the uterus is less than 12 weeks' size, freely mobile and without adnexal pathology, vaginal hysterectomy should be possible, irrespective of descent. The uterine size and the experience of the surgeon will determine whether it can be easily done.

Whilst descent in a multipara is more evident, there is always sufficient descent in a nullipara to permit satisfactory vaginal hysterectomy. In the author's series, 146 married nullipara had vaginal hysterectomy for dysfunctional uterine bleeding, fibroids, adenomyosis or severe mental handicap — there were no failures.

From this series, two facts emerge: nullipara do have uterine descent in the form of downward mobility, and vaginal hysterectomy can be performed in the absence of uterine prolapse, even in nulliparous women who had an intact hymen before an examination under anaesthesia.[38] Dealing with a normal-size uterus in a nullipara is comparable to dealing with an enlarged uterus in a multipara — relative space is the important criterion.

Previous abdominal surgery

Previous pelvic surgery per se is not a contraindication to vaginal hysterectomy as the nature of the previous operations is the deciding factor.

These operations can be broadly divided into four categories:

1. Operations performed on the uterus are the most important — caesarean section, hysterotomy and myomectomy demand extra care, but do not constitute an absolute contraindication unless they have been performed repeatedly in the past. In the author's series there were 214 patients with previous caesarean section with 1 trauma to the bladder and ureter. Ventrofixation, an obsolete operation, contraindicates vaginal hysterectomy, though on 6 occasions it was successfully performed without resorting to the abdominal route. However, this was achieved after much patience and perspiration.

2. Sling operations for prolapse also make vaginal hysterectomy difficult. Only a very experienced vaginal surgeon will be able to cope without resorting to abdominal hysterectomy.

3. Operations performed on the tubes, ovaries and broad ligament tissues give rise to a few flimsy adhesions reaching close to the upper pedicle, which are easily separable and do not hinder surgery. They should not be a contraindication.

4. Operations performed on structures or organs other than the genital tract, such as adhesiolysis, or operations involving the intestines, gall bladder, urinary tract (but nor the bladder) are not contraindications.

Encountering any adhesion that holds the uterus inseparably or fear of traumatizing a hollow organ should be an indication to abandon the vaginal route and complete the operation abdominally.

Previous vaginal operations

An earlier vaginal operation per se is not a contraindication to vaginal hysterectomy. However, it warns the surgeon to exercise extra care. The operations come under the following categories:

1. Operations on the vaginal epithelium and around it, e.g. anterior colporrhaphy, vaginal wall cyst,
2. Cervical amputation.
3. Fothergill's operation — a combination of points 1 and 2 above.
4. Operations through the vagina and where the peritoneum is entered, e.g. surgery on the tube and/or ovary,
5. Sites slightly away from the site of hysterectomy, e.g. posterior colpoperineorrhaphy, Bartholin's cyst.

Cervical amputation is a relative contraindication to vaginal hysterectomy. It distorts the anatomy considerably and thus to attempt vaginal hysterectomy after a previous Fothergill's operation is to invite bladder or rectal injury. The other categories merit special attention.

Cervical polyp/fibroid

Quite often a cervical polyp or myoma extrudes from the cervical lip or from within the cervical canal, fills the vagina partly or wholly and obscures speculum examination. It can be the cause of continuous excessive bleeding resulting in marked anaemia. Such patients need extra care and are often subjected to abdominal hysterectomy.

The speculum findings per se in such a case will suggest that the vaginal route is not possible and an abdominal hysterectomy is necessary. However, gaining access to the vaginal angle and opening the vagina by the abdominal route will not be easy. Bringing out a necrotic and infected polyp through the peritoneal cavity is also not desirable. Mattingly & Thompson[24] consider abdominal hysterectomy to be contraindicated as

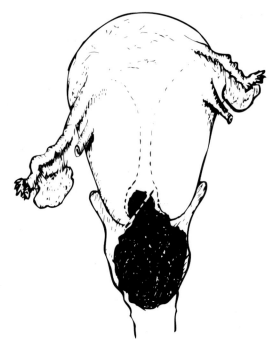

Fig. 18.1 The cervical polyp/fibroid fills almost all of the vagina and apparently contraindicates vaginal hysterectomy. Polypectomy close to its base (dotted line), followed by examination under anaesthesia will favour vaginal hysterectomy. The inset shows the difference.

there is an increased risk of infection as well as ureteral damage due to the dilated cervix, which is close to the ureter.

The prima facie case against vaginal hysterectomy can change radically in favour of such a procedure if polypectomy or myomectomy is done vaginally and then an assessment under anaesthesia follows (Fig. 18.1). The patulous and distended vagina makes it easier to do a vaginal hysterectomy, though the patulous wide open cervix will need an extra traction suture to close it. Until the uterine vessels are secured, there may be more oozing than usual, because of increased vascularity. Twenty-four cases of such large polyps were thus treated by the author. There was no difficulty and all hysterectomies were successfully completed vaginally. It is advantageous to perform the hysterectomy at the same sitting as it avoids repetition of anaesthesia and hospitalization, besides being more convenient as all preparations for hysterectomy have been made.

For those who would avoid abdominal hysterectomy, fearing infection or damage to the ureters, or vaginal hysterectomy because of a patulous dilated cervix, a re-evaluation at 8–12 weeks after vaginal polypectomy or myomectomy can be done. The involuted pelvic findings usually then favour a vaginal hysterectomy

Carcinoma-in-situ of cervix

Severe dysplasia and carcinoma-in-situ CIN grade III need careful attention and treatment as a lapse can spell disaster. It must be accepted that hysterectomy is excessive treatment for most patients,[39] Routine hysterectomy for carcinoma-in-situ cannot be recommended but patients who do not want children and who have involved margins of cone may be treated by hysterectomy.[40]

Among several modalities of therapy, hysterectomy has a definite place for those who have completed child-bearing. This should be by the vaginal route. There is no need for oophorectomy for CIN. A definitive size or length of vaginal cuff can be removed vaginally, in contrast to additional dissection which is involved if the abdominal route is taken.[41-43]

Mitchell[44] feels that vaginal hysterectomy is an excellent operation for carcinoma-in-situ when the involved areas in the cervix have been diagnosed by cone and the adjacent tissue mapped by colposcopy either within 48 hours or after 8 weeks. Vaginal hysterectomy can be employed with great advantage in the treatment of carcinoma-in-situ.[14] Navratil did 339 hysterectomies for carcinoma-in-situ between 1946 and 1964 and 76.4% were vaginal hysterectomies.

If the chosen treatment is hysterectomy, it should be by the vaginal route.

Endometrial malignancy

The right mode of treatment is total abdominal hysterectomy with bilateral salpingo-oophorectomy combined with pre- and postoperative radiotherapy. However, sometimes one is confronted with a patient who has endometrial carcinoma and has other high risks, e.g. morbid obesity, hypertension, diabetes or impaired cardiorespiratory status. Such a patient, if assessed under anaesthesia by an experienced vaginal surgeon, can be favourably operated by the vaginal route.

According to Jeffcoate,[37] when the patient is obese or diabetic or has any other condition which makes hysterectomy dangerous, there is much to be said in favour of vaginal hysterectomy which gives results almost as good as those of abdominal hysterectomy, even if the tubes and ovaries are not always removed simultaneously. Ingiulla[45] performed vaginal hysterectomies in 460 out of 573 corpus cancer cases: survival rates were 73.2% compared with 71.4% of the abdominal group.

The vaginal route is favoured for endometrial cancer as opposed to the abdominal one by many authorities.[13,14,46-48a]

If the cases are correctly selected, and liberal Schuchardt's incision is taken if necessary, the disadvantage of vaginal hysterectomy is overcome.[14]

Postmenopausal bleeding

In cases with persistent or recurrent menopausal bleeding in the absence of a cause, hysterectomy can be carried out easily by the vaginal route and this involves little risk and upset.[37]

The treatment of choice in these patients is hysterectomy and bilateral oophorectomy. Postmenopausal patients are ideal candidates for prophylactic oophorectomy[48b] — more so if they have recurrent vaginal bleeding. If there is no contraindication, hysterectomy should be by the vaginal route, provided the operator is well-versed with performing oophorectomy at vaginal hysterectomy.

High-risk cases for anaesthesia

Patients with interstitial pulmonary fibrosis or those with markedly restricted pulmonary function, impaired cardiac status complicated by hypertension, obesity or diabetes may be better treated by radiotherapy for ablation of ovarian function or hysteroscopic endometrial ablation, rather than by hysterectomy. However, if hysterectomy has to be performed, the anaesthetist prefers the gynaecologist to take the vaginal route, thus avoiding abdominal surgery and sparing the use of muscle relaxants. A low spinal anaesthesia is used and the surgeon tries to be quick as possible.

Patients with endometrial carcinoma, carcinoma-in-situ of the cervix, atypical endometrial hyperplasia and third-degree uterine prolapse require a hysterectomy rather than ablation.

EXAMINATION UNDER ANAESTHESIA

This singularly important examination should form an integral part of the management of a patient needing a hysterectomy. Every vaginal hysterectomy should be preceded by an examination under anaesthesia and abdominal hysterectomy should not be considered unless there is a contraindication to vaginal hysterectomy. All patients scheduled for abdominal hysterectomy should be examined under anaesthesia provided there are no contraindications to a vaginal hysterectomy. For an experienced gynaecologist, it is an assurance against an occasional lapse or error of judgement. For the inexperienced, it is sound practice, aids learning and removes any misconception. Sometimes surprises may surface in the form of misjudged uterine size, missed adnexal pathology or the presence of an ovarian cyst instead of a fibroid. Vaginal surgery, particularly vaginal hysterectomy, can only be learnt and further mastered, if the findings of an examination under anaesthesia are combined with judgement from increasing experience.

The important points are:

1. Exclude a contraindication to vaginal hysterectomy.

2. Assess uterine mobility, size and descent. The mobility in all directions is to be tested — anteroposterior, side-to-side and downwards. This, along with pelvic examination, gives an idea as to the availability of free space on all sides of the uterus during surgery. Adequate uterus-free pelvic space or operative space around the uterus facilitates vaginal surgery and is important in the assessment of the technical feasibility of vaginal hysterectomy. This is a new surgical concept. A 10–12 weeks' size uterus, enlarged transversely and/or in an anteroposterior direction, thereby reducing the uterus-free space, poses a technical problem.

3. Determine the descent of the cervix when traction is applied with a vulsellum on both lips. As a rule, there is descent, even in a nullipara, which is sufficient to permit a vaginal hysterectomy.

4. In patients with a history of previous surgery or adnexal pathology, further evaluation is necessary. A vulsellum is applied to each lip of the cervix separately. The vulsellum on the anterior lip pulls the cervix towards the perineum to evaluate the anterior vaginal mucosal findings whilst the vulsellum on the posterior lip pulls the cervix towards the symphysis to assess the posterior vaginal mucosa findings. The descent of the cervix, shallowness or depth of the fornix and the free movement of the vaginal mucosa can thus be ascertained. Sufficient descent, a deep fornix and free vaginal mucosa are favourable indications for a vaginal hysterectomy. Shallow lateral fornices diminish the space for surgery. If the vaginal mucosa is tautly held back at the site of bladder and rectal reflections, caution is needed whilst opening the pouch. Puckering or retraction of the posterior vaginal mucosa at the site of the posterior pouch indicates pelvic inflammatory disease or endometriosis. The latter may form a dimple at the site.[48c] An outpouring of chocolate-like material when the pouch is opened at the operation confirms this.

5. An inability to visualize the cervix on introducing a full-length Sims speculum and visualization only after an anterior vaginal wall retractor is used forms a contraindication for vaginal hysterectomy unless traction on both cervical lips and individually on each lip indicates otherwise.

6. Under certain circumstances, each point needs careful assessment. In the presence of fibroids, it is important to determine the size of the uterus as well as the site of the fibroids, multiplicity and accessibility, in case debulking is required.

7. For all women undergoing a diagnostic dilatation and curettage who are likely to need a hysterectomy, evaluation for the route of hysterectomy should begin by an examination under anaesthesia done at the same time.

DESCENT, PROLAPSE, AND MOBILITY

These three, though repeated, need to be understood and differentiated between. Descent and prolapse are relative terms, as descent in excess is prolapse. Under anaesthesia, when traction is applied to the cervix with a vulsellum, there is descent akin to first-degree prolapse. This is not unusual and is physiological, being of a greater degree in a multipara. In contrast, prolapse is pathological and is present even when the patient has not been anaesthetized.

The uterus is mobile in four directions:

1. Downwards — tested by traction and evident as descent.
2. In an anteroposterior direction — tested by moving the uterus to and fro by pressure separately applied anteriorly and posteriorly.
3. In a sideways direction — tested by pressing on the lateral walls of the uterus, first in one direction and then the other.
4. In an upward direction, never used vaginally.

Mobility upwards is not tested but can be appreciated at bimanual examination by pushing the cervix upwards along with either forward or backward direction, giving fundal movement accordingly and indicating uterine mobility upwards.

Free mobility is physiological, whilst restricted mobility is pathological. There cannot be prolapse without descent and descent implies downward mobility. When downward mobility or descent is combined with antero-posterior mobility under anaesthesia, a retroverted uterus can be ante-verted and vice versa. Testing anteroposterior mobility and side-to-side mobility gives an idea as to the uterus-free pelvic space. This estimation, along with the degree of descent, is a better guideline than the distance between the ischial tuberosities which Nichols[49] recommends. The latter is as fallacious as external pelvimetry in obstetrics.

FAVOURABLE FINDINGS UNDER ANAESTHESIA

1. Absence of any contraindication.
2. Mobility of the uterus in all planes.
3. Uterine descent (even in the absence of prolapse).
4. Adequate uterus-free pelvic space around the uterus.
5. Free vaginal mucosa around the site of both pouches.
6. Normal cervical length of portio vaginalis with deep fornices.

As a rule, the cervix descends under anaesthesia irrespective of parity.

UNFAVOURABLE FINDINGS UNDER ANAESTHESIA

1. Uterus more than 12 weeks' size.
2. Restricted uterine mobility.
3. Adnexal pathology.
4. Shallow lateral fornices.
5. Cervix flush with the vaginal mucosa.

6. Short cervix and shallow fornices; bladder and/or rectum almost on the cervical lip.
7. Loss of mobility of the vaginal skin or obvious restriction at the site of the anterior or posterior pouches.

The first three are contraindications to the vaginal route while the others make for a less favourable situation which can be overcome by an experienced committed surgeon.

TENTATIVE VAGINAL HYSTERECTOMY

Even in experienced hands, there are times when it is felt that, though difficult, perhaps a vaginal hysterectomy may succeed. A trial by the vaginal route is undertaken with full preparations to switch over to an abdominal route, if necessary. It is best to discuss this in advance with the patient and her relatives. Failure to do so can result in the patient losing confidence in the surgeon.

Likely to fall into this category are:

1. Those with 10–14 weeks' size uterus with fibroids or adenomyosis with diminished uterus-free space,
2. Those who have had two or more earlier caesarean sections,
3. Nulliparous women with an enlarged uterus,
4. Those who have had previous surgery for prolapse or suspension,
5. Those with doubtful adnexal pathology.

At any stage of the operation, if the situation warrants a change to an abdominal hysterectomy, there should not be any hesitation to do so nor a false sense of pride. Failure to take a prompt decision can cause additional problems such as sepsis, increased blood loss due to difficulties encountered, as well as prolongation of surgery and anaesthesia. An action taken in the patient's best interests invites admiration and the operator should not feel he or she has failed. It is comparable to a trial forceps delivery in obstetrics. Such a plan will considerably reduce the number of abdominal hysterectomies, enhance the operator's experience and sharpen his or her judgement.

Pelvic inflammatory disease and endometriosis do not unequivocally preclude undertaking a vaginal hysterectomy as long as the surgeon is ready and willing to complete the procedure through a transabdominal incision, if necessary.[21]

Advantages

The advantages usually outweigh the disadvantages. In most cases, the hysterectomy is in fact completed vaginally, without unnecessary surgical procedures. The many difficult steps at abdominal hysterectomy, such as severing the uterosacral and Mackenrodt's ligaments, opening the vagina and securing the angles, have already been completed vaginally, thus facilitating the abdominal procedure, should a switch-over be necessary.

The loss of time, slightly prolonged anaesthesia or the chance of mild sepsis should not deter the operator from attempting a procedure which is scientifically indicated and is in the best interests of the patient. The attendant morbidity of abdominal hysterectomy, particularly the development of incisional hernia, can be lessened.

FAILED VAGINAL HYSTERECTOMY

There are times when a vaginal hysterectomy fails and a switch-over to the abdominal route is required for its completion. The reasons may be:

1. Omission of examination under anaesthesia.
2. Unsuspected abnormality such as adnexal pathology.
3. Error of judgement, e.g. unduly large uterus.
4. Overconfidence.
5. Lack of experience and/or necessary confidence.

Patience, perseverance and confidence grow with experience. If vaginal hysterectomy is attempted after a thorough examination under anaesthesia, the chances of a switch-over to the abdominal route are very uncommon. In the author's series of more than 3800 vaginal hysterectomies spanning 25 years, 104 were tentative vaginal hysterectomies with only 4 requiring the abdominal route. This is most encouraging; otherwise all 104 would have been operated abdominally.

Nichols[50] has noted: 'There are times when the surgeon feels that the patient should have a vaginal hysterectomy but his courage fails him and he gives himself the benefit of doubt'.

When to switch over to the abdominal route

1. A band of inaccessible fixation is holding up the uterus and preventing descent.
2. Unsuspected adnexal pathology, e.g. ovarian tumour or endometriosis.
3. Underestimated uterine size.
4. Inaccessible myoma.
5. Inability to open the uterovesical peritoneum.
6. If a ligature slips, resulting in haemorrhage.
7. Diffident and/or inexperienced operator.

Technical points

1. The endeavour should be to learn intelligently and acquire mastery to discover the planes of cleavages so as to open both pouches.

2. If bladder separation is difficult:
   a. use a bladder sound;
   b. attempt to dissect the bladder angle, uterocervico broad ligament space;
   c. dissect safely to take off the serosal layer of the uterus reverse intrafascial method;
   d. reach the uterovesical peritoneum from behind the uterus.
3. Be familiar with the bladder and rectal bulge.
4. Any or both pouches, if required, can be opened after the uterine vessels are secured or even a step or two later.
5. If opening the pouch of Douglas is difficult, the cervix should be held up towards the pubic symphysis and tissue from the back of the cervix pushed upwards and backwards. It is vital to keep feeling the cervix directly, whilst further dissection is done. Tactile sensation is important — feel the tissues frequently!
6. The presence of a dimple at the site of the pouch of Douglas may indicate the presence of ovarian endometriosis.
7. In cases of pelvic inflammatory disease, if a firm band is felt posterolateral to the uterus, when cut, it provides descent.
8. If, on reaching the upper pedicle or after its severance, the uterus does not descend, the likely reasons are intestinomental adhesions or sling of previous surgery for prolapse or suspension. This is a serious consideration for changing the route.
9. Debulking is required when:
   a. clamp or suture on the lateral connections is not possible;
   b. the top of the fundus cannot be felt by the fingers from one of the two spaces — it will not be possible to deliver the fundus from either of the spaces. The preference is for the posterior space as it is easier;
   c. there is a myoma. Myoma enucleation is gratifying surgery and an ideal debulking method. The best myoma to enucleate is the most accessible and the largest. A posterior wall myoma is easier than an anterior one. The crux lies accessible to the lowermost part of a large myoma when working within the uterine wall. Surprisingly, bleeding is scant.
10. Downward traction through a suture on intact tissue will bring otherwise inaccessible tissue within reach for the next suture, after which the former can be cut medially. This method will provide a higher reach (Fig. 18.2).

UTEROCERVICAL BROAD LIGAMENT SPACE

If the presence of anterior adhesions prevents access to the uterovesical peritoneum, it can still be gained by the lateral window approach. The adhesions are between the bladder and lower uterine segment and are denser in the middle. However, the lateral area is free — a uterocervico

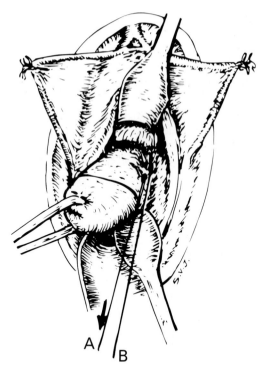

Fig.18.2   Traction on suture A gives access to inaccessible tissue for the next suture (B), and so on.

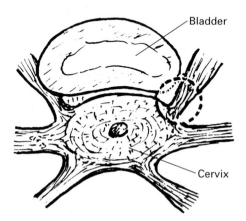

Fig. 18.3   At the lateral angle of the uterovesical junction there is slightly more room, a window or uterocervico broad ligament space (circle of dotted lines), to enter the uterovesical space and begin bladder separation.

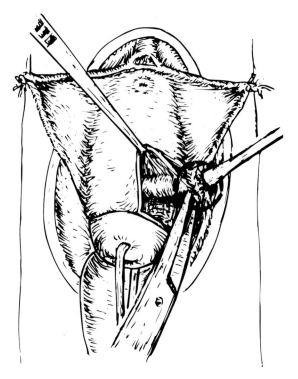

Fig. 18.4   Sharp dissection near the lateral uterocervical margin to find the uterovesical space succeeds in entering the lateral window or uterocervico broad ligament space (circle of dotted lines).

broad ligament space which has not been described earlier (Fig. 18.3). Whilst an attempt to find the uterocervico broad ligament space is being made, sharp dissection near the lateral margin of the uterocervical junction will enable the operator to enter it (Fig. 18.4). This surgically created space aids the operator and will provide access to the uterovesical fold of the peritoneum. It continues laterally between the two leaves of the broad ligament. A finger placed here, whilst probing medially, gives the plane of cleavage. The bladder is then pushed medially and upwards, thus separating it. Dissection is continued medially till the other end is reached. Uncommonly, such as in the case of a patient with two previous caesarean sections, a similar dissection is required from the other end either to meet in the centre or to go completely around.

The space is bound anteriorly by the bladder and the anterior leaf of the broad ligament. It is bound posteriorly by the uterocervical surface and the posterior leaf of the broad ligament. The contents are the loose areolar tissue, lateral uterocervical margin and the uterine vessels (Fig. 18.5).

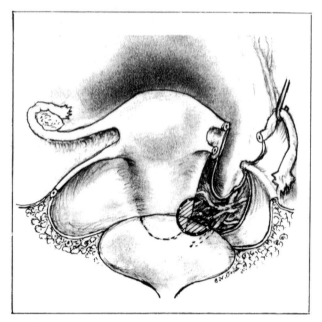

Fig. 18.5 Entry from the lateral angle near the uterovesical junction on the lateral uterocervical border helps to get a window space or uterocervico broad ligament space (circle of dotted lines) to begin bladder separation medially. Contents are well seen.

SUTURING TECHNIQUE

First described by Halban in 1932[51] this method replaces the use of a clamp with a direct suture. It has many advantages in that it is easier to use than a clamp and saves time. Since it does not occupy any space, it is particularly useful in nulliparae and where the uterus is enlarged. There is less tissue reaction, infection and postoperative pain. There are also fewer chances of injury to the ureter.

In my personal series this suturing technique was employed in all cases. It was extremely helpful when space was at a premium.

DEBULKING

This is required for an enlarged uterus when all accessible tissue has been cut and no further uterine descent is possible. Restricted mobility, less space and strong ligaments are responsible. If the fundal top cannot be reached by the fingers passed from behind or in front of the uterus, then debulking will be needed for further surgery. If the fundal top can be well felt, it is invariably possible to deliver the fundus from one of the two spaces after the uterine and ascending vessels have been secured.

Debulking a myomatous uterus is gratifying surgery, in contrast to debulking an adenomyotic uterus. It is not necessary to remove many or all of the myomas. The most accessible, largest myoma is the one that is selected. Posterior wall myomas are more easily accessible than anterior wall ones and, therefore, removable. As long as the operator can reach even a bit of a large myoma and grasp it, then it can be separated bit by bit, till the whole of the myoma is cut in toto or has been morcellated. If a large myoma cannot be removed as a whole, it can be debulked by morcellation. Once the fundus is accessible, the debulking can be stopped.

If the enlargement is due to adenomyosis, the bulging uterine wall or adenomatous area can be debulked by morcellating myometrial chunks. Once a large amount is removed, further access for surgery will ensue. Alternatively, Lash's method[25a] of coring can be used for non-myomatous uteri,[25b] but is rarely required if morcellation and the dechunking are used. It was used in 236 cases in the author's series without resorting to Lash's technique, by enucleating the myoma or morcellating myometrial chunks. When there is a vertically enlarged uterus and the uterocervical length is increased without an increase in anteroposterior or transverse diameters, then vertical bisection is preferred. This was amply performed by Kovac[25] by the coring method.

OOPHORECTOMY AT VAGINAL HYSTERECTOMY

The sole purpose of removing the ovaries prophylactically is to prevent ovarian malignancy or any benign problem arising in the conserved ovaries. The debate on preservation versus removal dates from the 19th century, when Lawson Tait, father of surgery, was accused of 'spaying' women (cited in Studd 1989[33]); the controversy appears to be unending.

In a study undertaken by Jacobs & Oram,[52] it was found that 85% of members and fellows of the Royal College of Obstetrics and Gynaecology remove the ovaries in postmenopausal women and 59% in women aged 49 years or older. Tindall[53] recommends removal after 47 years of age. It is essential to fulfil prerequisites and rule out any contraindications.

Studd[33] has shown a clear advantage of prophylactic oophorectomy, including a 47% chance of further surgery when ovaries are preserved at hysterectomy for endometriosis.[54] Studd is of the opinion that prophylactic oophorectomy should be offered to all women over 40 years having abdominal hysterectomy and should only be performed after full discussion and consent. In a personal communication, J. Donald Woodruff has said that the ovaries should be removed in patients over the age of 40 years if the abdomen must be opened for any pelvic pathology.[55] Also, they should be removed whether the hysterectomy is vaginal or abdominal.

Capen[56] suggests the selective removal of ovaries through the vagina in selected patients and the surgeon must be skilled. In a study of hysterectomy among women of reproductive age, less than 2% had their ovaries removed when the hysterectomy was vaginal and 35% at abdominal hysterectomy.[19]

There is no place for risky surgical acrobatics, and only if transvaginal oophorectomy or salpingo-oophorectomy can be performed safely and under vision, should it be done.[49] It is often easier to remove the ovary only, leaving the tube in situ.[57]

The cervix and ovaries are prone to disorders which can be malignant. The ovaries are worse because of their inaccessibility for screening and diagnosis and the added disadvantage of the poor prognosis of ovarian carcinoma. To leave behind the ovaries at hysterectomy is to lose an opportunity for prophylactic removal and is as dangerous, if not worse, as leaving behind the cervix at abdominal hysterectomy. Indeed, in cases with a high risk of ovarian malignancy, leaving behind the ovary makes the hysterectomy incomplete.

Routine oophorectomy was possible in 702 of 740 vaginal hysterectomies in women older than 45 years of age with a past or family history indicating removal.[30] The decision was based on the rationale that if the patient was undergoing abdominal hysterectomy and her ovaries were to be removed, the same principle would apply to vaginal hysterectomy. There were no major complications. It is strongly suggested that the selection of the vaginal route for hysterectomy should not deprive a woman of prophylactic oophorectomy, nor should the lack of expertise in performing oophorectomy at vaginal hysterectomy be the reason to adopt the abdominal route with its increased morbidity. It is apparent as well as appropriate that a beginner will not attempt to do this, but a stage must come in every gynaecologist's career when he or she should be able to remove the ovaries at vaginal hysterectomy with ease. The earlier this expertise is attained, the better. The ideal is to begin learning in postmenopausal patients with third-degree uterine descent.

Being able to perform oophorectomy at vaginal hysterectomy gives added advantage when such a need arises unexpectedly. This may be the case when a vaginal hysterectomy is performed for menorrhagia and during surgery the removed uterus shows endometrial malignancy. It is also applicable in patients who are at high risk for ovarian cancer but due to previous incisional hernia repair cannot be operated abdominally and must be subjected to a vaginal hysterectomy.

URETER AT VAGINAL HYSTERECTOMY

Of ureteral injuries occurring during hysterectomy, two-thirds occur during abdominal hysterectomy and one-third at vaginal hysterectomy. This is borne out in Everett & Mattingly's series of 1500 major pelvic operations, where 60% of ureteral injuries were from abdominal operation and 40% from vaginal hysterectomy.[58] Injury at straightforward vaginal hysterectomy is rare. It is vital, however, to remain close to or hugging the lateral margin of the uterus and cervix.

The ureter is at risk in vaginal hysterectomy when:

1. the uterosacral and Mackenrodt's ligaments are clamped without retracting the bladder, particularly the lateral angles;

2. the uterine clamp slips;

3. too much traction is applied to the cervix, without a retractor in the uterovesical space, thus bringing the ureteral knee closer;

4. the anatomy is distorted due to previous caesarean section, when the bladder is displaced to one side, bringing one of the ureters medially;

5. in procedentia, if the uterovesical space is not secured before the ligaments are clamped.

MORBIDITY AND MORTALITY

The mortality of vaginal hysterectomy at most centres is less than 0.1%,[37] Dicker[19] had one death in 810 cases. At King's College, in the last 15 years, there have been no deaths following hysterectomy,[33] neither did Pratt[59] have any. There were no fistulae in Pratt's 1000 cases, but 3 patients required a laparotomy for retroperitoneal bleeding. Copenhaver[46] reported a series of 1000 vaginal hysterectomies with and without repairs, without any damage to the bowel. In the author's personal series of 3800 vaginal hysterectomies, there was 1 death, 4 bladder injuries, 1 rectal injury, 1 ureteral injury, 1 ileal loop injury and 2 patients required a laparotomy.

DISCUSSION

When a hysterectomy is to be undertaken, it should be the endeavour of every gynaecologist to consider first the vaginal route; only when there is a contraindication to this should the abdominal route be resorted to. Since the commonest gynaecological operation is hysterectomy, there is ample opportunity to learn and perfect the art of vaginal surgery.

It is mandatory for every gynaecologist to attain such a degree of operating skill by the different routes since the reasons for or against doing hysterectomy vaginally are the advantages or disadvantages to the patient, who is the only one to be considered.[57]

If the technique is learnt in simple cases, the operator's confidence will grow and fears diminish, whilst the judgement for indications and contra-indications will sharpen. Then a time will come when the number of vaginal hysterectomies will increase and consequently, the number of abdominal hysterectomies will decrease.

The operative treatment of dysfunctional uterine bleeding, adenomyosis and fibroids should be by the vaginal route. After all, debulking is a part of surgical exercise. Does one give up on even the toughest abdominal hyster-ectomy? Then why should one flinch from flimsy adhesions at vaginal hysterectomy? It is often said that the pelvic findings are not in favour of a vaginal hysterectomy, but it is seldom admitted that the gynaecologist in question does not favour the vaginal route!

As the frontiers of science advance, operative techniques are scaling new heights through operative laparoscopy and hysteroscopic endometrial ablation. However, many gynaecologists will continue to treat a large

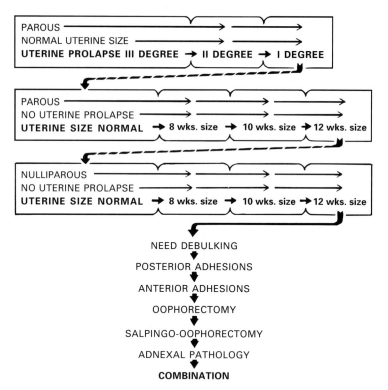

Fig. 18.6 Flow chart showing the stages for developing operative technique in vaginal hysterectomy starting from a straight forward normal-size parous uterus with third-degree descent to more difficult presentations and more complex procedures.

number of patients by hysterectomy. It will be in the best interest of the patient if the vaginal or gynaecological route is mastered.

Developing expertise in operative technique must begin from a very favourable normal-size parous uterus with third-degree descent to gradually less favourable and finally, what is considered unfavourable to difficult as shown in Fig. 18.6.

ACKNOWLEDGEMENT

The author wishes to thank Dr V. Karani MD for her untiring help in the compilation of this manuscript.

REFERENCES

1. Langenbeck J C M. Geschichte einer von mir glucklich verrichteten extirpation der ganzen gebarmutter. N Biblioth Chir Ophthalm 1819–1820 1: 551
2a. Soranus. Quoted by Senn N. The early history of vaginal hysterectomy. JAMA 1895; 25: 476–482
2b. Czerny. Zur laparo-hysterotomie. Wien Med Presse 1879; 20: 1265–1268

3. Koeberle cited in Studd J W W. Hysterectomy and menorrhagia, Baillieres Clin Obstet Gynaecol 1989; 3: 415–424
4. Jackson A R. Vaginal hysterectomy for cancer. JAMA 1885; 5: 169–171
5. Schauta F. Die hauptindication der vaginalen total-exstirpation ist und bleibt des carcinoma uteri, Wien Med Bl 1890; 13: 551–553
6. Doyen (1939) Cited in Green-Armytage V B. Vaginal hysterectomy: new technique — follow-up of 500 consecutive operations for haemorrhage. J Obstet Gynaecol Br Empire 1939; 46: 848–856
7. Green-Armytage V B. Vaginal hysterectomy: new technique — follow-up of 500 consecutive operations for haemorrhage. J Obstet Gynaecol Br Empire 1939; 46: 848–856
8. Palmer A C. Discussion on the role of vaginal hysterectomy in treatment of prolapse. Proc R Soc Med 1948; 41: 676
9. Howkins J. Discussion on the role of vaginal hysterectomy in treatment of prolapse. Proc R Soc Med 41: 676–677
10. Stallworthy J. The present status of hysterectomy. Practitioner 1957; 178: 291–297
11. Stallworthy J. Donald Fothergill meeting. J Obstet Gynaecol Br Commonwlth 1961; 68: 1061–1065
12. Watson P S. Late results in vaginal hysterectomy. J Obstet Gynaecol Br Commonwlth 1963; 70: 29
13. Van Bastiaanse B M A. In: Atti del symposium internazionale su i virilismi in ginecologis e su la terapia del cancero del corpo dell'utero. Florence: Scientifiche Salpietra, 1962
14. Navratil E. The place of vaginal hysterectomy. J Obstet Gynaecol Br Commonwlth 1965; 72: 841–846
15. Mitra S. Radical vaginal hysterectomy and extraperitoneal pelvic lymphadenectomy for cancer of the cervix. J Obstet Gynaecol Br Empire 1955; 62: 672–675
16. Mitra S. Extraperitoneal lymphadenectomy and radical vaginal hysterectomy for cancer of the cervix (Mitra technique). Am J Obstet Gynecol 1959; 78: 191–196
17. Purandare B N. Vaginal hysterectomy with review of author's 203 cases. J Obstet Gynecol 1946; 7: 77–80
18. Babcock W W. The technique for vaginal hysterectomy. Surg Gynecol Obstet 1932; 54: 193–199
19. Dicker R C, Scally M J, Greenspan J R et al. Hysterectomy among women of reproductive age — trends in USA 1970–78. JAMA 1982; 248: 323–327
20. Howkins J, Stallworthy J. Vaginal hysterectomy and hysterocolpectomy. In: Bonney's gynaecologic surgery. 8 ed. London: Bailliere Tindall, 1974: pp 226–254
21. Moore J G. Vaginal hysterectomy with intra pelvic adhesions — clinical problems. In: Nichols D H, ed. Injuries and complications of gynecologic surgery. 2 ed. Baltimore, Md: Williams & Wilkins, 1988: pp 102–107
22. Krige C F. Vaginal hysterectomy and genital prolapse repair. A contribution to the vaginal approach to operative gynaecology. Johannesburg: Witwaterstand University Press, 1965
23. Weaver R T, Johnson F L. Vaginal hysterectomy. Am J Obstet Gynecol 1951; 62: 1117–1123
24. Mattingly R F, Thompson J D. (eds) Te Linde's operative gynecology. 8 ed. Philadelphia: J B Lippincott 1985: pp 225–230, 548–555
25a. Lash A F. A method for reducing the size of uterus in vaginal hysterectomy. Am J Obstet Gynecol 1941; 42: 452–459
25b. Kovac S R. Intramyometrial coring as an adjunct to vaginal hysterectomy. Obstet Gynecol 1986; 67: 131–136
26. Hawksworth W, Roux J P. Vaginal hysterectomy. J Obstet Gynecol Br Empire 1958; 65: 214–228
27. Centaro A, de Laurentiis G, Morresi G. Riv Obstet Ginec 1965; 19: 587
28. Gray L A. Vaginal hysterectomy. Ann Surg 1954; 139: 666–678
29. Richter K, Lakomy W. Ueber die scheidenlange nach der abdominalen and vaginalen uterusexstirpation. Zentralbl Gynakol 1953; 75: 1921–1925
30. Sheth S S. The place of oophorectomy at vaginal hysterectomy. Br J Obstet Gynecol 1991; 98: 662–666
31. Thom M, White P J, Studd J W W et al. Prevention of and treatment of

endometrial disease in climacteric women receiving oestrogen therapy. Lancet 1979; i: 455–457
32. Noble A D. Management of menorrhagia. Br Med J 1985; 291: 296–297
33. Studd J W W. Hysterectomy and menorrhagia. Bailliere's Clin Obstet Gynecol 1989; 3: 415–424
34. Sheth S S, Asher L I. Clinical evolution of vaginal hysterectomy. J Obstet Gynecol India, 1966; 6: 534–539
35. Burke W C Jr. Vaginal hysterectomy for epithelioma of the cervix. New York Med J. 1883; 37: 103
36. Edwards E A, Beebe R A. Vaginal hysterectomy. Surg Gynecol Obstet 1949; 89: 191–199
37. Jeffcoate. Hysterectomy and its aftermath. In: Jeffcoate's principles of gynecology. Revised by Tindall V R. London: Butterworths, 1987: pp 706–709
38. Sheth S S, Malpani A. Vaginal hysterectomy for the management of menstruation in mentally retarded women. Int J Gynaecol Obstet 1991; 35: 319–321
39. Jordan J A. The management of premalignant conditions of the cervix. In Studd J, ed. Progress in obstetrics and gynecology, vol 2. Edinburgh: Churchill Livingstone, 1982
40. Copplesonn M. Cervical intraepithelial neoplasia gynecologic oncology. Fundamental principles and clinical practice. New York: Churchill Livingstone, 1981: pp 457–464
41. Navratil E. In: La prophylaxie en gynécologic et obstétrique. Tome I. Conférences et rapports du congress international de gynécologic et d'obstétrique. George, Geneva: Librairie de Université, 1954
42. Kempers R D, Hunter J S Jr, Welch J S. Indications for vaginal hysterectomy. Obstet Gynecol 1959; 13: 677–682
43. Smith L R, Pratt J H. Vaginal hysterectomy in the geriatric patients. Obstet Gynecol 1959; 14: 84–91
44. Mitchell G W. Benign and malignant disease of the breast. In: Mattingly R F, Thompson J D, eds Te Linde's operative gynecology. 8th ed. Philadelphia: J B Lippincott 1985: pp 183–202
45. Ingiulla C. Vaginal hysterectomy for treatment of carcinoma endometrium. Am J Obstet Gynecol 1968; 100: 541–543
46. Copenhaver E H. Vaginal hysterectomy — an analysis of indications and complications among 1000 operations. Am J Obstet Gynecol 1962; 84: 123–128
47. Gray L A. Prolapse of the uterus and vagina and various operations. In: Vaginal hysterectomy. 2nd ed. Springfield, Il: Charles C. Thomas, 1963: pp 44–61
48a. Pratt J H, Symmonds R E, Welch J S. Vaginal hysterectomy for carcinoma of the fundus. Am J Obstet Gynecol 1964; 88: 1063–1071
48b. Sheth S S, Malpani A. Routine prophylactic oophorectomy at the time of vaginal hysterectomy in postmenopausal women. Arch Gynecol Obstet 1992; 251: 87–91
48c. Sheth S S. Vaginal dimple: a sign to diagnose endometriosis. J Obstet Gynecol 1991; 2: 292
49. Nichols D H. Update on surgery. Contemp J Obstet Gynecol 1987; 29: 92–109
50. Nichols D H. Clinical problems, injuries and complications of gynaecologic surgery. 2 ed. Baltimore, Md: Williams & Wilkins, 1988: pp 102–107, 130–132
51. Halban J. Gynakologische operations. Lehre, Vienna, UR Bau & Schwarzenberg, 1932
52. Jacobs I, Oram D. Prevention of ovarian cancer. A survey of the practice of prophylactic oophorectomy by Fellows and Members of the Royal College of Obstetricians and Gynaecologists. Br J Obstet Gynecol 1989; 111: 756–765
53. Tindall V R. Hysterectomy and its aftermath. Jeffcoate's principles of gynecology, Revised by Tindall V R. 5 ed. London: Butterworths, 1987: pp 706–709
54. Montgomery J C, Studd J W W. Oestradiol and testosterone implants after hysterectomy for endometriosis. Contrib Gynecol Obstet 1987; 16: 241–246
55. Woodruff D J. Personal communication, 1986
56. Capen C, Irwin H, Margin J, Masterson B. Vaginal removal of the ovaries in association with vaginal hysterectomy. J Reprod Med 1983; 28: 589–593
57. Cohen J. Abdominal and vaginal hysterectomy — new techniques based on time and motion studies. 1st ed. London: Heinemann Medical; 1972: 72–132
58. Everett H S, Mattingly R F. Urinary tract injuries resulting from pelvic surgery. Am J Obstet Gynecol 1956; 71: 502
59. Pratt J H. A personal series of 1000 vaginal hysterectomies. South Med J 1980; 73: 1360

19. The role of transvaginal sonography in gynecologic oncology

J. Carter   L. B. Twiggs

Transabdominal sonography has dramatically altered the practice of obstetrics and gynecology. Unfortunately image resolution is not as good as we would like. With the introduction of transvaginal sonography (TVS) image resolution has improved dramatically. The transducer is closer to the pelvic organs and so higher frequencies can be used, reducing attenuation of the sound beam, resulting in improved overall image quality.[1]

From our earliest days in medical school we are drilled with the concept of performing a thorough and accurate physical examination. Even more so, in our specialty of obstetrics and gynecology, we rely heavily on the accuracy of our vaginal examination. But just how accurate is the vaginal examination? In a prospective study[2] we have determined that over 40% of our vaginal examinations were inaccurate when compared to TVS. Similarly, Andolf & Jorgensen[3] found ultrasound superior to clinical examination in terms of sensitivity (83 and 67%, respectively), whereas specificity was similar for both methods (96 and 94%, respectively).[4] Granberg & Wikland[5] were able to detect normal postmenopausal ovaries by bimanual palpation in only 30% of cases, compared to 87% in other series, by ultrasound.[6-8]

What about the accuracy of transabdominal sonography (TAS) compared to TVS? TAS and TVS were compared by Tessler et al in 108 non-pregnant patients.[9] The studies were independently obtained by two radiologists and interpreted on the basis of identical clinical information. Overall TVS was superior in 65 cases (60.2%), equal in 39 (36.1%) and inferior in 4 (3.7%). They concluded that TVS should replace TAS in the initial assessment of gynecologic disorders. Similarly, Lande et al[10] in comparing TAS and TVS found that TVS added diagnostically useful information in 89% patients with cystic adnexal masses, and in 66% of patients with tubo-ovarian abscess. Additional clinical information can also be obtained by TVS. By using variations in pressure with the probe, precise localization of pelvic tenderness can be determined, under direct real-time visualization.

OVARY

TAS has been utilized as a screening tool for the early detection of ovarian

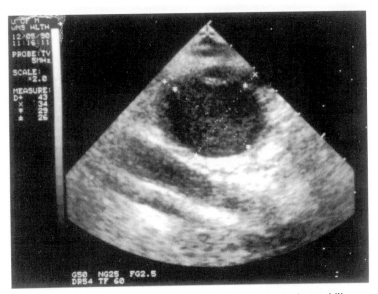

Fig. 19.1 A normal ovary lying in its characteristic position over the internal iliac artery and vein.

cancer with mixed results.[11–14] Other results using TVS have been encouraging.[15,16] Included in these reviews are prospective analyses of at-risk patients for ovarian carcinoma. The pick-up rate is in the order of 2–3%. The combination of a pelvic examination by an experienced gynecologist, a TVS and a CA-125 has not been reported as most of the studies have been conducted by radiologists using TAS.

The ovaries are usually identified in their characteristic location, lying on the pelvic side wall just medial to the internal iliac vein (Fig. 19.1). This anatomical relationship is useful to remember in patients whose ovaries are difficult to visualize. By careful scanning in this location, most ovaries can usually be identified.[17] There are many influencing factors governing ovarian size. These include age, parity, obesity, menstrual status and use of hormone replacement therapy. Premenopausal ovarian volume is influenced greatly by the stage of the menstural cycle. Preovulatory volume varies between 5.1 and 6.2 cm³, while the postovulatory volume averages about 3.2 ± 1.7 cm³.[18] Due to the enormous fluctuation in size of the ovary, three-dimensional measurements are preferred over two-dimensional measurements. By applying the formula for a prolate ellipse ovarian volume is determined:

$$\text{Volume} = (\pi/6) \times D_1 \times D_2 \times D_3$$

where the maximum transverse (D_1), anteroposterior (D_2) and longitudinal (D_3) diameters are measured.[19]

Ovarian volumes in postmenopausal women tend to be half that of premenopausal women. Higgins et al[20] determined mean normal postmenopausal ovarian volumes to be 2.9 cm³, but with a very wide range of 0.4–7.8 cm³. Goswamy et al[21] calculated ovarian volumes on 2246 postmenopausal women and found the right ovarian volume to average 3.58 cm³ (s.d. 1.40; range 1.00–14.01 cm³) and left ovarian volume to average 3.57 cm³ (s.d. 1.37; range 0.88–10.90 cm³). All ovaries assessed as of normal morphology by ultrasound were found to be so at subsequent laparotomy. Regression analysis of their data revealed that the most important predictors of ovarian volume was the number of years since the menopause. Other factors significantly affecting volume include weight, parity, age at menopause and a history of breast cancer. After the menopause there is a sharp decrease in ovarian volume, and an early menopause is associated with smaller ovaries throughout the remainder of life. In scanning ovaries in postmenopausal women it is useful to remember that some ovaries are highly placed in the pelvis and gentle abdominal manipulation may be needed to move them closer to the vaginal probe. Also bowel shadowing may obscure the view: fasting patients for a few hours may reduce this problem.[22,23]

Ovarian morphology and size were studied by Campbell et al.[24] The volume difference between the right and left ovaries averaged 1.48 ± 19 cm³. They concluded that an ovary with a volume more than twice normal, and/or twice the size of its fellow should be regarded as suspicious.

OVARIAN CARCINOMA

Epithelial ovarian cancer is now the leading cause of death from gynecologic malignancies. It is unusual in young women; its incidence rises after age 40 to the eighth decade, where a plateau occurs. As the symptoms and signs of patients with ovarian cancer are often overlooked or ignored until advanced-stage disease is present, Goswamy et al[25] believe that ovarian cancer screening should begin in all women aged over 45 years by TVS.

It is unfortunate that in those women who do present for regular pelvic examination, due to the inherent inaccuracy of the examination, errors are made. As discussed above, even in our own hands, clinical impression of the vaginal examination was incorrect in 40% of cases. To examine adequately a postmenopausal women, who may be obese or have a stenotic atrophic vagina, may even further increase the inaccuracies in this subgroup of women.

Many of us have been indoctrinated with the philosophy of 'the palpable postmenopausal ovary syndrome'. For a number of reasons this concept is outdated. To screen properly for ovarian cancer, detection should occur prior to the lesion being clinically palpable (Fig. 19.2). A 1.0 cm cancer lesion has been present for 30 tumor doublings and has been present for 60% of its lifespan, and has approximately 10⁹ cells present. Also, even

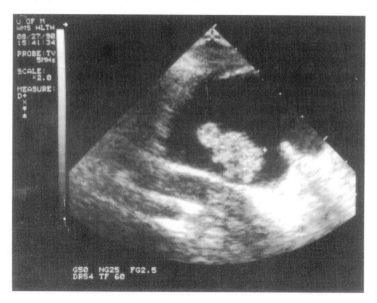

Fig. 19.2 A small, non-palpable carcinomatous ovary surrounded by ascites.

though the mean postmenopausal ovarian volume is in the order of 3.0 cm³, the range varies considerably, with the maximum volume in the order of 7.8 cm³, which is easily clinically palpable. TVS allows accurate determination of ovarian volume in these patients, and importantly, an assessment of the internal architecture or morphology of the ovary. Schoenfeld et al[26] identified 29 postmenopausal women by TVS with unilateral simple cysts with no separations or solid components, diameters less than or equal to 5 cm and with no free fluid in the pelvis. All underwent surgical exploration, with the finding of benign histopathology in all. Rubin & Preston[27] published a 4-year experience with adnexal masses in postmenopausal women using TAS, and only 1 in 32 patients whose masses were less than 5 cm had an endometroid carcinoma 3 cm in size. Perhaps if TVS were used, this patient too could have been identified on other criteria. Nevertheless, it appears from these preliminary data that small (<5 cm) unilocular postmenopausal cysts have a low incidence of malignant disease. Andolf and colleagues[28] used ultrasound for detection of ovarian enlargement in 805 women aged between 40 and 70 years, in 99% of whom the ovaries and/or their vessels could be identified. Various ovarian lesions were found in 35 women, including five mucinous and serous cystadenomas, one carcinoma, two borderline tumors and a cancer of the caecum, none of which were detected by manual or pelvic examination.

A multimodal prospective study reported by Jacobs and colleagues[29] of screening for ovarian cancer amongst apparently healthy postmenopausal women revealed that over 1000 women were screened with vaginal examination, CA-125 estimation and abdominal ultrasound. The specificity for ovarian cancer of serum CA-125 measurement and vaginal examination was 97.0 and 97.3% respectively. By combining serum CA-125 measurement and ultrasound, and vaginal examination and ultrasound, specificities of 99.8 and 99.0% respectively were achieved. By combining all three tests, 100% specificity was achieved, indicating that although no individual screening test has acceptable specificity for ovarian cancer, the combination of the three achieved an acceptable specificity.[29]

In a large ovarian cancer screening program using TAS, Campbell et al[24] obtained a positive result in 338 screens (2.3%) out of a total of over 14 000 screens. They were able to identify 5 patients with early-stage primary ovarian cancer and 4 patients with metastatic ovarian cancer. Their overall false-positive rate was 2.3%, with a specificity of 97.7%. The predictive value of a positive result on screening was 1.5%. The odds that a positive result on screening indicated the presence of an ovarian tumour, any ovarian cancer or primary ovarian cancer were about 1:2, 1:37 and 1:67 respectively.

UTERINE CORPUS

The uterine corpus is an important structure in TVS. It serves as a useful anatomical landmark for targeted organ imaging. Once identified, its relationship with intrapelvic structures and masses can be determined.[30, 31] The endometrial appearance varies throughout the menstrual cylce. In the proliferative phase, the endometrial thickness increases and appears either iso- or hypoechoic. During the midcycle or periovulatory period, a characteristic trilaminar appearance occurs, while in the luteal phase, increasing tortuosity of the endometrial glands and glycogen accumulation result in a hyperechoic endometrium.

The thickness of the endometrium is measured from the echogenic interface of the junction of endometrium and myometrium. This measurement represents two layers of endometrium. The hypoechogenic halo is not included in the measurement, as this represents the inner layers of compact and vascular myometrium. The average thickness of the endometrium is greater in the secretory phase (3.6 ± 1.4 mm) than in the proliferative phase (2.9 ± 1.0 mm; $P \leq 0.05$).[32]

Endometrial atrophy in the postmenopausal period results in a thin hypoechoic endometrium on TVS. Five millimeters has been found to be the distinct cut-off point, below which all postmenopausal endometrium is inactive and normal.[33, 34] In a group of postmenopausal women, Schoenfeld and colleagues[26] assessed the thickness and structure of the uterine mucosa. Abnormal or suspicious endometrial patterns occurred in a thick and hyperechoic endometrium. Within the group of patients with sonographically suspicious endometria according to the above criteria, 81% were found to have endometrial cancer or adenomatous hyperplastic changes. In only 19% did the histological findings not confirm the ultrasonographical assessment. Within the group with sonographically normal endometrium, 98% had normal histological findings of atrophic endometrium.[35]

Fleischer et al[36] correlated the sonographic appearance of the endometrium with histopathologic findings in 38 patients who underwent hysterectomy. The thickness was accurately assessed within ±1 mm in 33 patients.

CARCINOMA OF THE ENDOMETRIUM

Endometrial cancer is now the most common gynecological malignancy, but is one of the least common causes of cancer deaths in women. This is due to the fact that most patients present early in their disease with abnormal bleeding. There still exists a group of patients — probably about 5% in total — who are asymptomatic, the diagnosis being made at operation for other reasons. A preoperative diagnosis in these patients may alter the surgical approach, including performing a radical hysterectomy and pelvic node dissection.[37] Even in the group where a preoperative diagnosis of endometrial cancer has been made, determination of endometrial tumor volume, depth of myometrial invasion and cervical extension may also alter the surgical approach.

Endometrial hyperplasia in postmenopausal women appears as a thickened, hyperechoic endometrium with an intact subendometrial halo. Microinvasive endometrial carcinoma may have similar ultrasonic features. Once invasion is established, the subendometrial halo, consisting of compact myometrium, is lost. This is the first ultrasonic feature of invasion seen sonographically. With more advanced myometrial invasion, a distinct tumor–myometrial interface can be visualized. Myometrial invasion may also produce a thickened and irregular central endometrial interface with echogenic or hyoechoic patterns combined with infiltration of hyperdense structures within the myometrium (Fig. 19.3).[38-40]

In an attempt to standardize measurements of myometrial invasion, Schoenfeld et al[26] measured invasion from the endometrial lumen to the most distant tumor interface. This distance was then divided by the total thickness of the uterine myometrium. If the lumen could not be discerned, the extent of myometrial invasion was estimated by dividing the total anteroposterior uterine distance by the total endometrial width. Myometrial invasion was suspected if this ratio exceeded 30%.

Myometrial invasion was accurately measured sonographically in 70% in a group of patients with endometrial cancer, within 10% of the actual measurement on the gross surgical specimen.[41] Preoperative assessment of myometrial invasion by TVS in a group of 25 patients with histologically proven endometrial cancer was determined by Gordon et al,[42] who found that in 84% of cases, TVS correctly predicted the depth of myometrial invasion within 15% of the actual measurement. TVS was found to be

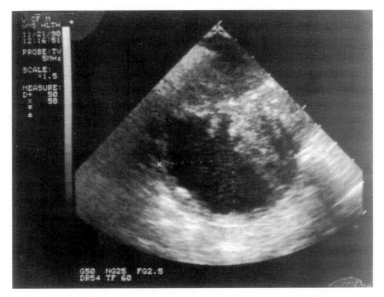

Fig. 19.3 A cystic carcinoma of the uterine corpus, with deep myometrial invasion.

accurate in 16 cases, with 3 misdiagnoses representing overestimation of deep invasion in superficially invasive tumors. Therefore the sensitivity of TVS in detecting deep invasion was 100%, the specificity was over 80%, and the accuracy was 84%.[26] Cacciatore et al[43] used preoperative ultrasound to stage 93 patients with endometrial cancer and were able to predict correctly myometrial invasion in 80%. Sonographic staging was accurate in 91% of cases.

CARCINOMA OF THE CERVIX

Preinvasive cervical cancer is common, with over 200 000 cases of cervical intraepithelial neoplasia occurring yearly in the USA and 50 000 new cases of carcinoma-in-situ diagnosed. Despite the early diagnosis and treatment of these preinvasive lesions, invasive cervix cancer remains the third most common gynecological malignancy in women, causing about 7000 deaths annually. Treatment of early-stage disease involves radical surgery to remove the tumor and adjacent parametria. Radical hysterectomy is usually combined with pelvic node dissection to give additional staging information regarding nodal spread. There is also evidence to suggest that cytoreduction improves the prognosis.[44]

The staging of cervix cancer is currently clinical, with patients allocated to different stages on preoperative vaginal examination. Due to the inaccuracies of the vaginal examination, and confusing inflammatory infiltration, up to 30% of cervix tumors are incorrectly staged.[45] In the search for a solution to the staging problem, pretherapeutic operative evaluation (staging

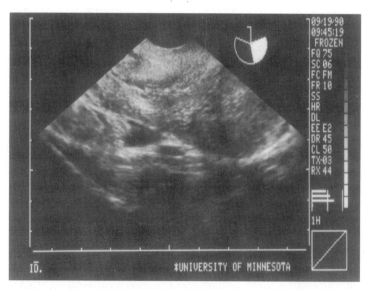

Fig. 19.4 A large, exophytic carcinoma of the uterine cervix, showing a clear demarcation between normal and tumor tissue.

laparotomy) has been advocated.[46,47] This procedure, though, may be associated with significant added morbidity.[48]

Prognostic factors for cervix cancer include patient age, stage, histological type, depth of invasion, tumor volume and presence of lymph node metastasis. At present, there are no large series of TVS as an adjunct in the clinical staging of cervix cancer. Cervical tumor size and depth of invasion have been evaluated by transrectal sonography (TRS),[49] most carcinomas being hypoechoic to the surrounding cervical tissue, although some appeared hyperechoic (Fig. 19.4). The maximal depth of invasion was graded according to whether the carcinoma was confined to the inner, middle or outer third of the cervical wall. In a study of 41 patients who underwent radical hysterectomy for cervical carcinoma, TRS correctly predicted the depth of cervical invasion in 85% of cases[49]. There were 4 cases where the extent of stage I carcinoma was overestimated, i.e. apparent extension of the carcinoma to the outer third of the cervix which was not confirmed histologically. There were only 2 cases in which the histologically verified depth of invasion was greater than the sonographic impression.

As mentioned above, the spread of cervical carcinoma to the parametria is a crucial factor in terms of clinical staging as well as treatment planning. When primary irradiation is elected, parametrial involvement can be tracked as a means of monitoring therapeutic response. Normal parametria should appear equal on both sides, exhibit smooth margins and taper off laterally in width (Fig.19.5). Sonographic changes suggestive of infiltration include a lateral disparity with unilateral shortening or widening and

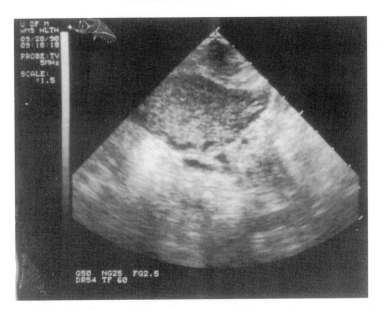

Fig. 19.5   Normal parametria, showing smooth tapering margins.

especially the presence of irregular parametrial margins. Additionally a shift of the cervix toward the affected side should raise suspicion of extrauterine spread.

Advanced-stage disease is diagnosed by distal vaginal spread or spread to the pelvic side walls. The pelvic side wall appears as a highly echogenic structure which delimits the field of view through acoustic absorption. Once disease has spread to the pelvic side walls, the pelvic ureter is usually obstructed with resultant hydroureter, hydronephrosis and renal failure. TVS is able to diagnose ureteric obstruction in these patients.

GESTATIONAL TROPHOBLASTIC DISEASE

TAS and TVS are important in the management of patients with gestational trophoblastic disease. With an enlarged uterus rising out of the pelvis, TAS is preferred. Complete molar pregnancy has a characteristic 'honey-combed' sonographic appearance. Partial hydatidiform mole has an abnormal conceptus with persistent embryonic or fetal elements and a placenta with a mosaic of normal-appearing villi alternating with areas of focal villous swelling and trophoblastic hyperplasia and is usually associated with autosomal trisomy. The uterus is enlarged in 30% of cases, normal for the period of amenorrhea in 30% and small for dates in 30%. Ovarian enlargement by thecalutean cysts is common.

Evacuation of molar pregnancy may be fraught with the danger of perforation, hemorrhage and incomplete evacuation. Suction curettage performed under continuous ultrasonic control is an invaluable technique to minimize the dangers of this procedure.

In managing patients with persistant disease postevacuation, TVS allows a closer view of the myometrium and uterine cavity. Localized disease within the myometrium is almost impossible to detect by computed tomography (CT) scan and TAS. TVS, preferably with color flow Doppler, provides a more accurate method of determining localized disease and response to treatment. Small localized foci of trophoblast can be imaged, and response to chemotherapy monitored. Schneider and associates[50] report such a patient. TVS was able to demonstrate a 2×2 cm intramural nodule. After chemotherapy this nodule showed liquefaction and subsequent resolution by TVS, paralleling the decline in beta human chorionic gonadotropin titres.

Duplex Doppler has also been utilized to assess the uterine circulation in patients with invasive mole and choriocarcinoma.[51] Those tumors requiring chemotherapy had a very low impedence to flow, suggesting the trophoblast in invasive mole and choriocarcinoma has a greater tendency to form large low-resistance channels within the myometrium compared to normal pregnancy.

RECURRENT GYNECOLOGIC MALIGNANCY

Despite the current radical surgical approach to gynecological cancer, and adjuvant chemo- and radiotherapy, recurrence remains a major problem and the cause of significant morbidity and resultant mortality. The majority of recurrences of cervix and endometrial cancers occur within the pelvis within 2–3 years of primary treatment. Current detection relies on vaginal examination (with its inherent inaccuracies) and vaginal vault cytology, supplemented usually by expensive CT scanning.

Although cell proliferation occurs continuously in human tumors, evidence indicates that it does not take place more rapidly in cancers than in their normal tissue counterparts. It is not the speed of cell proliferation but the failure of the regulated balance between cell loss and cell proliferation that differentiates tumor tissues from normal. When tumors are extremely small, growth follows an exponential pattern, but later seems to slow. Gompertzian growth means that as a tumor mass increases, the time required to double the tumor's volume also increases. If it is assumed that a tumor begins from a single malignant cell, then a 1 mm mass will have undergone approx 20 tumor doublings; a 5 mm mass will have undergone approx 27 tumor doublings; and a 1 cm lesion will have undergone approx 30 tumor doublings, and have been present for 60% of its life-span, and have approximately 10^9 cells present.

Thus clinical techniques recognize tumors late in their growth, and metastatic disease may well have occurred long before there is obvious evidence of the primary lesion. Also in late stage of tumor growth a very few doublings in tumor mass make a dramatic impact on the size of the tumor. Once a tumor becomes palpable (1 cm diameter), only three more doublings would produce an enormous tumor mass (8 cm diameter).

TVS may eliminate the subjectivity of the vaginal and rectal examination and provide a more objective assessment. A central recurrence typically appears as a hypoechoic, usually irregular area on the vaginal stump whose echo pattern usually resembles that of the primary tumor. Suspicious areas on the pelvic wall usually have more sharply defined borders, especially when the lesion is a carcinomatous lymph node (Fig. 19.6).[26]

DUPLEX DOPPLER SONOGRAPHY

Ultrasound has recently assumed a useful role in vascular diagnosis. The vessel wall and lumen can be visualized with B-mode ultrasound while the Doppler mode permits flow to be demonstrated and measured. The Doppler effect describes the change in frequency of ultrasound scattered by red cells moving within a vessel. If the ultrasound signal is transmitted along the axis of the vessel, then the velocity of the red cells can be related to the shift in Doppler frequency. If the signal approaches the vessel at an angle, then the frequency of the reflected signal is reduced in proportion to the cosine of that angle. The signal reflected from a moving interface contains frequency as well as amplitude information; therefore it is possible to process and display these data to show the relative motion of the target toward or away from the ultrasound transducer. The Doppler frequency

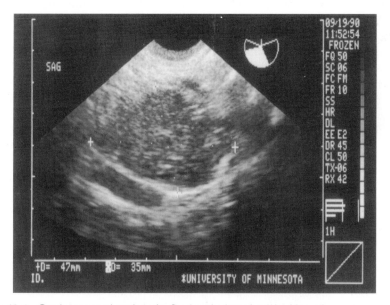

Fig. 19.6 Carcinomatous lymph node, fixed to the lateral pelvic side wall.

information may be presented for analysis as an audible signal, and/or in graphic form as a time-varying plot of the frequency spectrum of the returning signal. This is done using a fast Fourier transform to perform the frequency analysis. If the angle of the vessel axis to the ultrasound beam can be measured, accurate calculation of flow velocity is possible. The contour of the maximum Doppler shifted frequency corresponds to the variation in blood flow velocity over the cardiac cycle. This waveform shape is dependent on both the condition of the proximal circulation and on that of the distal receiving bed.[52] With a given pressure waveform at the entrance of an arterial segment, however, the time–velocity waveform shape will vary with the impedance of the receiving circulation, and this is apparent from the many different waveforms in the adjacent branches of the aorta in spite of the common origin. In color flow imaging, a color converter assigns colors based on the direction and variance of detected frequency shifts. Flow variance or turbulence in these images appears green, mixed with the red or blue that indicates flow direction. The velocity of flow is indicated by the brightness of each color displayed.

In 1971 Folkman and colleagues[53] proposed that the increasing cell population in a malignant tumor must be preceded by the production of new vessels to supply their metabolic needs. Numerous studies of experimentally induced tumors and angiographic findings in human tumors show that tumor vessels display characteristics that enable a presumptive diagnosis of malignancy to be made.[54,55] These pathologic vessels have an irregular course, and fail to branch and decrease in size, as do normal vessels. There is also an increase in arteriovenous malformations and so-called 'tumor lakes' where angiographic dye collects.[56] These abnormal vessesl do not have normal smooth muscle walls, the site of peripheral resistance and hence exhibit low resistance flow.[57] Doppler ultrasound has been able to differentiate benign from malignant tumors with a high level of specificity by assessment of its vascular supply and intratumoral blood flow.[58]

The assessment of pelvic flow involves the ultrasonic visualization of the uterus and ovaries. The uterine artery is then identified, just lateral to the cervix, in the base of the broad ligament. The maximum auditory and visual signal is obtained, and from this flow velocity waveform a spectral tracing provides the angle-independent estimator of velocity. There are a

Table 19.1 Indices of downstream resistance in common use for analysis of arterial flow velocity waveform

Index	Variable
Pulsatility index (PI)	A–B/mean
Resistance index (RI)	A–B/A
Systolic diastolic ratio	A/B

A = Peak systolic Doppler shift frequency; B = end diastolic shift frequency; mean = mean maximum Doppler shift frequency over the cardiac cycle.

number of these estimators, but the one most commonly used in gynecology is the pulsatility index (PI). Other estimators include the resistance index (RI) and the A/B ratio. These indices are ratios of the maximum Doppler shifted frequencies in systole and diastole (Table 19.1). A high PI generally reflects an increased impedance distally with resultant decreased flow, whereas a low PI reflects lowered impedance and an increased flow. In a similar fashion ovarian flow is estimated from the ovarian artery at the hilum of the ovary or within the ovarian stroma.

Flow during the normal menstrual cycle has been extensively studied. During the proliferative phase the uterine vessels appear similar to other arteries in the body with a prominent notch and little or no end diastolic velocity.[59] During the luteal phase there is a low diastolic flow, which is not continuous (i.e. during part of diastole there is no flow). Near the end of the secretory phase changes in the vessel compliance begin and an end diastolic component is usually present.

Studies have demonstrated that the flow velocity in the ovarian artery is dependent on serum hormone levels (i.e. on the phase of the menstrual cycle) and on the site of the dominant follicle.[60,61] In the luteal phase, the ovary containing the dominant follicle has a flow–velocity profile of low resistance flow, and increased diastolic flow. The ovary not containing the dominant follicle has low or absent flow during part of the diastole. This is also the flow pattern in both ovaries during the follicular phase of the cycle.[62, 63]

Using transvaginal color Doppler, Kurjak et al[64] determined the normal flow pattern of pelvic vessels. Diastolic flow was absent or small and the value of the RI was >0.05. In abnormal flow patterns, there is a high diastolic flow and the RI was <0.50. A statistically significant difference could not be shown between the left and the right uterine artery, even in patients with unilateral pelvic masses. They were able to show color flow inside the endometrium and myometrium in all cases of endometrial carcinoma. The peripheral impedance was very low in such cases with RI of 0.38 ± 0.06. Similarly, in all cases of adnexal malignancy, color flow was detected inside the tumor. Newly formed vessels showed very prominent blood flow with high velocity (20–60 cm/s) and very low resistance (RI = 0.25–0.45). Demonstration of small vascular branches inside the solid part of the tumor was a regular finding.

The accuracy of ultrasound assessment of flow was assessed by Taylor et al.[65] In a group of patients scheduled for laparotomy, Duplex assessment of flow was compared with an ultrasound probe applied directly to pelvic vessels at laparotomy. The ovarian arteries demonstrated qualitatively and quantitatively distinct flow patterns compared with the internal and external iliac arteries. The mean PI for the ovarian artery (1.58, s.d. 0.54, $n = 33$) was significantly lower than that for the internal iliac artery (2.81, s.d. 0.93, $n = 28$, $P < 0.001$) or the external iliac artery (5.59, s.d. 2.74, $n = 24$, $P < 0.001$).

Ultrasonic assessment of intratumoral flow in patients with benign pelvic masses such as fibroids, benign ovarian cysts etc. reveals that uterine artery blood flow has a high pulsatility (RI = 0.82 + 0.05). A regular finding in patients with malignant adnexal tumors was the demonstration of small vascular branches that ramify throughout the solid part of the tumor. All cases showed an almost identical velocity waveform characteristic with low pulsatility (RI = 0.33 + 0.08) and high velocity. Uterine artery flow velocity waveforms in a group of control patients showed a high pulsatility and a low or absent diastolic flow (RI = 0.84 + 0.08).[66] Hata et al[67] assessed uterine and tumor vascularity in 8 normal subjects and 97 patients with gynecologic pathology using real-time two-dimensional and pulsed-wave Doppler. Each arterial blood flow velocity waveform was classified into two types. The resistance indices of normal and abnormal flows were >0.7 and <0.7 respectively. Abnormal flows were not detected in normal patients. Typically abnormal flows were documented in all cases of endometrial carcinoma, ovarian carcinoma and trophoblastic disease. Doppler signals were not detected in 18/36 (50%) cases with cervical carcinoma, and abnormal flows were noted in only 6 (16.7%). All cases of cervical carcinoma with abnormal flows were stage IIB or greater. Doppler ultrasonic findings were consistent with those of pelvic angiography in the cases of trophoblastic disease.

Bourne et al[68] using this reasoning tried to assess whether changes in the intraovarian vasculature or blood flow impedance could be used to identify potentially malignant masses. They confirmed that malignant ovarian tumors showed clear evidence of neovascularization and PI values were significantly lower than for patients with benign pelvic pathology (PI = 0.3–1.0 versus 3.1–9.4, respectively). In a follow-up study[69] they described the use of transvaginal ultrasonography and color flow imaging in detecting endometrial cancer in postmenopausal women. They measured the impedance to uterine arterial and intratumoral blood flow and found that a PI of 2.00 would give a detection rate of 99.0% with a false-positive rate of 2.6%. In contrast, measurement of endometrial tumor thickness in the same group of patients (taking a cut-off value of 5 mm as the upper limit of normal) yielded a rate of detection of cancer of 99%, but a false-positive rate of 41%.

Probably the most vascular of all gynecologic tumors, and hence the most amenable to such investigations, are the gestational trophoblastic tumors. Shimamoto et al[70] demonstrated rapid blood flow within hypoechoic regions of invasive hydatidiform moles. After chemotherapy these areas disappeared, following the regression of the beta human chorionic gonadotropin curve. Long et al[71] assessed the uterine circulation in 38 patients with invasive mole or choriocarcinoma. Their results indicate that the uterine circulation in women with trophoblastic tumors requiring chemotherapy has a very low impedence to flow and is markedly different from that found in the non-pregnant state. This suggests that the trophoblast in invasive mole and choriocarcinoma has a greater tendency to form large low-resistance channels within the myometrium than in a normal pregnancy.

REFERENCES

1. Modica M M, Timor-Tritsch I E. Transvaginal sonography provides a sharper view into the pelvis. J Obstet Gynecol Neonatal Nurs 1988; 17: 89–95
2. Carter J, MacDonald L et al. Just how accurate is the vaginal examination? (Submitted J Reprod Med 1992)
3. Andolf E, Jorgensen C. A prospective comparison of clinical ultrasound and operative examination of the female pelvis. J Ultrasound Med 1988; 7: 617–620
4. Andolf E, Jorgensen C. A prospective comparison of transabdominal and transvaginal ultrasound with surgical findings in gynecologic disease. J Ultrasound Med 1990; 9: 71–75
5. Granberg S, Wikland M. A comparison between ultrasound and gynecologic examination for detection of enlarged ovaries in a group of women at risk for ovarian carcinoma. J Ultrasound Med 1988; 7: 59–64
6. Fleischer A C, Gordon A N, Entman S S. Transabdominal and transvaginal sonography of pelvic masses. Ultrasound Med Biol 1989;15: 529–533
7. Mendelson E B, Bohm-Velez M, Joseph N, Neiman H L. Gynecologic imaging; comparison of transabdominal and transvaginal sonography. Radiology 1988; 166: 321–324
8. Leibman A J, Kruse B, McSweeney M B. Transvaginal sonography: comparison with transabdominal sonography in the diagnosis of pelvic masses. AJR 1988; 151: 89–92
9. Tessler F N, Schiller V L, Perrella R R, Sutherland M L, Grant E G. Transabdominal versus endovaginal pelvic sonography: prospective study. Radiology 1989; 170: 553–556
10. Lande I M, Hill M C, Cosco F E, Kator N N. Adnexal and cul-de-sac abnormalities: transvaginal sonography. Radiology 1988; 166: 325–332
11. Timor-Tritsch I E, Bar-Yam Y, Elgali S, Rottem S. The technique of transvaginal sonography with the use of a 6.5 MHz probe. Am J Obstet Gynecol 1988; 158: 1019–1024
12. Schwimer S R, Lebovic J. Transvaginal pelvic ultrasonography. J Ultrasound Med 1984; 3: 381–383
13. Campbell S, Goswamy R, Goessens M, Whitehead M. Real-time ultrasonography for determination of ovarian morphology and volume. A possible early screening test for ovarian cancer? Lancet 1982; 2: 425–426
14. Campbell S, Royston P, Bhan V, Whitehead M I, Collins W P. Novel screening strategies for early ovarian cancer by transabdominal ultrasonography. Br J Obstet Gynaecol 1990; 97: 304–311
15. Andolf E, Jorgensen C, Svalenius E, Sunden B. Ultrasound measurement of the ovarian volume. Acta Obstet Gynecol Scand 1987; 66: 387–389
16. Andolf E, Jorgensen C, Astedt B. Ultrasound examination for detection of ovarian carcinoma in risk groups. Obstet Gynecol 1990; 75: 106–109
17. Rottem S, Levit N, Thaler I et al. Classification of ovarian lesions by high frequency transvaginal sonography. J Clin Ultrasound 1990; 18: 359–363
18. Granberg S, Wikland M. Comparison between endovaginal and transabdominal transducers for measuring ovarian volume. J Ultrasound Med 1987; 6: 649–653
19. Rodriguez M H, Platt L D, Medearis A L, Lacarra M, Lobo R A. The use of transvaginal sonography for evaluation of postmenopausal ovarian size and morphology. Am J Obstet Gynecol 1988; 159: 810–814
20. Higgins R V, Van Nagell J R, Donaldson E S et al. Transvaginal sonography as a screening method for ovarian cancer. Gynecol Oncol 1989; 34: 402–406
21. Goswamy R K, Campbell S, Royston J P et al. Ovarian size in postmenopausal women. Br J Obstet Gynaecol 1988; 95: 795–801
22. Van Nagell J R, Higgins R V, Donaldson E S et al. Transvaginal sonography as a screening method for ovarian cancer. A report of the first 1000 cases screened. Cancer 1990; 65: 573–577

23. Meire H B, Farrant P, Guha T. Distinction of benign from malignant ovarian cysts by ultrasound. Br J Obstet Gynaecol 1978; 85: 893–899
24. Campbell S, Bhan V, Royston P, Whitehead M I, Collins W P. Transabdominal ultrasound screening for early ovarian cancer. Br Med J 1989; 299:1363–1367
25. Goswamy R K, Campbell S, Whitehead M I. Screening for ovarian cancer. Clin Obstet Gynecol 1983; 10: 621–643
26. Schoenfeld A, Levavi H, Hirsch M, Pardo J, Ovadia J. Transvaginal sonography in postmenopausal women. J Clin Ultrasound 1990; 18: 350–358
27. Rubin M C, Preston A L. Adnexal masses in post-menopausal women. Obstet Gynecol 1987; 70: 578–581
28. Andolf E, Svalenius E, Astedt B. Ultrasonography for early detection of ovarian carcinoma. Br J Obstet Gynaecol 1986; 93: 1286–1289
29. Jacobs I, Stabile I, Bridges J et al. Multimodal approach to screening for ovarian cancer. Lancet 1988; 153: 268–271
30. Mendelson E B, Bohm-Velez M, Joseph N, Neiman H L. Endometrial abnormalities: evaluation with transvaginal sonography. AJR 1988; 150: 139–142
31. Malpani A, Singer J, Wolverson M K, Merenda G. Endometrial hyperplasia: value of endometrial thickness in ultrasonographic diagnosis and clinical significance. J Clin Ultrasound 1990; 18: 173–177
32. Fleischer A C, Kalemeris G C, Entman S S. Sonographic depiction of the endometrium during normal cycles. Ultrasound Med Biol 1986; 12: 271–277
33. Goldstein S R, Nachtigall M, Snyder J R, Nachtigall L. Endometrial assessment by vaginal ultrasonography before endometrial sampling in patients with postmenopausal bleeding. Am J Obstet Gynecol 1990; 163: 119–123
34. Nasri M N, Coast G J. Correlation of ultrasound findings and endometrial histopathology in postmenopausal women. Br J Obstet Gynaecol 1989; 95: 1333–1338
35. Schurz B, Metka M, Heytmanek G, Wimmer-Greinecker G, Reinold E. Sonographic changes in the endometrium of climacteric women during hormonal treatment. Maturitas 1988; 9: 367–374
36. Fleischer A C, Kalemeris G C, Machin J E, Entman S S, James A E. Sonographic depiction of normal and abnormal endometrium with histopathologic correlation. J Ultrasound Med 1986; 5: 445–452
37. Osmerw R, Volksen M, Schauer A. Vaginosonography for early detection of endometrial carcinoma? Lancet 1990; 335:1569–1571
38. Chambers C B, Unis J S. Ultrasonographic evidence of uterine malignancy in the postmenopausal uterus. Am J Obstet Gynecol 1986; 154: 1194–1199
39. Scott W W, Rosenshein N B, Siegelmann S S, Sanders R C. The obstructed uterus. Radiology 1981; 141: 767–770
40. Breckenridge J W, Kurtz A B, Ritchie W G M, Macht E L. Postmenopausal uterine fluid collection: indicator of carcinoma. AJR 1982; 139: 529–534
41. Fleischer A C, Dudley B S, Entman S S, Baxter J W, Kalemeris G C, James A E. Myometrial invasion by endometrial carcinoma: sonographic assessment. Radiology 1987; 162: 307–310
42. Gordon A N, Fleischer A C, Reed G W. Depth of myometrial invasion in indometrial cancer: preoperative assessment by transvaginal ultrasound. Gynecol Oncol 1990; 39: 321–327
43. Cacciatore B, Lehtovirta P, Wahlstrom T, Ylostalo P. Preoperative sonographic evaluation of endometrial cancer. Am J Obstet Gynecol 1989; 160: 133–137
44. Potish R A, Downey G O, Adcock L L, Prem K A, Twiggs L B. The role of surgical debulking in cancer of the uterine cervix. Int J Rad Oncol Biol Phys 1989; 17: 979–984
45. Zander J, Baltzer J, Lohe K J, Ober K G, Kaufmann C. Carcinoma of the cervix: an attempt to individualize treatment. Am J Obstet Gynecol 1981; 139: 752–759
46. Potish R A, Twiggs L B. An analysis of adjuvant treatment strategies for carcinoma of the cervix. Am J Clin Oncol 1989; 12: 430–433
47. Twiggs L B, Potish R A, George R J, Adcock L L. Pretreatment extraperitoneal surgical staging in primary carcinoma of the cervix uteri. Surg Gynecol Obstet 1984; 159: 243–250
48. Oakley G J, Downey G O, Twiggs L B, Adcock L L, Carson L F, Potish R A. Operative morbidity of surgical staging in carcinoma of the uterine cervix: impact of nodal metastases and influence on recurrence. (Submitted Obstet Gynecol 1992)

49. Bernaschek G, Deutinger J, Kratochwil A. Endosonography in obstetrics and gynecology. Berlin: Springer-Verlag, 1990: 97–122
50. Schneider D F, Bukovsky I, Wwinraub Z, Golan A, Caspi E. Transvaginal ultrasound diagnosis and treatment follow-up of invasive gestational trophoblastic disease. J Clin Ultrasound 1990; 18: 110–113
51. Long M G, Boultbee J E, Begent R H J, Hanson M E, Bagshawe K D. Preliminary Doppler studies on the uterine artery and myometrium in trophoblastic tumours requiring chemotherapy. Br J Obstet Gynaecol 1990; 97: 686–689
52. Evans D H, Barrie W W, Asher M J, Bentley S, Bell P R F. The relationship between ultrasonic pulsatility index and proximal arterial stenosis in a canine model. Circ Res 1980; 46: 470–475
53. Folkman J, Merler E, Abernathy C, Williams G. Isolation of a tumor factor responsible for angiogenesis. J Exp Med 1971; 33: 275
54. Ney F G, Feist J N, Altemus L R, Ordinario V R. Characteristic angiographic criteria of malignancy. Radiology 1972; 104: 567–570
55. Gammill S L, Shipkey R B, Himmelfarb E H, Parvey L S, Rabinowitz J G. Roentgenology-pathology correlative study of neovascularity. AJR 1976; 126: 376–385
56. Strickland B. The value of arteriography in the diagnosis of bone tumors. Br J Radiol 1959: 32: 705–713
57. Kurkak A, Jurkovic D, Alfirevic Z, Zalud I. Transvaginal color Doppler imaging. J Clin Ultrasound 1990; 18: 227–234
58. Jellins J, Kossoff G, Boyd J, Reeve T S. The complementary role of Doppler to the B-mode examination of the breast. J Ultrasound Med 1983; 2: 29–37
59. Schulman H, Fleischer A, Farmakides G et al. Development of uterine artery compliance in pregnancy as detected by Doppler ultrasound. Am J Obstet Gynecol 1986; 155: 1031–1036
60. Baber R J, McSweeney M B, Gill R W et al. Transvaginal pulsed Doppler ultrasound assessment of blood flow to the corpus luteum in IVF patients following embryo transfer. Br J Obstet Gynaecol 1988; 95: 1226–1230
61. Steer C V, Campbell S, Pampiglione J S, Kingsland C R, Mason B A, Collins W P. Transvaginal colour flow imaging of the uterine arteries during the ovarian and menstrual cycles. Hum Reprod 1990; 5: 391–395
62. Taylor K J W, Burns P N, Wells P N T et al. Ultrasound Doppler flow studies of the ovarian and uterine arteries. Br J Obstet Gynaecol 1985; 92: 240
63. Thaler I, Manor D, Rottem S, Timor-Tritsch I E, Brandes J M, Itskovitz J. Hemodynamic evaluation of the female pelvic vessels using a high-frequency transvaginal image-directed Doppler system. J Clin Ultrasound 1990; 18: 364–369
64. Kurjak A, Zalud I, Alfirevic Z, Jurkovic D. The assessment of abnormal pelvic blood flow by transvaginal color and pulsed doppler. Ultrasound Med Biol 1990; 16: 437–442
65. Taylor K J W, Burns P N, Wells P N T, Conway D I, Hull M G R. Ultrasound Doppler flow studies of the ovarian and uterine arteries. Br J Obstet Gynaecol 1985; 92: 240–246
66. Kurjak A, Zalud I, Jurkovic D, Alfirevic Z, Miljan M. Transvaginal color Doppler for the assessment of pelvic circulation. Acta Obstet Gynecol Scand 1989; 68: 131–135
67. Hata T, Hata K, Senoh D et al. Doppler ultrasound assessment of tumor vascularity in gynecologic disorders. J Ultrasound Med 1989; 8: 309–314
68. Bourne T, Campbell S, Steer C, Whitehead M I, Collins W P. Transvaginal colour flow imaging: a possible new screening technique of ovarian cancer. Br Med J 1989; 299: 1367–1370
69. Bourne T H, Campbell S, Whitehead M I, Royston P, Steer C V, Collins W P. Detection of endometrial cancer in postmenopausal women by transvaginal ultrasonography and colour flow imaging. Br Med J 1990; 301: 369
70. Shimamoto K, Sakuma S, Ishigaki T, Makino N. Intratumoral blood flow: evaluation with color Doppler echography. Radiology 1987; 165: 683–685
71. Long M G, Boultbee J E, Begent R H J, Hanson M E, Bagshawe K D. Preliminary Doppler studies on the uterine artery and myometrium in trophoblastic tumours requiring chemotherapy. Br J Obstet Gynaecol 1990; 97: 686–689

20. The treatment of cervical intraepithelial neoplasia

A. Bigrigg   J. Browning

Cervical intraepithelial neoplasia (CIN) describes the histopathological condition where part or whole of the thickness of the cervical squamous epithelium is replaced by cells showing varying degrees of atypia. It encompasses dysplasia and carcinoma-in-situ (CIS). It is currently graded as CIN I, II or III according to the differentiation of basal, intermediate and superficial thirds of the epithelium, but the conditions are recognized as being part of a continuous process.

Dyskaryosis is a cytological term used to describe cells compatible with origin from CIN or carcinoma of the cervix. It is classified as mild, moderate or severe according to appearances suggesting origin from CIN I, II or III. The distinction between changes compatible with human papillomavirus (HPV) infection or CIN I is particularly difficult to make.

Cytological grading correlates poorly with subsequent histological diagnosis. This correlation can be substantially improved if the three cytological grades are merged to two.[1] The Bethesda system[2] divides abnormal smears into those showing high- and low-grade squamous intraepithelial lesions (SILs).

The exact rate and the course of progression from pre-cancer to invasive disease is not known. Indeed, because of ethical problems in the appropriate trial construction, this information will probably remain unknown. The existing knowledge is fraught with confounding factors:

1. Much old data exist, where a new disease process may have evolved.
2. Punch biopsy may be an unreliable end-point (see below)
3. Cone biopsy diagnosis, on the other hand, is reliable but affects treatment and so precludes proper observation.

Of 131 women in Auckland, New Zealand, who continued to have abnormal cytology after CIN III on cone biopsy, 18% had invasive lesions at 10 years and 36% at 20 years.[3] Robertson et al[4] have demonstrated a 46% regression of CIN I over a 2-year cytological follow-up without treatment.

At present we cannot identify which individuals with CIN have the potential for malignant progression. A blanket approach to treatment is therefore necessary.

Current opinion largely favours the treatment of patients with CIN II or III lesion, although conservatism may be justified for CIN I.

ASSESSMENT

Prior to treatment the cervix is usually assessed by a cervical smear, colposcopy and biopsy. Other methods include endocervical curettage, microcolpohysteroscopy and cervicography.

Cervical smears

Cervical smears may have a false-negative rate to 15% in detection of histologically confirmed CIN. Operator experience is of cardinal importance. However, the Aylesbury spatula with a long endocervical tongue and Cervex (plastic brush spatula) may improve the quality of pick-up over the conventional Ayre's spatula.[5]

The detection rate of abnormal cells in a given population is the best measure of sampling efficiency.[6] The presence of endocervical cells provides evidence that the endocervix has been sampled but for a low-risk population of over 20000 women Mitchell & Medley[7] have shown that the incidence of CIN is not significantly different between a group whose smears showed endocervical cells and those whose smears lacked them. The endocervical brush (cytobrush) has a greater pick-up of endocervical cells and should perhaps be used in conjunction with a conventional spatula for screening the high-risk population who have had previous surgery.

The taking of two simultaneous smears or repetition of the first smear at 6-month intervals decreases the false-negative rate but incurs extra laboratory costs. Good-quality control at the laboratory is mandatory. This can be extended to individual smear-takers if a computerized cervical screening programme is in operation.[8]

Colposcopy

Binocular microscopy of the cervix is used to examine the whole transformation zone and to define and biopsy abnormal epithelium. Visual diagnosis on the basis of epithelial, vascular and acetic or iodine stain characteristics is demonstrably inaccurate (37.5% correct diagnosis) when compared with biopsy of the whole transformation zone.[9] In a 10-year period in British Columbia 10% of invasive carcinoma and 16% of microinvasive carcinoma was misdiagnosed at colposcopy.[10]

Diagnostic biopsy

Two methods in common use are punch biopsy and low-voltage diathermy loop excision biopsy. Punch biopsy tends to crush and may not include stroma. A low-voltage diathermy loop biopsy requires more sophisticated equipment but can control haemorrhage and produces samples of greater size. Prendiville et al[11] have shown that the artefactual damage is minimal. As larger biopsies can be taken the diagnosis of microinvasion or invasion is more easily made. The false-negative rate of small biopsies is of concern (54%) particularly if microinvasive or invasive lesions are missed.[9] Buxton and colleagues[12] describe undercalling by punch biopsy in 47% of cases and notes: 'These findings have important implications both for patient management and for trial design and must cast doubt on the results of studies in pre-invasive disease using directed punch biopsies as an end point'.

Endocervical curettage

This technique is more widely used in the USA than the UK. The endocervical canal is sampled to exclude glandular or squamous dysplasia or carcinoma. Wright et al[13] reported the use of endocervical curettage after large loop excision of the transformation zone. In only 1 of 155 patients was information obtained that would have altered the clinical outcome. If adenocarcinoma or a skip lesion is suspected, a large cone biopsy is indicated in any case.

Microcolpohysteroscopy

In 1984 Soutter and associates[14] reported the use of microcolpohysteroscopy to define the extent of endocervical involvement of CIN when the upper limit of the lesion could not be seen at colposcopy. They demonstrated good correlation between microcolpohysteroscopy and histological measurements. This technique is currently not widely used, although Hallam et al[15] have harnessed it to tailor the depth of large loop excision.

Cervicography

This is a photographic screening technique whereby a technician may take a colpophotograph after applying acetic acid. Its main value is in teaching and screening. If allied to cervical cytology, it may increase screening sensitivity.[16]

TREATMENT

Treatment has hitherto been either by a local destructive method or by excision. Local destructive therapy was attractive as it could be performed under local anaesthetic as an outpatient procedure. It was acceptable where colposcopic assessment was satisfactory. If colposcopy was unsatisfactory (entire transformation zone not visible) then cold knife cone biopsy or hysterectomy was preferred.

This dichotomy has been blurred with the emergence of large loop excision of the transformation zone (LLETZ) and laser cone biopsies. These procedures can be performed as outpatient procedures and excisional histology is available.

Destructive methods

These may be used when the following criteria apply:

1. The entire lesion is visualized within the transformation zone.
2. There is no suggestion of microinvasive or invasive cancer.
3. There is no suspicion of endocervical glandular disease.
4. The cytology and histology correspond.

These methods are cryotherapy, electrocoagulation diathermy, cold coagulation and laser vaporization. The aim of local destructive therapy is to ablate to a depth where all CIN within gland crypts would be destroyed without unnecessarily destroying normal tissue. Anderson & Hartley[17] measured the depth of crypt involvement with CIN in 343 cone biopsies. They showed that destruction to a depth of 3.8 mm would eradicate 99% of involved tissues. Boonstra and colleagues[18] consider 4 mm to be an adequate depth. Most colposcopists aim for a depth of destruction or excision of at least 5 mm, although accurate assessment of this depth is difficult (Table 20.1).

Cryotherapy

Cryonecrosis is effected by crystallization of intracellular water. Freeze–thaw–freeze techniques produce best results. Tissue is destroyed to a depth of 4–5 mm. There is some concern as to the adequacy of this technique. It can, however, be performed with little or no analgesia. Charles & Savage assessed the literature and found that cure rates varied from 27 to 96%.[19]

Electrocoagulation diathermy

This destroys tissue by a combination of fulguration and coagulation.

Table 20.1 Destructive methods of treatment of CIN

	Cryocautery	Electrocoagulation diathermy	Cold coagulation	Laser vaporization
Depth of destruction	2–5 mm	7–10 mm	3–4 mm	5–7 mm
Analgesia required	None/Local	General/Local	Local	Local
Success rates (at 1 year)	27–96%[19]	88–97%[20, 21]	94%[22]	94%[23]

Temperatures of over 700°C are produced, making it relatively painful. It is therefore usually performed under general anaesthesia. Discharge and bleeding may occur postoperatively but cervical stenosis appears uncommon. Tissue destruction is to at least 7 mm and cure rates of 88–97% are quoted.[20,21]

Cold coagulation

In this method the tissue is destroyed by application of a thermasound heated to 120°C to the cervical surface. Treatments of approximately 20 seconds are given to five overlapping areas. The equipment is simple to use and inexpensive. Local anaesthesia only is required. A cure rate of 94% may be achieved.[22]

Laser vaporization

Laser energy boils intracellular water, producing steam and exploding the cell. The carbon dioxide laser is theoretically and practically well-suited to cervical treatment. Power density and dwell time may be varied and the power may be pulsed or continuous. Laser equipment is expensive but vaporization techniques are easy to learn.

Depth of destruction can be controlled. The procedure can be performed under local anaesthetic. Primary and secondary haemorrhage may occur.

Laser vaporization remains a method of choice when CIN extends on to the vaginal fornices.

Excisional methods

Some form of excisional treatment is mandatory for the patient with an unsatisfactory colposcopy (see above). There is also a trend to low-morbidity excisional methods (LLETZ or laser cone) replacing the destructive techniques previously described.

Excisional methods offer advantages over destructive methods in terms of defining the nature of the lesion and completeness of excision.

Present published series of LLETZ and laser cones have shown the consistent finding of unexpected microinvasive or invasive carcinoma even when the lesions would have been considered suitable for destructive therapy. The incidence varies from 0.5 to 1.0%.[24–28]

When a histological specimen is produced it is also possible to judge completeness of excision. Incomplete excision is an important indicator of patients at high risk of recurrence. Bigrigg et al[24] recorded a 5.3% incomplete excision rate in their series of 1000 patients and one-third of these had recurrent CIN. Incomplete excision does not necessarily infer the presence of residual disease since it may be destroyed by the effect of the loop/laser, by subsequent attempts at haemostasis with the ball electrode, or it may spontaneously regress.

Cold knife cone biopsy

The first knife conization was performed by Lis Franc in 1815.[29] It is performed under general anaesthetic. Prior to excision Lugol's iodine is used to identify the iodine-negative ectocervix and haemostatic sutures may be placed in the cervix. Ideally a truncated cone or cylinder should be removed rather than a true cone which may transect gland crypts, leaving residual disease. A Beaver (bent-blade) knife may be helpful. Following excision haemostasis is usually obtained by suture. The inverting Sturmdorf suture should be avoided because of risk of cervical stenosis and burying of residual abnormal epithelium. Subsequent colposcopy may prove very difficult after cone biopsy with suturing where the new squamocolumnar junction is invisible in a high canal position.

Laser conization

This was described by Dorsey & Diggs in 1979.[30] It is performed under colposcopic control and only local anaesthesia is required. The initial circumferential cut is to some 7 or 8 mm depth. A small hook is then used to facilitate the inward movement of the beam to truncate the cone at the endocervical canal. Suturing is avoided where possible and by enlarging the laser spot, bleeding can be controlled by laser coagulation.

Baggish et al[23] compared laser conization and laser evaporization. They found few disadvantages to conization, apart from adding an average of 4 minutes to operating time.

Comparison of laser and cold knife cone biopsy. The therapeutic efficiency of both techniques of cone biopsy is similar to that of hysterectomy[23,31]

The frequent complications are those of haemorrhage, infection and cervical stenosis. Uterine perforation and pelvic abscess may occur (see Table 20.2).

Intra- and postoperative bleeding is a greater problem with cold knife

Table 20.2 Comparison of laser and cold knife cone biopsy

	Laser cone	Knife cone
Therapeutic efficiency[32-34]	93–96%	90–94%
Visibility of whole transformation zone after treatment[32]	66%	38%
Cervical stenosis after treatment[35]	7–25%	26–36%
Infection rate[34]	2.3%	6.8%
Peri- and postoperative bleeding[32,34]	1.8–5.0%	14.6–17%
Blood loss[34]		
Mean perioperative	1.6 ml	16.3 ml
Mean in first 24 hours	6.8 ml	80.0 ml

cone biopsy than laser cone or indeed any of the destructive techniques. This is because there is no coagulation element in the excision technique.

It is difficult to compare infection rates because of heterogeneity of diagnostic criteria; however, Larsson[34] reports infection more commonly after cold knife cone biopsy than after laser cone. Cervical stenosis may cause painful or absent menstruation with haematometra and also makes adequate cytological and colposcopic follow-up difficult. Bostofte et al[32] report that 12 weeks after surgery a cotton-wool probe could be inserted in the cervical canal for cytological sampling in 93% of women after laser cone but only 74% after cold knife cone. Four patients (6.8%) in the laser group and 2 (3.3%) in the cold knife group developed dysmenorrhoea due to stenosis of the cervical canal. Also, the complete transformation zone was more likely to be completely visible after laser than knife cone.

Cervical stenosis and infection may theoretically cause infertility. Hammond & Edmonds (1990)[36] postulate that the lack of cervical mucus may have a deleterious effect. No study, however, has ever shown that any treatment for CIN — except hysterectomy — has an effect on subsequent fertility.

Pregnancy complications have largely been confined to patients undergoing cold knife conization[37-39] Mid-trimester loss, increased rate of preterm labour, low birth weight and cervical dystocia leading to caesarean section are all described. All these trials can be criticized because of lack of proper controlled construction. It seems, however, that patients undergoing cold knife cone biopsy probably have a slightly increased risk of such complications compared to those undergoing destructive techniques. This may be related to the amount of destroyed tissue. No information is currently available about pregnancy following laser cone.

Operative times for the two techniques appear to be similar.[32] A major advantage of laser conization is that it can be performed as an outpatient procedure under local anaesthetic.

Laser cones also have the advantage of being performed under magnification through the microscope and the disadvantage that the specimen may have greater thermal artefact, making histological interpretation more difficult.

Large loop excision of the transformation zone

Large loop excision of the transformation zone is commonly known as LLETZ, low-voltage diathermy loop excision or loop electrosurgical excision procedure. Invention of new names is unhelpful and the authors will use the original acronym of LLETZ.

Original description of LLETZ. Prendiville et al first described large loop excision of the transformation zone in 1989.[27] Their report was confined to description of the technique for women in whom the transformation zone was fully visible and confined to the cervix. The technique can be used as

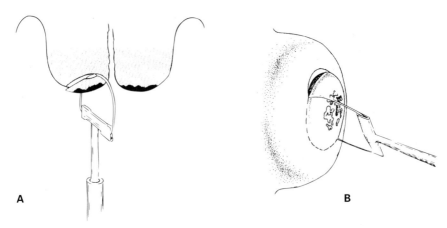

Fig. 20.1 (A and B) Two views of large loop excision of the transformation zone.

an alternative to cone biopsy and this was described by Mor-Yosef et al in 1990.[40] LLETZ is performed under colposcopic guidance. The loop is advanced into the cervix just lateral to the transformation zone until the required depth has been achieved. It is then taken slowly across the cervix enveloping the transformation zone (Fig. 20.1). It is withdrawn just beyond the other lateral margin of the transformation zone. The loop is moved slowly so the current will jump ahead of the wire, producing a clean cut with only superficial coagulative effect. If the wire is pushed across the cervix too forcefully there will be deeper coagulation but less cutting effect.

The transformation zone varies in shape and size, as does the depth of excision required, depending on the position of the squamocolumnar junction. Loop dimensions can be varied in width and depth. The transformation zone can be excised in one or more pieces. The authors prefer to use a loop of no greater diameter than 2 cm. The larger the loop, the more difficult it is to manipulate and there is a tendency to 'drag' in the tissue; it is necessary to increase the power used and possibly a greater amount of tissue is damaged.

If using the loop to excise tissue to a depth of 2 cm or more, the procedure can be performed in two stages with a wider initial excision at the ectocervix and a smaller-loop excision higher in the endocervical canal.

The diathermy power required depends on the amount of tissue in contact with the wire. The aim is to use sufficient power to cut through the tissue whilst minimizing tissue damage. Power should be going through the wire when it is initially brought into contact with the tissue. The diathermy machine used must have a steep power versus impedance curve. The improved technology of the diathermy machines is one of the main reasons why LLETZ is so much more successful today than the electrical conization procedures described earlier this century.

The loop itself consists of an insulated shaft connected to an insulated horizontal arm to which the hard stainless steel wire is attached. The wire is very thin (about 0.02 mm diameter), and reusable.

The procedure is performed under local anaesthetic. This is injected directly around the transformation zone, into the stroma underlying the transformation zone, or as a paracervical block.

Prior to Prendiville's description of LLETZ,[27] Cartier[42a] had described small loops for cervical biopsy and excision. He used a pure cut current which does not produce haemostasis and will not effect such a rapid passage. The tissue remains in contact with the wire longer and there is increased desiccation. In a non-controlled trial, Wright et al compared the effectiveness of using small-diameter (0.5–0.6 cm) wire loop electrodes against large-diameter (1.5–2.0 cm) electrodes. The small loop produced an 80% cure rate as opposed to 90% with the large loop. The tissue specimen was also less acceptable for pathological interpretation.[41]

Pathological techniques. When the transformation zone is removed in more than one piece, processing it can be difficult unless a technique such as that described by Codling et al[42b] is used. With this method the strips of cervix are pinned on to a corkboard in the correct orientation as they are removed. Another pin indicates the 12 o'clock position. The strips are then processed in a single specimen. Accompanying the specimen is a detailed diagram showing the area of abnormality at colposcopy.

Wright et al[41] have compared the histological changes in the cervical epithelium and stroma following carbon dioxide laser conization and loop excision. The type and extent of injury were almost identical although slightly greater carbonization was seen in the laser specimens. The artefact was assessed by direct measurement using a grid (Fig. 20.2).

Complications of LLETZ. Most patients will have vaginal bleeding and discharge for up to 2 weeks. In a small proportion this will persist for 12 weeks.[43] Secondary haemorrhage severe enough to require hospital admission occurred in only 6 out of 1000 patients in one series.[24]

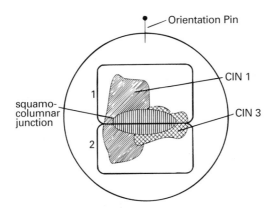

Fig. 20.2 Diagram of colposcopic appearance of the cervix.

The transformation zone is visible in 73–90% of patients after treatment.[26,43] Luesley et al report an incidence of 1.3% cervical stenosis, defining this as the inability to pass a Hegar 3 probe into the endocervix. All patients with stenosis had an excision deeper than 14 mm.[26]

Long-term side-effects are still incompletely documented. The longest follow-up to date is 22 months.[44] Bigrigg et al described 44 pregnancies from a group of 1000 women who underwent LLETZ following satisfactory colposcopy. Such pregnancies had an apparently normal course.[45]

Various studies have report therapeutic success rates up to 1 year of between 95 and 97%.[24–27] Bigrigg and associates report a recurrence rate of 0.7% in the second year following treatment. Ninety-four per cent follow-up was obtained. This is similar to the dysplasia rate in the back-ground population[44]

Comparison of laser versus LLETZ. In a controlled trial, 199 patients with histologically confirmed CIN II and III were randomized to treatment by carbon dioxide laser vaporization or LLETZ.[25] The women in the LLETZ group experienced less perioperative haemorrhage, less discomfort, and operative time was greatly reduced. There was no significant difference between the recurrence of CIN in the two groups. At 6-month follow-up recurrence rates of 8.2% (CIN II) and 7.5% (CIN III) were observed in the laser group, and 5% (CIN II) and 5.3% (CIN III) in the LLETZ group.

Other advantages of LLETZ include low initial capital outlay and portability of machinery. Laser carries a danger to the eyesight of patients and staff and necessitates the use of protective goggles.

There have been no randomized trials to date comparing laser cone excision and loop diathermy cone excision. Information relating the incidence of complications to the depth of LLETZ conization is also lacking.

Hysterectomy

In the past even radical hysterectomy and radiotherapy have been considered appropriate treatment for preinvasive disease.[46] Abdominal or vaginal hysterectomy is acceptable therapy for CIN but would normally only be performed if there was other coexisting gynaecological disease.

If the lesion extends into the vaginal vault, hysterectomy with excision of a demarcated cuff is appropriate. Complete excision is obtained more easily via the vaginal than abdominal route. The vault should be oversewn or sutured in a suitable manner to allow subsequent colposcopy.

Following hysterectomy for CIN follow-up is mandatory. Recurrences or de novo preinvasive disease (vaginal intraepithelial neoplasia) has been reported up to 20 years later, although most recurrences occur in the first 2 years.[31] Recurrence may be treated surgically or by laser vaporization, laser excision or knife excision.

Some patients, especially those with recurrent disease, request hysterectomy to rid themselves completely of their anxiety about the cervix. They

Table 20.3   Subsequent development of microinvasive or invasive carcinoma

Source	Method	Number of Patients	Incidence of microinvasive or invasive cancer
Coppleson (1976)[47]	Hysterectomy	8898	0.4%
Coppleson (1976)[47]	Cold knife cone biopsy	5442	0.3%
Gordon & Duncan (1991)[22]	Cold coagulation	1628	0.1%
Pearson et al (1989)[48]	Laser vaporization	4222	0.2%

must be informed of the extra morbidity and mortality with this procedure compared to others in common use and the possibility of subsequent invasive carcinoma even after hysterectomy (Table 20.3).

Combination techniques: excision and destruction

In large lesions where CIN extends from the cervix on to the vagina, a combination of excisional techniques for the transformation zone and laser vaporization for the periphery of the lesion is increasingly being used.

NEGATIVE HISTOLOGY

Negative histology occurs in this context when an excision biopsy specimen shows no evidence of expected CIN. The reasons for this may be:

1. False-negative histology.
2. False-positive cytology, colposcopy or punch biopsy.
3. Complete excision with initial biopsy.
4. Altered immune response as a reaction to biopsy, causing regression.
5. Time delay allowing spontaneous resolution between decision to treat and treatment.

It has previously been shown in this chapter that cytological, colposcopic and histological allocations all carry error and intraoperator error is common, especially in the cytopathological reporting of low-grade lesions.

Negative histology has been a major feature in all the published series on LLETZ (Table 20.4). There has been a tendency to associate negative

Table 20.4   Negative histology reported with LLETZ (no CIN found)

Series	Negative histology
Bigrigg et al (1990)[24]	4.7%
Luesley et al(1990)[26]	27.0%
Murdoch et al(1991)[43]	41.0%
Prendiville et al(1989)[27]	8.0%
Whiteley et al (1990)[49]	7.5%

histology exclusively with LLETZ. This is not the case. Skehan et al[9] reported a 20% rate in their series of laser cones. The same phenomenon has undoubtedly led to unnecessary treatment with destructive therapies. It is only with the development of excisional methods that the evidence is apparent rather than destroyed. It would appear that the problem cannot be obviated by prior punch biopsy. Murdoch and colleagues[43] in a series of 600 LLETZ procedures report an overall negative histology rate of 41%. Preliminary punch biopsies were taken in approximately 50% of cases. The negative histology rate was 38% in those who did not have prior punch biopsy and 43% in those who did. A punch biopsy was taken in cases when the colposcopist was less sure of what he or she was seeing. The lower the grade of referral cytology, the higher the negative histology grade.

Negative histology rates of 27–41% are not acceptable and must be improved. This may be achieved by better cooperation by pathologists and clinicians and more conservative treatment of borderline and mildly dyskaryotic lesions.

TREATMENT IN PREGNANCY

The pregnant patient with an abnormal smear should undergo colposcopy. The necessity for biopsy depends on the index of colposcopic suspicion of a microinvasive or invasive lesion. Treatment should be avoided if possible Iatrogenic bleeding is particularly distressing for a patient when pregnant. Although cold knife conization or wedge biopsy was previously performed, a small loop biopsy is ideal. Colposcopy should be repeated approximately every 3 months to ensure the lesion is not progressing. This is not more likely because of the pregnancy. It is therefore safe to leave treatment even of CIN III until after delivery, Van Nagell et al[50] described the major complication rate in 66 pregnant women having cone biopsies to be 7.5% compared to 3.4% in 529 non-pregnant patients. Conization during pregnancy was responsible for 5% fetal loss.

Antenatal smears may be difficult to interpret and some become negative in the postpartum period. The management dilemmas of a positive smear in pregnancy are best avoided by abandoning opportunistic antenatal smears and establishing a good population screening programme.

CHEMICAL TREATMENT

5-Fluorouracil, thymopetin and interferon have all been used in the treatment of CIN, but are not currently used as primary agents.

PREVENTION

Cervical cytology screening is the mainstay of any cervical carcinoma prevention programme. Good compliance will be optimized by a well-organized call and recall, preferably computerized, programme. Opportunistic screening is ineffective, resulting in the same relatively low-risk individuals being screened repeatedly. There is little increment in the benefit from screening a low-risk population more than once every 3 years, although women who have already had treatment for CIN should have yearly cytology.[51] Screening rates in excess of 90% are possible in stable communities with cooperation between pathologists, gynaecologists and general practitioners. Community-based nurses can be trained to take good-quality smears.

The patient should be counselled as to the harmful effects of smoking and the benefit of stopping.[52]

There should also be an explanation of the increased risks of multiple sexual partners with a view to either minimizing these or using barrier contraception. The male partner with genital warts or sexually transmitted disease should be investigated and treated.

SINGLE-VISIT DIAGNOSIS AND TREATMENT

Most patients can expect to visit the colposcopy clinic at least three times after having a cervical smear requiring referral. Diagnosis takes place at the first visit, treatment at the second and follow-up colposcopy at the third. Such a system is time-consuming for the patient and clinician. It leads to anxiety over a longer period for the patient and is costly.

Bigrigg et al[24] described single-visit diagnosis and treatment system. The cornerstones of this system are LLETZ and post-treatment cytological screening rather than colposcopy.

Prior to her clinic visit the patient should be suitably prepared both mentally and physically. Information about cervical smears, colposcopy and possible treatment should be sent to the patient. Included with this information may be a questionnaire. When this is returned the patient can then be sent an appointment for the middle of her menstrual cycle. Colposcopy is optimal at this stage. If the patient is taking the oral contraceptive pill, using an intrauterine contraceptive device, or is postmenopausal, a course of ethinyloestradiol (10 days 20 μg) prior to the appointment will increase the rate of satisfactory colposcopy[53,54] Johnson and colleagues[55] used Lamicel to improve exposure of the transformation zone but this needs to be passed intracervically and takes 3–4 hours to work.

Treatment without prior histological diagnosis can be performed if the patient has been referred with a dyskaryotic smear and the lesion is seen within the transformation zone. Excisional methods of treatment are preferable as the entire histology of the transformation zone will be available. The false-negative histology rate associated with single-visit LLETZ treatment (4.7%) is gratifyingly low.[24] Gordon & Duncan[22] treated 90% of patients referred with severe dyskaryosis by cold coagulation on their first clinic visit. They concede that 30 out of 1628 (1.8%) may have initially received inappropriate treatment.

In 1988 Posner & Vessey[56] showed that patient anxiety is greater during the wait for colposcopy and is only marginally less waiting for treatment at a second visit. It therefore seems reasonable to minimize the period between referral and treatment as much as possible. A single-visit system will reduce waiting lists and completely eliminate the wait between diagnosis and treatment.

Although post-treatment colposcopy is often recommended, supporting evidence that it is better than cytology is lacking. Lopes et al[57] in 1990 show that there was only one recurrence detected in 1000 colposcopic post-laser examinations that was not diagnosed on the first post-treatment smear. Murdoch et al from the same centre reported that in 600 colposcopic examinations after large loop excision 3 cases of residual disease were missed that were diagnosed cytologically. Cervical cytology in the same group was falsely negative only once.[43] There is no need for colposcopy again after treatment if excision was complete and cytological surveillance is negative.

Single-visit diagnosis and treatment are therefore safe and acceptable for most patients. A more cautious approach may be justified in women with low-grade lesion and an incomplete family.

PSYCHOLOGICAL CONSIDERATIONS

Marteau et al[58] show that anxiety levels among women about to undergo colposcopy were higher than in women the night before surgery and similar to those found following an abnormal result at antenatal serum alpha-fetoprotein screening for fetal abnormality. The women were as concerned about undergoing colposcopy as they were about what might be wrong with them. There was no relationship between the anxiety scores and the seriousness of referral.

Campion et al[59] have shown significant changes in patients' attitudes towards sex and towards their sexual partners.

These studies emphasize the need for sensitive handling and to provide as much information before, during and after treatment as possible (both verbal and written). Clinicians need to treat the whole patient as well as the whole transformation zone!

CONCLUSIONS

1. There has been a trend away from the radical hysterectomy or radiotherapy once advocated for treatment of CIN to cold knife cone biopsy and thence to conservative outpatient colposcopic treatment.

2. Colposcopy, even with directed biopsy, has a significant error rate: microinvasive and invasive lesions may be missed

3. Destructive therapies such as cold coagulation and laser vaporization should be supplanted by a method that excises the whole of the trans-

formation zone and has it available for histological scrutiny. Such methods are LLETZ and laser conization; the former is less expensive.

4. A single-visit diagnosis and treatment regime is applicable to many patients.

5. A knowledge of the natural history of low-grade lesions may allow a rational, more conservative approach to their treatment.

ACKNOWLEDGEMENTS

We are grateful to Josie Schoonderwoerd, Ron Jones and our other colleagues at Green Lane/National Women's Hospital, Auckland.

REFERENCES

1. Bigrigg M A, Codling B W, Pearson P, Read M D, Swingler G R. Specificity of cervical cytology in predicting the histological degree of dysplasia. J Exp Clin Cancer Res 1990; 9: 73
2. National Cancer Institute Workshop. The 1988 Bethesda system for reporting cervical/ vaginal cytological diagnoses. JAMA 1982; 262: 931–934
3. McIndoe W A, McLean M R, Jones R W, Mullins P R. The invasive potential of carcinoma in situ of the cervix. Obstet Gynecol 1984; 64: 451–458
4. Robertson J H, Woodend B E, Crozier E H, Hutchinson J. Risk of cervical cancer associated with mild dyskaryosis. Br Med 1988; 297: 18–21
5. Wolfendale M. Cervical samplers. Br Med J 1991; 302: 1554–1555
6. MacGregor J E. What constitutes an adequate cervical smear? Br J Obstet Gynaecol 1991; 98: 6–7
7. Mitchell H, Medley G. Longitudinal study of women with negative cervical smears according to endocervical status. Lancet 1991; 337: 265–267
8. Codling B, Bigrigg A. Cervical screening and Government policy. Br Med J 1989; 299: 855
9. Skehan M, Soutter W P, Lim K, Krausz T, Pryse-Davies J. Reliability of colposcopy and directed punch biopsy. Br J Obstet Gynaecol 1990; 97: 811–816
10. Benedet L L, Anderson G H, Boyes D A. Colposcopic accuracy in the diagnosis of micro-invasion and occult invasive carcinoma of the cervix. Obstet Gynecol 1985; 4: 557–562
11. Prendiville W, Davies R, Berry P L. A low-voltage diathermy loop for taking cervical biopsies: a qualitative comparison with punch biopsy forceps. Br J Obstet Gynaecol 1986; 93: 773–776
12. Buxton E J, Luesley D M, Rollason T P, Shafi M I, Redman C W E. Colposcopically-directed punch biopsy: an inaccurate and misleading investigation? Br J Obstet Gynaecol 1992; 99: 268–270
13. Wright T C, Gagnon S, Richart R N, Ferenczy A. Treatment of cervical intra-epithelial neoplasia using the loop electrosurgical excision procedure. Obstet Gynecol 1992; 79: 147–153
14. Soutter W P, Fenton D W, Gudgeon P, Sharp F. Qualitative microcolpohysteroscopic assessment of the extent of endocervical involvement by cervical intra-epithelial neoplasia. Br J Obstet Gynaecol 1984; 91: 712–715
15. Hallam N, Edwards A, Harper C et al. Diathermy loop excisions: a series of 1000 patients: an update. Proc Br Soc Colposcopy Cytopathol 1991
16. Wilkinson E J. Pap smears and screening for cervical neoplasia. Clin Obstet and Gynaecol 1990; 33: 824
17. Anderson M C, Hartley R B. Cervical crypt involvement by intra-epithelial neoplasia. Obstet Gynecol 1980; 55: 546–550
18. Boonstra H, Aalders J G, Koudstaal J, Oosterhuis J W, Janssens J. Minimal extension

and appropriate topographic position of tissue destruction for treatment of cervical intra-epithelial neoplasia. Obstet Gynecol 1990; 75: 227–231

19. Charles E H, Savage E W. Cryosurgical treatment of intra-epithelial neoplasia. Obstet Gynaecol Surv 1980; 35: 539–548
20. Woodman C B J, Jordan J A, Mylotte M J, Gustafeson R, Wade-Evans T. The management of cervical intra-epithelial neoplasia by coagulation electrodiathermy. Br J Obstet Gynaecol 1985; 92: 751–755
21. Chanen W, Rome R M. Electrocoagulation diathermy for cervical dysplasia and carcinoma in situ: a 15-year survey. Obstet Gynecol 1983; 61: 673–679
22. Gordon H K, Duncan I D. Effective destruction of cervical intra-epithelial neoplasia (CIN) 3 at 100°C using the Semm cold coagulator: 14 years experience. Br J Obstet Gynaecol 1991; 98: 14–20
23. Baggish M S, Dorsey J H, Adelson M. A ten-year experience treating cervical intra-epithelial neoplasia with the CO_2 laser. Am J Obstet Gynecol 1989, 161: 60–68
24. Bigrigg M A Codling B W, Pearson P, Read M D, Swingler G R. Colposcopic diagnosis and treatment of cervical dysplasia at a single clinic visit. Lancet 1990, 336: 229–231
25. Gunasekera P C, Phipps J H, Lewis B V. Large loop excision of the transformation zone (LLETZ) compared to carbon dioxide laser in the treatment of CIN: a superior mode of treatment. Br J Obstet Gynaecol 1990; 97: 995–998
26. Luesley D M, Cullimore J, Redman C W E et al. Loop diathermy excision of the cervical transformation zone in patients with abnormal cervical smears. Br Med J 1990; 300: 1690–1693
27. Prendiville W, Cullimore J, Norman S. Large loop excision of the transformation zone (LLETZ): a new method of management for women with cervical intra-epithelial neoplasia. Br J Obstet Gynaecol 1989; 96: 1054–1060
28. McIndoe G A J, Robson N S, Tidy J A, Mason W P, Anderson M C. Laser excision rather than vaporisation: the treatment of choice for cervical intra-epithelial neoplasia. Obstet Gynecol 1989; 74: 165–168
29. Lis Franc M J. Memoire sur l' amputation du col de l'uterus. Gaz Med Par 1834; ii: 385
30. Dorsey J H, Diggs E S. Microsurgical conisation of the cervix by carbon dioxide laser. Obstet Gynecol 1979; 54: 565–570
31. Hellberg D, Nilsson S. Twenty years experience of follow-up of the abnormal smear with colposcopy and histology and treatment by conisation or cryosurgery. Gyn Oncol 1990; 38: 166–169
32. Bostofte E, Berget A, Larsen J F, Pedersen P H, Rank F. Conisation by carbon dioxide laser or cold knife in the treatment of cervical intra-epithelial neoplasia. Acta Obstet Gynecol Scand 1986; 65: 199–202
33. Tabor A, Berget A. Cold knife and laser conisation for cervical intra-epithelial neoplasia. Obstet Gynecol 1990; 76: 633–635
34. Larsson G. Conization for preinvasive and early invasive carcinoma. Acta Obstet Gynecol Scand (suppl) 1983; 114: 1–40
35. Kristensen G B, Jensen L K, Holund B. A randomised trial comparing two methods of cold knife conisation with laser conisation. Obstet Gynecol 1990, 76: 1009–1013
36. Hammond R H, Edmonds D K. Does treatment for cervical intra-epithelial neoplasia affect fertility and pregnancy? Br Med J 1990; 301: 1344–1345
37. Leiman G, Harrison N A, Rubin A. Pregnancy following conisation of the cervix: complications related to cone biopsy. Am J Obstet Gynecol 1980; 136: 14–18
38. Jones J M, Sweetnam P, Hibbard B M. The outcome of pregnancy after cone biopsy of the cervix: a case-controlled study. Br J Obstet Gynaecol 1979; 86: 913–916
39. McCann S W, Mickal A, Crapanzano J T. Sharp conisation of the cervix. Obstet Gynecol 1969; 22: 470–475
40. Mor-Yosef S, Lopes A, Pearson S, Monaghan J M. Loop diathermy cone biopsy. Obstet Gynecol 1990; 75: 884–886
41 Wright T C, Richart R M, Ferenczy A. Comparison of specimens removed by CO_2 laser conization and loop electrosurgical excisional procedures. Obstet Gynecol 1992; 79: 147–153
42a. Cartier R. Practical colposcopy. 2nd ed. New York: S. Karger, 1984: pp 146–150, pp 202–212
42b. Codling B W, Bigrigg A, Pearson P, Read M D, Swingler G R. Histological

interpretation of tissue removed by diathermy loop excision. J Obstet Gynecol 1991; 11: 221–223

43. Murdoch J B, Grimshaw R N, Monaghan J M. Loop diathermy excision of the abnormal cervical transformation zone. Int J Gynaecol Cancer 1991; 1: 105–111
44. Bigrigg A, Codling B, Sheenan A, Pearson P, Read M, Swingler G. Description of long and short term complications after treatment of cervical intra-epithelial neoplasia (CIN) with low voltage loop diathermy. Int J Obstet Gynecol 1991; 5: 438
45. Bigrigg M A, Codling B W, Pearson P, Read M D, Swingler G R. Pregnancy after cervical loop diathermy. Lancet 1991; 337: 149
46. Galvin G A, Te Linde R W. The present status of non-invasive cervical carcinoma. Am J Obstet Gynecol 1949; 37: 15–32
47. Coppleson M. Management of pre-clinical carcinoma of the cervix. In: Jordan J A, Singer A, eds. The cervix uteri. London: Saunders, 1976: p 453
48. Pearson S E, Whittaker J, Ireland D, Monaghan J M. Invasive cancer of the cervix after laser treatment. Br J Obstet Gynecol 1989; 96: 486–488
49. Whiteley P F, Olah K S. Treatment of cervical intraepithelial neoplasia: experience with low voltage diathermy loop. Am J Obstet Gynecol 1990; 162: 1272–1277
50. van Nagell J R, Parker J C, Hicks L P, Conrad R, England G. Diagnostic and therapeutic efficacy of cervical conisation. Am J Obstet Gynecol 1975; 124: 134–139
51. Paul C, Bagshaw S, Bonita R et al 1991 cervical screening recommendations: a working group report. NZ Med J 1991; 104: 291–295
52. Berggren G, Sjostedt S. Pre-invasive carcinoma of the cervix uteri and smoking. Acta Obstet Gynecol Scand 1983; 62: 593–598
53. Prendiville W J, Davies W A R, Davies J O, Shepherd A M. Medical dilation of the non-pregnant cervix: the effect of ethinyl oestradiol on the visibility of the transformation zone. Br J Obstet Gynaecol 1986; 93: 508–511
54. Saunders N, Anderson D, Gilbert L, Sharp F. Unsatisfactory colposcopy and the response to orally administered oestrogen: a randomised double-blind placebo controlled trial. Br J Obstet Gynaecol 1990; 97: 731–733
55. Johnson N, Crompton A C, Wyatt J, Buchan P C, Jarvis G J. Using Lamicel to expose high cervical lesions during colposcopic examinations. Br J Obstet Gynaecol 1990; 97: 46–52
56. Posner T, Vessey M. Prevention of cervical cancer: the patient's view. England: Hollen St Press, 1988
57. Lopes A, Mor-Yosef S, Pearson S, Ireland D, Monaghan J M. Is routine colposcopic assessment necessary following laser ablation of cervical intra-epithelial neoplasia? Br J Obstet Gynaecol 1990; 97: 175–177
58. Marteau T M, Walker P, Giles G, Smail M. Anxieties in women undergoing colposcopy. Br J Obstet Gynaecol 1990; 97: 859–861
59. Campion M J, Brown J R, et al. Psychosexual trauma of an abnormal cervical smear. Br J Obstet Gynaecol 1988; 95: 175–181

21. Surgery for recurrent gynaecological cancer

J. H. Shepherd   K. F. Tham

Recurrent cancer for the patient is a failure of treatment. It presents a management dilemma to the clinician which is made no easier by the patient's expectations. Surgery in many cases offers the only realistic hope for a complete eradication of disease, and represents the last chance for survival. It is now more than 40 years since Brunschwig[1] described a one-stage abdominoperineal operation for the complete excision of the pelvic viscera for advanced carcinoma. Since then pelvic exenterative procedures have gradually gained widespread acceptance due to a steady decrease in mortality and morbidity, together with an improvement in survival. A total pelvic exenteration classically involves removal of the bladder, uterus, ovaries, vagina, rectosigmoid, anus, pelvic lymphatics and the soft tissues of the pelvis. In an anterior exenterative procedure the anorectum is preserved, while the bladder is preserved in a posterior exenteration.

INDICATIONS FOR PELVIC EXENTERATION

Pelvic exenterative surgery is performed for recurrent and sometimes advanced primary tumours of the pelvis. The tumour sites include those of the cervix, corpus uteri, vulva, vagina, ovary, bladder, colon, rectum, prostate and urethra. Gynaecological cancers form the majority of suitable cases, by virtue of their central position in the pelvis. With the exception of ovarian cancer they have a tendency to remain localized within the pelvis and to spread by continuity along tissue planes to neighbouring organs, before metastasizing to more remote areas. Of the gynaecological cancers by far the commonest indication for exenterative surgery is cervical cancer which has recurred after radiotherapy, accounting for between 60 and 80% of all cases.[2–8]

The main justification for pelvic exenterative surgery is generally accepted to be potential curability. However it has been suggested that palliative pelvic exenteration may bring about benefits which are worthwhile and comparable to those obtained in aggressive surgery for advanced ovarian malignancy.[9] The comparison may not be totally valid because in ovarian cancer effective chemotherapy is available after optimal surgery, while in recurrent cervical cancer no consistently effective postoperative therapy exists.[10] Deckers et al[11] believed that the elimination of symptoms such as pain, fistulae, pelvic sepsis, haemorrhage and malodorous areas of tumour necrosis are worthwhile objectives in the patient with advanced pelvic malignancy, significantly improving the quality of life for the patient and her family. Another series noted a lack of serious morbidity, short hospital stay and an acceptable 5-year survival of 23% in patients with metastatic nodal disease after palliative exenterative procedures.[9] In some cases dissection may have proceeded beyond the point of no return before unresectable tumour is found, and the pelvic exenteration becomes an unintentional palliative procedure by default. Very occasionally an exenterative procedure is carried out for radiation necrosis without histological evidence of recurrence.

The main arguments against palliative exenteration are the limited survival of patients with metastatic disease, and the mortality and the sometimes extreme morbidity associated with these procedures. The majority opinion appears to be that palliative exenteration is a futile exercise, with a high complication rate and a poor quality of life between surgery and death, especially in those with gross residual local or distant disease.[5,10,12,13]

DIAGNOSIS OF RECURRENT CERVICAL CANCER

When all the stages of cervical cancer are considered, about one in three patients will have recurrent or persistent disease following therapy. Recurrent disease is defined as evidence of a histologically proven tumour mass after initial treatment has led to the complete eradication of disease on clinical, surgical and pathological grounds. Improvement in radiation techniques over the years has generally led to a decline in the number of patients presenting with recurrent cervical cancer. Cervical screening has decreased the incidence of primary invasive cervical cancer itself, while surgery is curative in the majority of cases detected early.

The clinical presentation of the patient with recurrence is often insidious. Weight gain in the absence of significant leg oedema and fluid accumulation is a reassuring sign. Clinically it may be difficult to distinguish recurrent cancer on pelvic assessment from changes due to radiation fibrosis, previous surgery and a pelvic mass from adherent bowel loops. A smear for cytology is taken at each visit, though interpretation is difficult, especially in the first 3 months after completion of radiotherapy. This is due to the 'radiation effect', which produces distortion in cytological appearances.

Histological confirmation is essential, and an examination under anaesthesia is carried out with Trucut needle biopsies taken from the parametria and other suspicious areas. Lopez et al[14] noted a high diagnostic yield of almost 90% and minimal morbidity in the assessment of recurrent cancer after radiation with transvaginal parametrial needle biopsies. The associated complications include bleeding and pelvic sepsis, which are uncommon. Cystoscopy and proctosigmoidoscopy are often performed at the same time, and biopsies taken if necessary.

PELVIC EXENTERATION: PATIENT SELECTION

Proper selection of patients has been one of the main factors contributing to the decreasing mortality and morbidity of exenterative procedures.[15] The age of the patient should not by itself be an absolute contraindication to surgery,[5,16] though an upper limit of 70 years has been suggested.[6,17] It has been noted that the mortality rate in geriatric patients was only slightly increased compared to younger age groups.[5] However it does not seem reasonable to subject an obese patient in her 80s and beyond, with multiple medical problems, to a lengthy morbid operative procedure, and the prolonged period of postoperative rehabilitation that is required.

It is generally accepted that metastases outside of the pelvis are an absolute contraindication to pelvic exenteration. The triad of unilateral leg oedema, sciatic pain and ureteric obstruction is ominous and pathognomonic of pelvic side wall involvement and unresectable disease. Leg oedema suggests venous and lymphatic obstruction of the iliac vessels and channels, and sciatic pain implies neural sheath involvement of the sacral plexus.

Evaluation by chest X-ray, computer tomography (CT) with contrast enhancement, intravenous urography, lymphography, renal and liver function tests are done as part of the preoperative assessment and to exclude metastastic disease. Occasionally radioimmunoscintigraphy is helpful in defining the nature of suspicious areas seen on CT scans. Bone metastasis in recurrent cervical cancer is uncommon, with an incidence estimated at 1.8%,[18] and radionuclide bone scans are not part of the usual investigations when the patient is asymptomatic.

Scalene lymph node biopsy has been carried out prior to surgery so that patients with positive nodes would be excluded.[19] This however is not a routine procedure, and Manetta et al[20] demonstrated that none of 24 patients with recurrent cervical cancer being evaluated for exenterative surgery had metastases to the scalene nodes on biopsy.

Patients with major psychotic illnesses should be excluded. The stress of pelvic exenteration has been identified as threefold.[21] First is the feeling of inevitability and helplessness when the diagnosis of recurrent cancer is made. Then there is the trauma of undergoing yet another surgical procedure, of a significantly greater magnitude than what she has gone through so far. Unrealistic expectations, high anxiety levels and denial tendencies are unfavourable parameters. The third stress factor is the sense of mutilation with severe distortion in the perception of body and sexual image. In a retrospective questionnaire and interview survey of 74 women who had undergone major mutilating gynaecological surgery, 80% were found to have felt anxious and depressed. A third were distressed at the loss of reproductive function, and there was a significant degree of sexual dysfunction.[22] The reduction of libido and inhibition of sexual activity in the patient with a colostomy are well-established. In most series there will be a proportion of women who prefer death to mutilation.[21,22]

Cases where the recurrence is central and mobile, with no clinical and radiological evidence of fixation and parametrial involvement, are candidates for exploratory laparotomy. However fixation can be caused at times by radiation and fibrosis from previous surgery, as well as by pelvic inflammatory conditions. This issue often can only be decided upon at laparotomy. When the diagnostic investigations indicate disease outside of the pelvis an attempt should always be made to obtain histological confirmation with guided needle biopsies, before the patient is excluded from consideration for exenterative surgery.

The final decision to proceed to exenterative surgery is made at laparotomy. The entire abdomen is explored for extrapelvic disease, and sampling of the para-aortic nodes and pelvic lymphadenectomy carried out for frozen section analysis. Apparent fixation of the tumour mass to the pelvic side wall must be resolved by dissection and frozen section examination before a decision is made to discontinue the procedure. True tumour involvement of the pelvic side walls, positive high common iliac and para-aortic nodes, and extrapelvic spread are all contraindications to continuation of surgery. Generally about 40–50% are found to be unsuitable for exenteration at laparotomy.[2,3,8]

It is uncertain if positive pelvic nodes should be an absolute contraindication to exenterative surgery. It was noted that a significantly lower 5-year survival rate was associated with involved pelvic nodes[12,13,23,24] and survival was so brief and difficult in these patients that pelvic exenteration was contraindicated. Others believed that surgery is worthwhile even when pelvic nodes are involved,[9,25] especially in patients with only microscopic and not gross disease in the involved nodes.[25] The average 5-year survival for patients with positive pelvic nodes in one particular series was 26.3%,[26] and though the prognosis was generally poor, some individual long-term survivals could be achieved and it was difficult to predict which patient would do so. Positive nodes, especially microscopic disease, should not be an absolute contraindication in the presence of other favourable factors. Other contraindications to exenterative surgery that have been suggested include positive peritoneal cytology and fixation of small bowel to the specimen by infiltrating cancer.[23] However Symmonds et al[5] did not consider extension to the cul-de-sac or invasion of an adherent loop of bowel contraindications to exenteration.

In summary, generally about 25–80% of patients with recurrent pelvic cancer being evaluated for exenterative surgery will be found to be unsuitable at the initial assessment. Of those who proceed to an exploratory laparotomy another half will be excluded because of the findings at operation.[2,3,8,12] The patient who is a candidate for exenterative surgery will

Table 21.1   Pelvic exenteration: patient selection

Clinical features
Age/medical conditions
Symptomatology
Psychiatric illnesses

Investigations
Chest X-ray
Computed tomography (CT) of abdomen/pelvis
Intravenous urography
Lymphography
Radioimmunography

Operative procedures
Examination under anaesthesia
Cystoscopy and proctosigmoidoscopy
Guided needle biopsies
  Parametrium
  Bladder
  Rectum
  Pelvis
  Distant sites
Exploratory laparotomy
  Intraoperative biopsies
  Pelvic lymphadenectomy
  Para-aortic node sampling

have a central resectable recurrent cancer which involves the bladder or the rectum, negative para-aortic nodes, and no evidence of intraperitoneal spread or distant metastasis. The factors involved in the selection of patients for exenterative surgery are summarized in Table 21.1.

PELVIC EXENTERATION: URINARY RECONSTRUCTION

Prior to 1950 urinary diversion consisted mainly of ureterosigmoidostomy and the wet colostomy, with significant problems of faecal contamination of the urinary tract, ascending infection and difficulties in application of the external appliance. Bricker[27] in 1950 popularized the use of the ileal conduit as a form of urinary diversion after anterior or total pelvic exenteration. Since then various other segments of the bowel have been used, including the jejunum, transverse and sigmoid colon as an incontinent urinary conduit. However the patient is still left with an incontinent stoma with the constant need for an external appliance. This led to the development of the continent pouch, and the evolution of bladder substitutes where transurethral voiding takes place. In choosing the most appropriate form of urinary diversion or reconstruction for the patient we have to consider her wishes, age, general health, expected life expectancy, and the surgical expertise of the surgeon.

Incontinent urinary diversion

The use of the jejunal conduit has been largely abandoned because of significant electrolyte imbalances associated with its use. This results from the greater absorptive and secretory capacity of the jejunal mucosa, giving rise to the jejunal conduit syndrome characterized by hyponatraemia, hypochloraemia, hyperkalaemia, azotaemia and acidosis. This syndrome is reported in up to 50% of patients, and the occurrence of this complication can be minimized by the construction of the shortest possible conduit and the use of prophylactic oral electrolyte therapy.[28] The use of jejunal conduits should be considered only in patients with normal renal function, and when other intestinal segments could not be used because of a compromised blood supply due to previous irradiation or surgery.

An isolated segment of sigmoid colon was first used by Mogg[29] in 1965 in the treatment of neurogenic urinary incontinence. Ureterosigmoid urinary diversion has since been performed in patients after exenterative surgery for recurrent gynaecological malignancies, with favourable results and no significant difference in conduit morbidity or patient mortality when compared to ileal conduit procedures.[12,30] Use of the sigmoid colon in total exenteration is a time-saving procedure which has the advantage of obviating the need for a small bowel anastomosis, which is especially important in patients who have had irradiation. The ureterosigmoid anastomosis takes place at the proximal end of the isolated segment of sigmoid colon, avoiding the more heavily irradiated portion of the bowel. In anterior exenteration where there is no resection of the rectosigmoid the use of the ileal conduit is still favoured. The ileal conduit has the advantages of ease of construction and of being a time-tested procedure. The main disadvantage of an ileal conduit is that the ileum is in a relatively fixed position in the abdominopelvic cavity, and often receives a radiation dose close to or exceeding its tolerance level. In the construction of both the ileal and sigmoid conduits the intestinal segment is kept as short as possible so that there is minimal contact between urine and mucosa, and the conduit in effect does not act as a reservoir. In order to avoid utilizing irradiated bowel altogether the transverse colon has been used as a conduit for urinary diversion,[31,32] with a reported lower complication rate compared to ileal or sigmoid colon conduits.[33,34]

Long- and short-term complications are associated with incontinent urinary diversion procedures, and are summarized in Table 21.2. In addition to the complications mentioned the patient often encounters significant psychological problems with having to wear an external bag constantly. The overall complication rate generally varies from 30 to 60%,[30,31] and in some series the rate was as low as 8%.[12] The two most important factors in the development of a urinary leak and fistula are previous pelvic radiotherapy and sepsis with abscess formation.[4,35] Chronic urinary infection and ascending pyelonephritis are decreased by reimplanting the ureters by an antirefluxing submucosal tunnel technique, and the use of long-term urinary antiseptic or antibiotic therapy.

The management of anastomotic leaks in the first instance is con-

Table 21.2   Incontinent urinary diversion: complications

Leaks/Fistulae
   Anastomotic
   Ureteral
   Conduit
Ureter
   Obstruction
   Stenosis
Stoma
   Necrosis
   Stenosis
   Retraction
   Prolapse
   Parastomal hernia
Infection
   Acute pyelonephritis
   Chronic pyelonephritis
   Pelvic sepsis/abscess
Chronic renal failure
Electrolyte/metabolic imbalances
Calculus formation

servative, with percutaneous nephrostomy and the antegrade passage of ureteral catheters. If spontaneous closure does not occur with conservative measures or if the conduit becomes non-viable, surgical revision is required. Superficial stomal necrosis and retraction can be managed expectantly, while more extensive cases require surgical revision or even replacement of the urinary conduit.

Ureteral stents have been used to decrease the complication rate.[4,23,36] Use of a stent facilitates a precise anastomosis, and the risk of leakage and fistula at the anastomotic site is decreased. The stents keep the ends of the ureters open, and prevent obstruction to urine flow from tissue oedema. Placement of the stents is not technically difficult or time-consuming, and no additional surgery is required for removal as they are usually expelled spontaneously in the postoperative period. The risks of the use of stents include renal parenchymal damage, stent obstruction and the introduction of infection into the upper urinary tract.

Continent urinary diversion

Continent as opposed to incontinent urinary diversion has been developed to improve the quality of life after an exenterative procedure, and patient acceptance is significantly higher. The presence of a wet stoma and the necessity of a constant external appliance have been shown to place significant restrictions on the patient's lifestyle.[37] Continence is defined as the patient having absolute control of the timing of expulsion of urine from the reconstructed reservoir. The main principles involve the construction of a reservoir from a segment of bowel, with disruption of the tubular structure to eliminate the intermittent high-pressure spikes characteristic of any bowel segment. The continence mechanism is created by a number of different and rather ingenious ways, often utilizing the principle of Laplace's law which states that the pressure in a smaller-diameter lumen is higher than that in a lumen of larger diameter with which it is in continuity. Hence the caecum and ascending colon are often used for the reservoir, and the smaller luminal ileum or appendix as the conduit and stoma. Reinforcing sutures are frequently used as an additional safeguard against failure and incontinence.

The Kock pouch was first introduced in 1975,[32] and this consisted of two loops of ileum anastomosed together, with continence provided by intussuscepted nipple valves. The incidence of nipple failure with the Kock pouch generally is 10–20%. The Mainz pouch involves the construction of a reservoir consisting of the detubularized caecum, ascending colon and two loops of the ileum. Continence in the Mainz pouch is achieved by an ileoileal intussusception nipple technique.

The Indiana pouch utilizes an ileocolonic reservoir, and the ureters were tunnelled submucosally for an antirefluxing anastomosis. Reconfiguration of the caecum and a segment of the ascending colon was performed to prevent the generation of high-pressure contractions which may lead to incontinence. The incontinence mechanism was created by plicating the terminal ileal segment along with the ileocaecal valve. The Indiana pouch has the advantage of using the ascending colon, which is outside of the irradiation field, for the construction of the reservoir. Penalver et al[38] described a modified technique in 1989, where the caecum and ascending colon were mobilized and the transverse colon transected to create a colonic reservoir. This segment of bowel was then detubularized to eliminate the transient high-pressure transmissions of the colon. The continence mechanism was created by tapering the distal ileum, and the insertion of pursestring sutures at the ileocaecal valve which reinforced the intrinsically higher pressure in the lumen of the ileum. The low pressure in the reservoir and the muscular fibres of the colonic wall provided the antirefluxing mechanism at the ureterocolonic anastomosis.

The Mitrofanoff principle has been applied to create a continent urinary diversion after exenterative surgery.[39] The appendix was mobilized on its pedicle, and its blind end removed. One end was anastomosed to a detubularized pouch in a submucosal tunnel, and the other end brought to the surface as a stoma.

In patients with continent urinary diversions self-catheterization is necessary, and a dressing is applied to the stoma to prevent mucoid soiling between intubations. Complications with continent urinary diversions include problems associated with the reservoir such as leakage and fistula; stricture of the ileocaecal valve especially if reinforcing sutures have been placed;[40] stenosis of the ileal segment with difficulties in catheterization; infection and asymptomatic bacteriuria; and failure of the continence mechanism. Electrolyte imbalances are relatively infrequent because the intestinal mucosa of the intestinal pouches often show adaptive changes to the presence of urine, with decreased enzymatic activity and flattening of the epithelium.

Generally about 15–20% of patients would require reoperation for failure of continence and stoma problems, and for urinary leaks and fistulae. At least 4 weeks should lapse after surgery before intermittent catheterization of the reservoir is started. Other measures to decrease the incidence of leaks and fistulae are meticulous surgical technique, the use of surgical staplers, the control of infection, placement of a caecostomy tube, and careful postoperative saline irrigation of the reservoir to prevent distension with mucus. Rupture of the caecum has been reported after a continent ileocaecal urinary diversion.[41] The rupture was not related to suture line failure, and has been attributed to high wall tension and reduced compliance in the irradiated caecum.

Construction of a neobladder

The construction of a neobladder involves the fashioning of a bowel segment which stores urine and empties by either spontaneous micturition or by intermittent transurethral catheterization. Bowel segments used to construct the reservoir include the ileum, right colon or the rectosigmoid. Ileocolonic as well as ileocaecal pouches have been used. A 2–3 cm disc of the trigone together with the sphincter urethra are retained if there is no involvement by tumour, and this is anastomosed to the intestinal pouch. The continence mechanism is provided by the patient's own physiological sphincter, and an abdominal stoma is avoided altogether. Daytime continence may be maintained in up to 90% of patients, and nocturnal continence in 50% of all cases. Simultaneous reconstruction of the vagina and bladder performed together with an anterior exenterative procedure has been described.[42] Presently most of the data on the construction of a neobladder have been derived from studies on male patients,[43,44] and results in female patients may not be similar because of the differing anatomy of the urethra and sphincter mechanisms. The various forms of urinary reconstruction after exenterative surgery for gynaecological cancer are summarized in Table 21.3.

PELVIC EXENTERATION: VAGINAL RECONSTRUCTION

The construction of a neovagina is essential in the psychosexual rehabilitation of a select group of patients, after all or a significant part of the vagina has been removed in an anterior, posterior or total exenterative procedure. The presence of a neovagina enhances self-esteem and psychosexual readjustment even when the patient does not intend to be sexually active. Various techniques have been described, and vaginal reconstruction

Table 21.3   Pelvic exenteration: urinary reconstruction

Incontinent urinary diversion
   Ileal conduit
   Sigmoid colon conduit
   Transverse colon conduit
   Jejunal conduit
Continent urinary diversion
   Ileal pouch (Kock)
   Ileocaecal pouch (Mainz)
   Ileocolonic pouch (Indiana)
   Colonic pouch
   Mitrofanoff continent pouch
Construction of neobladder

Table 21.4   Pelvic exenteration: vaginal reconstruction

Delayed reconstruction
   Williams' vulvovaginoplasty
   McIndoe split-thickness skin graft (modified)
   Full-thickness skin graft

Concurrent reconstruction
   Gracilis myocutaneous graft
   Rectus abdominis myocutaneous graft
   Fasciocutaneous graft
   Pudendal-thigh graft

   Intestinal segments
   Omental J-flap

can be carried out as an interval procedure or concurrently with the exenterative surgery (Table 21.4).

Vaginal reconstruction can be performed as a delayed procedure because of a deliberate decision to do so, or when the patient is unable to decide at the time of the exenterative surgery. The William's vulvovaginoplasty procedure has the distinction of being simple, and the associated morbidity is minimal. The disadvantages are the awkward angle of the neovagina, and a significant amount of vulval tissue must remain if the procedure is to be used. Follow-up in these patients is often difficult in terms of access to the vaginal stump.[45]

A modification of the McIndoe method for vaginoplasty has been described as an interval procedure after exenterative surgery.[46] A split-thickness skin graft is placed over a granulation bed in the perineum 1–2 months after the initial exenterative surgery. A stent is required to immobilize the graft, and subsequently the patient has to use a dilator until regular sexual activity. Split-thickness skin grafts are more suited in patients where an anterior exenteration has been performed as the recto-sigmoid acts as a support for the graft. Full-thickness skin grafts taken from the labia, perineum or thigh can be fashioned into a vaginal tube and inverted into the pelvic cavity to create a neovagina. This is done as an interval procedure, and does not require a granulation bed for the graft to take.

Vaginal reconstruction done concurrently with the exenterative procedure has the advantages of avoiding the additional cost and anaesthetic exposure of a subsequent delayed operation. McCraw et al[47] in 1976 described the use of the gracilis myocutaneous graft to create a neovagina in patients who had previous irradiation. Bilateral or unilateral grafts are raised, and the grafts are transferred to the pelvis through a labial tunnel. The reconstruction is carried out concurrently, and the use of the gracilis flap is associated with neovascularization of the denuded pelvic floor. Neovascularization has important advantages in conveying blood elements, nutrients and antibiotics to the traumatized and denuded pelvic cavity. There is enhanced primary healing, and the advantage of an improved blood flow is especially important in patients who have had irradiation. The procedure does not usually prolong the operating time if it is done concurrently with another experienced surgical team working at the perineal end. No significant differences have been reported in operating time and blood loss between those who had the procedure and a control group who chose not to have any reconstruction.[48-50] There was also a lower incidence of complications and a generally shorter hospital stay due to improved healing brought about by the neovascularization and reinforcement of the pelvic floor by the neovagina. Neovascularization has also been associated with a decreased incidence of gastrointestinal fistulae.[50] Cosmetic results are often satisfying, with a high level of patient acceptance and good psychosexual rehabilitation.

There are short- and long-term complications associated with the use of the gracilis myocutaneous graft for vaginal reconstruction. Immediate and short-term complications include infection and necrosis of the graft resulting from the variable blood supply of the flap. Complications that occur later are stenosis of the neovagina, persistent labial oedema, graft prolapse, chronic discharge and abnormal thigh appearance and sensation. The incidence of graft prolapse was reported to be less with modifications of the standard technique such as using smaller flaps, anchoring the neovagina to the levator and retropubic fascia, and division of the neurovascular pedicle when mobility is limited.[49] Division of the neurovascular pedicle was not associated with an increased incidence of flap necrosis, presumably because of compensatory flow from the branches of the obturator artery through the more proximal portion of the gracilis muscle. A 'short' gracilis myocutaneous flap has been used for vulvovaginal reconstruction,[51] where the vascular pedicle from the medial femoral circumflex artery was deliberately sacrificed and viability of the pedicle maintained by branches of the obturator artery. This enabled a less bulky graft to be fashioned, and vaginal reconstruction was technically easier in the more restricted pelvic cavity when a low rectosigmoid anastomosis was being performed at the same time.[52]

Not all patients are candidates for the gracilis flap procedure. The flaps in obese patients are too thick and bulky for good cosmetic results, and in patients undergoing supralevator exenteration the long subcutaneous tunnel between the donor site in the thigh and the supralevator space leads to undue tension in the flap and a greater risk of necrosis.

A distally based rectus abdominis myocutaneous flap has been used for vaginal and pelvic reconstruction after exenterative surgery. The flap is based caudally on the inferior epigastric vascular pedicle to the rectus abdominis muscle. As with the gracilis graft there is revascularization with all the associated benefits. The bulk of the muscle and subcutaneous tissue fills the dead space of the pelvic cavity and prevents intestinal herniation through the pelvic inlet. The flap loss frequency is reported to be less with the rectus abdominis flap compared to the gracilis myocutaneous flap.[53] Primary healing may be expected and flap-related complications such as necrosis or herniation at the donor site are uncommon.[54,55] The epigastric donor site in this procedure does not interfere with the siting of colostomy and urinary conduit stomas, and an additional advantage is that the rectus abdominis donor site can be closed in continuity with the laparotomy incision.

Other forms of vaginal reconstruction performed with exenterative procedures include using a fasciocutaneous flap from the thigh,[56] and a neurovascular pudendal-thigh flap.[57] A partially sensate fasciocutaneous flap from the medial thigh can be raised without using the gracilis muscle as a vascular carrier, as there appears to be a constant suprafascial communicating vascular plexus. This flap offers an alternative to the gracilis myocutaneous flap when less bulky tissue is required for vaginal reconstruction. The blood supply however seems to be more variable, with the risk of total or partial flap necrosis.

The pudendal-thigh flaps are raised bilaterally in the groin crease lateral to the labial majora, and are then transposed to the midline and sutured together to form a skin-lined neovagina in the pelvic floor. In this procedure the neovagina apparently is sensate, retaining the same innervation of the erogenous zones of the perineum and upper thigh.

Intestinal segments have been used for the fashioning of a neovagina. Isolated segments of the caecum and ascending colon can be mobilized and brought down to the introitus on a vascular bundle derived from the right colic artery. The use of bowel segments for vaginal reconstruction suffers from the problems of contracture and often copious amounts of offensive discharge. Rarely the intestinal segment may detach from the introitus and retract up into the pelvic cavity.[23] Though extremely rare, patients have been known to develop cancer in the segments of small bowel used, and a case of an adenocarcinoma occurring in an irradiated caecal neovagina has been reported.[58] The patient has to wear a mould or dilators have to be used before regular sexual activity, and patient compliance is essential if satisfactory function is to be achieved.

In exenterative procedures the omentun is frequently mobilized and used as a lid to close off the pelvic inlet. The distal portion of the J omental flap could be made into a cylinder for a neovagina.[59] This cylinder was then sutured to the introitus, and lined by a split-thickness skin graft taken from the leg or buttock. The patient had to wear a vaginal mould to prevent contracture, and a second anaesthetic was necessary for assessment and fitting of the mould.

There is no doubt that the creation of a neovagina would contribute significantly to the psychosexual rehabilitation of a select group of patients after major exenterative surgery which is often mutilating. However in other patients vaginal reconstruction would not be appropriate because of age, marital status or personal inclination.

PELVIC EXENTERATION: PELVIC FLOOR RECONSTRUCTION

Exenterative surgery leaves a large defect in the floor of the pelvic cavity which is open to the outside through the perineum. This defect, together with the denuded areas, predisposes to infection and small bowel complications. Adherence of prolapsed loops of often irradiated small bowel results in bowel obstruction and fistula formation. In patients who require postoperative radiotherapy the immobile loops of small bowel in the pelvis lead to limitation of dosage and a higher incidence of complications. Reconstruction of the pelvic floor also confines infection to the pelvis to a certain extent, and is essential to prevent perineal herniation.

These complications have been well-recognized and various methods have been used to create a pelvic lid or floor (Table 21.5), with support given to the intra-abdominal contents to prevent prolapse. Originally a gauze pack was used for support to prevent herniation of the viscera through the perineum till they became adherent for self-support. Attempts were then made to create a floor at the brim of the pelvic cavity with isolated segments of sigmoid colon and ileum transfixed to the tissues at the brim. These pelvic 'lid' techniques were unsatisfactory because it soon became apparent that the pelvic cavity should be obliterated and the denuded floor covered to establish neovascularity.

Amnion-chorion grafts and collagen films have been used to exclude bowel from the pelvic cavity in the past. These materials however were found to be lacking in tensile strength. Human dura matter allografts have also been used for pelvic floor reconstruction.[3] This is a biological, non-viable and immunologically inert material which is well-incorporated into normal surrounding tissues without rejection reaction. The use of this material however has been associated with a high rate of small bowel fistulae.[60] The use of human dura allografts has also been reported in the repair of a large perineal hernia and prolapse of a myocutaneous neovagina after total exenteration.[61]

Other materials used include synthetic non-absorbable materials such as

Table 21.5 Pelvic exenteration: pelvic floor reconstruction

Omentum 'lid'/carpet
Peritoneum
   Peritoneal sac
   Peritoneal sling
   Peritoneal bag
   Free peritoneal graft
Synthetic absorbable mesh
   Polyglatin 910 (Vicryl) mesh
   Polyglycolic acid (Dexon) mesh
Allografts
   Amnion-chorion grafts
   Human dura mater grafts
Isolated intestinal segments
   Sigmoid segment
   Ileal segment
Synthetic non-absorbable materials
   Marlex
   Teflon
   Silastic prosthesis
   Steel mesh
Miscellaneous
   Ileocolonic urinary reservoir
   Pelvic pack
   Collagen films

Marlex, Teflon, Silastic prosthesis and even steel meshes. There were significant problems associated with the use of these synthetic materials such as infection, fistula formation and extrusion.

Stanley Way[62] in 1974 described the creation of a peritoneal 'sac' to encase the small bowel in a cul-de-sac of peritoneum. In this technique anterior and posterior flaps of peritoneum are developed at the beginning of the procedure. The flaps are then sutured together with a slowly absorbable suture (Dexon) at the end to form a sac which holds the entire bowel contents above the pelvic brim. A peritoneal sling or a free peritoneal graft isolated from the anterior peritoneum have also been used to close the pelvic floor.[2]

The omentum is a non-essential organ, has a rich blood supply and provides a strong, pliable and mobile membranous covering. Use of the omentum in the reconstruction of the pelvic floor fills the dead space with viable tissue and improves healing. It also assists in the resolution of infection and prevents adhesions of bowel loops to the pelvic floor. In some patients it has been long enough and detachment was not necessary to suture it to the sacral promontory to create a bag to retain the intestines. With progressive stretching this bag descends and fills the pelvic cavity eventually. Usually detachment is needed, and after division of the right gastroepiploic artery and vessels along the greater curvature of the stomach, the omentum is brought down into the pelvis. The blood supply is maintained by the left gastroepiploic artery, and the omentum is sutured to the pelvic brim and brought to lie upon the pelvic floor as a carpet. An omental pedicle graft based upon the right gastroepiploic artery can be used to cover and support an ureteroileal anastomosis when an urinary diversion is being perfomed.[63] The dependent portion of the omentum is then allowed to descend and to fill the pelvic cavity.

There can be mechanical problems associated with the use of the omentum to reconstruct the pelvic floor. It may not be strong enough to support and to elevate the intra-abdominal contents from the pelvic floor for any duration of time. In some patients despite maximal mobilization the omentum is not long enough to be used to carpet the pelvic floor, especially in thin patients and in patients who have had irradiation or previous surgery.

Buchsbaum et al[64] in 1985 reported on the use of a mesh made of polyglatin 910 (Vicryl) fibre for reconstruction of the pelvic floor. The mesh was sutured as a loose hammock across the pelvic brim, usually in conjunction with an omental lid or sling. The mesh has also been used on its own to form a pelvic lid when omentum was not available.[65] A mesh composed of another absorbable synthetic material (polyglycolic acid; Dexon) has been used to support small bowel away from the pelvis in patients receiving postoperative radiotherapy after exenterative procedures.[66] This allowed higher doses of radiotherapy without the associated hazard of radiation-induced bowel damage. These synthetic meshes provide a latticework for the deposition of granulation tissue and the formation of fibrosis. They add tensile strength to an omental floor, and contribute to a decrease in the incidence of bowel complications.[64–67] The main danger with the use of these meshes appears to be an increased risk of pelvic sepsis and abscess formation. There was an increased tendency to adhesion formation and pelvic abscesses when polyglycolic acid meshes were used in experimental surgery on canines.[68]

Pearlman et al[69] described the use of a continent ileocolonic urinary reservoir to fill and to line the pelvis. The reservoir was constructed from the distal ileum, the whole of the ascending colon and the proximal third of the transverse colon. This provided the necessary bulk for an expansile reservoir, and the complication rate of small bowel obstruction was reported to be more than halved.

PELVIC EXENTERATION: LOW RECTAL ANASTOMOSIS

After total or posterior exenterations patients are usually left with a permanent sigmoid end-colostomy. This has obvious effects on the perception of self-image and patients often experience significant difficulties in adapting to a permanent incontinent faecal stoma. In supralevator exenterative surgery the anal sphincters as well as the anorectal angulation are preserved. If as little as 3–4 of an anorectal stump can be preserved, a low rectal anastomosis can be performed to restore bowel continuity and to avoid a colostomy.[70] Low rectal anastomosis is facilitated by the use of the end-to-end circular surgical enteroentero anastomosis (EEA) stapler. The stapled anastomosis compared to one that is hand-sutured has a better blood supply, with less tissue inflammation and improved healing. Significant complications associated with low rectal anastomosis include the formation of fistulae and anastomotic leaks. Factors affecting the incidence of these complications include the degree of tension on the anastomotic line, vascularity of the two ends of bowel, the distance of the anastomosis from the anus, and whether the tissues used have been irradiated previously. In the presence of unfavourable factors and when the bowel has not been adequately prepared a defunctioning colostomy is indicated. Alternatively to avoid even a temporary colostomy the patient could be put on total parenteral nutrition postoperatively to minimize any stress on the anastomotic line and to improve healing. Often a portion of the omentum used to reconstruct the pelvic floor is utilized to form a wrap round the anastomotic site.

A low rectal anastomosis or end-to-end descending coloproctostomy is often associated with disabling diarrhoea and tenesmus in up to 70% of cases.[71] The construction of a rectal J-pouch with an end-to-side coloproctostomy may significantly relieve these symptoms without an increase in faecal incontinence. The J-pouch recreates the rectal bulb or reservoir, with a higher maximum pressure and an increased tolerable faecal volume.

PELVIC EXENTERATION: MORTALITY AND MORBIDITY

The mortality and morbidity associated with this formidable surgical undertaking have improved significantly. The factors which have contributed to this are summarized in Table 21.6. Improved perioperative monitoring and intensive care[3] have decreased complications due to haematological and fluid imbalances. Better antibiotic therapy has assisted in the control and prevention of infection.[5] Measures taken to decrease the incidence of pulmonary embolism after exenterative procedures include the routine use of heparin,[13] and prophylactic compartmentalization and plication of the inferior vena cava.[23] Postoperative hyperalimentation prevents malnutrition, and is an important factor in healing and infection control. The type of drains used for pelvic drainage has also been found to be important.[7]

Advances in surgical techniques that have made exenterative surgery safer and more acceptable include the use of surgical staplers, reconstruction of the denuded pelvic floor, and the evolution of reconstructive surgery for the lower urinary tract, vagina and bowel. Conduit methods of urinary diversion have drastically reduced the infection and metabolic complications associated with the wet colostomy and ureterosigmoidostomy. Innovations in the reconstruction of the vagina and pelvic floor bring viable, non-irradiated and vascularized tissue into large dead spaces, which improves healing and decreases the complication rate.

Table 21.6 Pelvic exenteration: factors contributing to decreased mortality and morbidity

---

Proper patient selection
Preoperative preparation
   Prophylactic antibiotics
   Prophylactic heparin
   Adequate bowel preparation
Improved anaesthesia/monitoring
Improved postoperative intensive care/monitoring
Changes in surgical techniques
   Urinary diversion/reconstruction
   Ureteral stents
   Pelvic floor reconstruction
   Vaginal reconstruction
   Surgical staplers
Hyperalimentation
Tertiary centres
Psychosexual/psychosocial rehabilitation
Accumulation of experience/audit

Ligation of the hypogastric arteries can be safely carried out if severe intraoperative haemorrhage occurs from damage to the hypogastric veins, as repeated suturing to attempt haemostasis may lead to the tearing of more pelvic vessels.[72]

Tertiary centres have been established where major and specialized surgery such as pelvic exenterations should rightly belong. A multidisciplinary approach with more emphasis on psychosocial and psychosexual aspects has helped in the eventual rehabilitation of the patient. There has been a gradual accumulation of clinical experience, with audits and reports leading to the identification of risk factors and further innovations in surgical techniques.

The operative mortality of pelvic exenterations presently is generally below 10% (Table 21.7). There is still considerable morbidity (Tables 21.8 and 21.9), and up to 84% of patients in one series were reported to require rehospitalization after pelvic exenterations.[74] Major morbidity associated with exenterative procedures usually involves the gastrointestinal and genitourinary tracts, and they can be acute or delayed. The late development of a fistula or obstruction may however be related to recurrent cancer, rather than as a direct consequence of surgery. The careful selection of suitable patients will lead to an improved survival and decreased morbidity.

Gastrointestinal complications

The two main gastrointestinal complications are small bowel obstruction and the formation of fistulae. The main factors related to small bowel obstruction are a denuded pelvic floor, sepsis and abscess formation, and the presence of a bowel anastomosis. A strong factor contributing to

Table 21.7   Pelvic exenteration: operative mortality

Authors	Number	%
Symmonds et al (1975)[5]	198	8.1
Morley & Lindenauer (1976)[2]	70	1.4
Rutledge et al (1977)[23]	296	13.5
Jakowatz et al (1985)[75]	104	2.9
Roberts et al (1987)[7]	38	5.3
Hatch et al (1988)[73]	69	2.9
Shingleton et al (1989)[16]	143	6.3
Anthopoulos et al (1989)[74]	20	5.0
Shepherd (1989)[8]	52	6.0
Soper et al (1989)[33]	69	7.2
Lawhead et al (1989)[13]	65	9.2
Morley et al (1989)[12]	100	2.0
Total	1224	5.8

Table 21.8   Pelvic exenteration: complications

General complications
Cardiovascular complications
  Cerebral thrombosis
  Myocardial infarction
  Disseminated intravascular coagulopathy
  Deep venous thrombosis and pulmonary
  embolism
  Thrombophlebitis
  Haemorrhage

Pulmonary complications
  Chest infection
  Atelectasis
  Consolidation

Wound complications
  Wound infection
  Wound dehiscence

Miscellaneous
  Malnutrition
  Metabolic imbalances

Gastrointestinal complications
Bowel obstruction
Enterocutaneous fistula
Enteroperineal fistula
Enterovaginal fistula
Rectovaginal fistula
Anastomotic leakage
Stoma necrosis/retraction
Intestinal bleeding

Urinary complications
Infection/pyelonephritis
Ureteral obstruction
Urinary leakage
Urinary stricture
Urinary fistula
Anastomotic leakage
Electrolyte imbalances
Stent obstruction
Stent renal parenchymal damage
Renal impairment/failure
Calculus formation
Incontinence
Stoma necrosis/retraction

Denuded pelvic floor complications
Sepsis/pelvic abscess
Small bowel obstruction
Bowel fistula
Perineal intestinal herniation

Vaginoplasty complications
Stenosis
Vaginal dehiscence
Partial/ total flap loss

Psychological maladjustment

Table 21.9 Pelvic exenteration: Overall reported incidence
of complications

Authors	Number	%
Morley & Lindenauer (1976)[2]	70	30.0
Jakowatz et al (1985)[75]	104	77.0
Shepherd (1989)[8]	52	19.0
Roberts et al (1987)[7]	38	55.3
Morley et al (1989)[12]	100	49.0
Anthopoulos et al (1989)[74]	20	84.0
TOTAL	384	47.0

Table 21.10 Pelvic exenteration: gastrointestinal complications

Authors	Number	Obstruction %	Fistula %
Symmonds et al (1975)[5]	198	12.0	13.0
Orr et al (1983)[34]	125	9.6	15.0
Averette et al (1984)[3]	92	16.3	5.4
Jakowatz et al (1985)[75]	104	10.0	10.0
Roberts et al (1987)[7]	38	21.0	26.3
Lawhead et al* (1989)[13]	65	6.1	4.7
Soper et al (1989)[33]	69	4.3	23.0
TOTAL	691	11.3	13.9

* Incidence within first 30 days post-surgery only.

gastrointestinal and genitourinary complications is prior radiotherapy.[3-5,7,33,75] The reported incidence of bowel obstruction varies from 4.3 to 21% (Table 21.10). The rate of reoperation for small bowel obstruction varies from 50 to 75%.[34,75] A certain proportion of cases with obstruction will resolve with conservative management, and surgical intervention is required if the patients do not respond and should not be delayed.

Intestinal fistulae may involve the large or small bowel and the perineum and vagina. The reported incidence of fistulae varies from 4.7 to 26% in different series (Table 21.10). The risk factors are similar to that for obstruction, and other significant factors include tension on the suture line and the adequacy of preoperative bowel preparation. Attempts at neo-vagina construction or extensive dissection in the vicinity of the recto-vaginal septum to obtain clear margins in anterior exenterations are also risk factors.[34] The management of intestinal fistulae consists of the correction of fluid balance, nutritional support with hyperalimentation, treatment of sepsis, radiographic localization of the fistula site if possible and reoperation. Rarely spontaneous closure of the fistula occurs with conservative measures. At reoperation resection of the affected segment with re-anastomosis may be difficult because of adhesions, sepsis and the presence of irradiated bowel. In these circumstances an intestinal bypass should be carried out, and occasionally the only feasible option is to perform a permanent diversionary procedure. Rarely repair of the fistula may be possible.

Overall, it has been reported that gastrointestinal complications account for about 60% of all reoperations for complications following pelvic exenterations.[34] Other complications in the patient with an intestinal anastomosis are pelvic sepsis and abscess formation from anastomotic leakage. The incidence of wound infection may also be higher, possibly from spillage and contamination during surgery.

Changes in surgical techniques which have led to a decrease in the incidence of gastrointestinal complications include reconstruction of the pelvic floor, use of non-irradiated tissues such as the transverse colon for urinary diversion or reconstruction and the use of surgical stapling devices. Routine postoperative hyperalimentation may decrease the incidence of gastrointestinal complications following exenterative surgery.[5,34]

Automatic surgical staplers have been shown to have certain advantages over the conventional suture technique. The devices commonly used are the thoracoabdominal (TA), gastrointestinal anastomosis (GIA) and the EEA instruments. The use of the EEA instrument has made possible low rectal anastomosis, sparing many patients the need for a permanent descending colostomy. Use of the surgical staplers in exenterative procedures was reported to be associated with a decreased operating time, blood loss and hospital stay when compared to the traditional two-layer suture technique.[76] The incidence of small bowel obstruction was also found to be significantly decreased with the use of staplers, without an increase in the occurrence of bowel strictures.[34] There is less trauma to the bowel, and the risk of peritoneal contamination is decreased.[4]

Genitourinary complications

These have already been discussed in the relevant sections. Reoperation for gastrointestinal and genitourinary complications following exenterative surgery carries a significant mortality and morbidity, and this is due to the presence of infection, tissue fragility, adhesions, poor nutritional status and low morale of the patient. Furthermore reoperation is sometimes performed in an acute situation, with a patient who has been inadequately prepared. The mortality rate of surgery in these circumstances varies from 8%[33] to as high as 50%.[34]

RECURRENT VULVAL CANCER

Over half of recurrences of vulval cancer occur at the local site, usually within 2 years of the initial treatment. Recurrence is more common in patients who had large primary tumours and metastatic disease in the groin nodes at the initial surgery. Surgery in recurrent local disease consists of wide local excision with adequate margins. When the recurrence is more extensive with involvement of the urethra, bladder, anus and rectum, exenterative procedures may be indicated. An anterior or posterior exenteration is performed most frequently, because if the geographic extent requires a total exenterative procedure, contraindications to surgery such as distant metastasis are usually present.[7] Cavanagh & Shepherd[77] noted that radical vulvectomy with pelvic exenteration was warranted in selected patients with primary stage 4 vulval cancer, with a corrected 5-year survival of 50%. Concurrent radiotherapy and chemotherapy may be used for patients with advanced primary and recurrent vulval cancer, avoiding the need for radical surgery in these patients.

Reconstruction of the vulva, and of the vagina if desired, is carried out with some of the techniques already described utilizing myocutaneous flaps from the anterior abdominal wall or thigh. In a report on the use of rectus abdominis myocutaneous flaps following radical excision of extensive vulval cancer, 94% of the grafts in 16 patients took with primary healing.[55]

RECURRENT UTERINE SARCOMAS

Pelvic exenteration can be carried out in a select group of patients with pelvic sarcomas. In the past the most frequent type of pelvic sarcoma requiring exenterative procedues was embryonal rhabdomyosarcoma in infants and young children. These tumours are now eminently treatable by combination radiation and chemotherapy, and radical surgery in almost all cases can be avoided. Pelvic exenterations for centrally recurring uterine sarcomas has been reported with comparable results to that for recurrent cervical cancer.[78]

RECURRENT OVARIAN CANCER

Surgery in recurrent ovarian cancer ranges from second-look procedures to pelvic exenterative operations. Surgical intervention is also required when intestinal obstruction occurs which does not respond to conservative therapy. Patients with recurrent ovarian cancer are not usually candidates for pelvic exenterations because of the nature of recurrence in the form of abdominal dissemination. Exenterative procedures have been carried out for patients with ovarian cancer that appears to be confined to the pelvis with isolated tumour masses.[8,13] Some cases are not true recurrences as complete eradication of disease has never been achieved by prior surgery or chemotherapy. When possible exenterative surgery has been associated with a significant increase in survival.[8] Eisenkop et al[79] described a modified posterior exenterative procedure which effectively removed all visible pelvic disease in patients with ovarian cancer. Complete extirpation of gross disease in even advanced disease was reported to be possible by en bloc resection of the pelvic organs in continuity with all pelvic peritoneum and a segment of the rectosigmoid, together with other debulking procedures.

RADICAL HYSTERECTOMY AS SALVAGE SURGERY IN RECURRENT CANCER

In place of pelvic exenterations radical hysterectomy has been carried out for a small central recurrence confined to the uterus, cervix and upper vagina without bladder or rectal involvement, and without lateral extension.[5,80] However the 5-year survival with this more conservative form of surgery appears to be significantly lower, with the occurrence of recurrences in the pelvis suggesting that surgical margins may have been compromised by avoiding exenterative surgery. Even with disease that appears to be confined, there may be subclinical extension into the adjacent parametria, bladder or rectum. There is also a significant incidence of major complications in the heavily irradiated bladder, ureters and bowel, and up to 30% of patients may require subsequent surgery for these complications.[80]

RECURRENCE AFTER PELVIC EXENTERATION

Favourable factors that decrease the risk of recurrence after pelvic exenterations for recurrent gynaecological cancers are the presence of small, mobile central masses without involvement of pelvic nodes or impingement upon the side walls. The best candidates are those who have recurrence diagnosed 1 year or more from the time of the initial radiotherapy. Clear margins on histological examination are also an important prognostic factor.[3,16,74]

CONCLUSIONS

Unfortunately in many cases of recurrent gynaecological cancer — especially that of the cervix after initial radiation therapy — the only form of salvage therapy that holds out the promise of a cure is ultraradical surgery with pelvic exenterations. The 5-year survival after pelvic exenterations is generally about 50% (Table 21.11). A specialized gynaecological

Table 21.11 Pelvic exenteration: 5 year survival

Authors	Number	%
Symmonds et al (1975)[5]	189	33.0
Morley & Lindenauer (1976)[2]	70	61.8
Rutledge et al (1977)[23]	296	42.1
Jakowatz et al (1985)[75]	104	27.0
Anthropoulos et al (1989)[74]	20	58.0
Hatch et al (1988)[73]	69	53.0
Lawhead et al (1989)[13]	65	23.0
Morley et al (1989)[12]	100	61.0
Shingleton et al (1989)[16]	143	50.0
TOTAL	1056	45.4

oncology unit with a multidisciplinary approach to patient management is required in order to attempt not only to save the patient but, more importantly, to improve her quality of life.

REFERENCES

1. Brunschwig A. Complete excision of pelvic viscera for advanced carcinoma. Cancer 1948; 1: 177–183
2. Morley G W, Lindenauer S M. Pelvic exenterative therapy for gynecologic malignancy. An analysis of 70 cases. Cancer 1976; 38: (suppl); 581–586
3. Averette H E, Lichtinger M, Sevin B-U, Girtanner R E. Pelvic exenteration: a 15-year experience in a general metropolitan hospital. Am J Obstet Gynecol 1984; 150: 179–184
4. Orr J W Jr, Shingleton H M, Hatch K D et al. Urinary diversion in patients undergoing pelvic exenteration. Am J Obstet Gynecol 1982; 142: 883–889
5. Symmonds R E, Pratt J H, Webb M J. Exenterative operations: experience with 198 patients. Am J Obstet Gynecol 1975; 121: 907–1005
6. Kraybill W G, Lopez M J, Bricker E M. Total pelvic exenteration as a therapeutic option in advanced malignant disease of the pelvis. Surg Gynecol Obstet 1988; 166: 259–263
7. Roberts W S, Cavanagh D, Bryson S C, Lyman G H, Hewitt S. Major morbidity after pelvic exenteration: a seven year experience. Obstet Gynecol 1987; 69: 617–621
8. Shepherd J H. Pelvic exenteration. Has it a role in 1987? A six year experience. Verh K Acad Geneeskd Belg 1989; 51: 31–44
9. Stanhope C B, Symmonds RE. Palliative exenteration — what, when, and why? Am J Obstet Gynecol 1985; 152: 12–16
10. McCullough W M, Nahhas W A. Palliative pelvic exenteration — futility revisited. Gynecol Oncol 1987; 27: 97–103
11. Deckers P J, Olsson C, Williams L A, Mozden P J. Pelvic exenteration as palliation of malignant disease. Am J Surg 1976; 131: 509–515
12. Morley G W, Hopkins M P, Lindenauer S M, Roberts J A. Pelvic exenteration, University of Michigan: 100 patients at 5 years. Obstet Gynecol 1989; 74: 934–943
13. Lawhead R A Jr, Clark D G, Smith D H, Pierce V K, Lewis J L Jr. Pelvic exenteration for recurrent or persistent gynecologic malignancies: a 10-year review of the Memorial Sloan-Kettering Cancer Centre experience (1972–1981). Gynecol Oncol 1989; 33: 279–282
14. Lopez M V, Kraybill W G, Fuchs G F, Johnston W D, Sala J M, Bricker E M. Transvaginal parametrial needle biopsy for detection of postirradiation recurrent cancer of the cervix. Cancer 1988; 61: 275–278
15. Jones W B. Surgical approaches for advanced or recurrent cancer of the cervix. Cancer 1987; 60 (suppl) : 2094–2103
16. Shingleton H M, Soong S J, Gelder M S, Hatch K D, Baker V V, Austin J M Jr. Clinical and histopathologic factors predicting recurrence and survival after pelvic exenteration for cancer of the cervix. Obstet Gynecol 1989; 73: 1027–1034
17. Talledo O E. Pelvic exenteration — Medical College of Georgia experience. Gynecol Oncol 1985; 22: 181–188
18. Peeples W J, Inalsingh C H A, Hazra T A, Graft D B S. The occurrence of metastasis outside the abdomen and retroperitoneal space in invasive carcinoma of the cervix. Gynecol Oncol 1976; 4: 307–312
19. Lee R B, Weisbaum G S, Heller P B, Park R C. Scalene node biopsy in primary and recurrent invasive carcinoma of the cervix. Gynecol Oncol 1981; 11: 200–206
20. Manetta A, Podczaski E S, Larson J E, De Geest K, Mortel R. Scalene lymph node biopsy in the preoperative evaluation of patients with recurrent cervical cancer. Gynecol Oncol 1989; 33: 332–334
21. Brown S B, Haddox V, Posada A, Rubio A. Social and psychological adjustment following pelvic exenteration. Am J Obstet Gynecol 1972; 114: 162–171

22. Crowther M E, Everett H, Corney R, Shepherd J H. Psychosocial and psychosexual adjustment of women with vulval and cervical carcinoma following radical surgery. Abst 21st British Congress of Obstetrics & Gynaecology, London 1989 July
23. Rutledge F N, Smith J P, Wharton J T, O'Quinn A G. Pelvic exenteration: analysis of 296 patients. Am J Obstet Gynecol 1977; 129: 881–890
24. Barber H R, Jones W. Lymphadenectomy in pelvic exenteration for recurrent cervix cancer. JAMA 1971; 215: 1945–1949
25. Creasman W T, Rutledge F. Is positive pelvic lymphadenopathy a contraindication to radical surgery in recurrent cervical carcinoma? Gynecol Oncol 1974; 2: 482–485
26. Rutledge F N, McGuffee V B. Pelvic exenteration: prognostic significance of regional lymph node metastasis. Gynecol Oncol 1987; 26: 374–380
27. Bricker E M. Bladder substitution after pelvic evisceration. Surg Clin North Am 1950; 30: 1511–1521
28. Klein E A, Montie J E, Montague D K, Kay R, Straffon R A. Jejunal conduit urinary diversion. J Urol 1986; 135: 244–246
29. Mogg R A. The treatment of neurogenic urinary incontinence using the colonic conduit. Br J Urol 1965; 37: 68–77
30. Stanhope C B, Symmonds R E, Lee R A, Williams T J, Podratz K C, O'Brien P C. Urinary diversion with use of ileal and sigmoid conduits. Am J Obstet Gynecol 1986; 155: 288–292
31. Schmidt J D, Buchsbaum H J, Nachtsheim D A. Long-term follow-up, further experience with and modifications of the transverse colon conduit in urinary tract diversion. Br J Urol 1985; 57: 284–288
32. Delgado G. Urinary conduit diversion in advanced gynecologic malignancies. Gynecol Oncol 1978; 6: 217–222
33. Soper J T, Berchuck A, Creasman W T, Clark-Pearson D L. Pelvic exenteration: factors associated with major surgical morbidity. Gynecol Oncol 1989; 35: 93–98
34. Orr J W Jr, Shingleton H M, Hatch K D, Taylor P T, Partridge E E, Soong S J. Gastrointestinal complications associated with pelvic exenteration. Am J Obstet Gynecol 1983; 145: 325–332
35. Lichtinger M, Averette H, Girtanner R, Sevin B-U, Penalver M. Small bowel complications after supravesical urinary diversion in pelvic exenteration. Gynecol Onçol 1986; 24: 137–142
36. Schlesinger R E, Ballon S C, Watring W C, Moone J G. The choice of an intestinal segment for a urinary conduit. Surg Gynecol Obstet 1979; 148: 45–51
37. Jones M A, Breckman B, Hendry W F. Life with an ileal conduit: results of questionnaire surveys of patient and urological surgeon. Br J Urol 1980; 52: 21–25
38. Penalver M A, Bejany D E, Averette H E, Donato D M, Sevin B-U, Suarez G. Continent urinary diversion in gynecologic oncology. Gynecol Oncol 1989; 34: 274–288
39. Woodhouse C R J, Malone P R, Cumming J, Reilly T M. The Mitrofanoff principle for continent urinary diversion. Br J Urol 1989; 63: 53–57
40. Mannel R S, Braly P S, Buller R E. Indiana pouch continent urinary reservoir in patients with previous pelvic irradiation. Obstet Gynecol 1990; 75: 891–893
41. Brand E. Cecal rupture after continent ileocecal urinary diversion during total pelvic exenteration. Obstet Gynecol 1991; 78: 570–572
42. Hendry W F, Christmas T J, Shepherd J H. Anterior pelvic reconstruction with ileum after cancer treatment . JR Soc Med 1991; 84: 709–713
43. Skinner D G, Lieskovsky G, Boyd S. Continent urinary diversion. J Urol 1989; 141: 1323-1327
44. Skinner D G, Sherrod A. Total pelvic exenteration with simultaneous bowel and urinary reconsturction. J Urol 1990; 144: 1433–1439
45. Hoffman M S, Fiorica J V, Roberts W S et al. Williams' vulvovaginoplasty after supralevator total pelvic exenteration. South Med J 1991; 84: 43–45
46. Morley G W, Lindenauer S M, Youngs D. Vaginal reconstruction following pelvic exenteration: surgical and psychological considerations. Am J Obstet Gynecol 1973; 116: 996–1003
47. McCraw J B, Massey F M, Shanklin K D, Horton C E. Vaginal reconstruction with gracilis myocutaneous flaps. Plast Reconstr Surg 1976; 58: 176–183
48. Lacey C G, Stern J L, Feigenbaum S, Hill E C, Braga C A. Vaginal reconstruction after

exenteration with use of gracilis myocutaneous flaps: the University of California, San Francisco experience. Am J Obstet Gynecol 1988; 158: 1278–1284

49. Copeland L J, Hancock K C, Gershenson D M, Stringer C A, Atkinson E N, Edwards C L. Gracilis myocutaneous vaginal reconstruction concurrent with total pelvic exenteration. Am J Obstet Gynecol 1989; 160: 1095–1101

50. Cain J M, Diamond A, Tamimi H K, Greer B E, Figge D C. The morbidity and benefits of concurrent gracilis myocutaneous graft with pelvic exenteration. Obstet Gynecol 1989; 74: 185–189

51. Soper J T, Larson D, Hunter V J, Berchuck A, Clark-Pearson D L. Short gracilis myocutaneous flaps for vulvovaginal reconstruction after radical pelvic surgery. Obstet Gynecol 1989; 74: 823–827

52. Berek J S, Hecker N F, Lagasse L D. Vaginal reconstruction performed simultaneously with pelvic exenteration. Obstet Gynecol 1984; 63: 318–323

53. Tobin G R, Day T G. Vaginal and pelvic reconstruction with distally based rectus abdominis myocutaneous flaps. Plast Reconstr Surg 1988; 81: 62–70

54. Skene A I, Gault D T, Woodhouse C R, Breach N M, Thomas J M. Perineal, vulval and vaginoperineal reconstruction using the rectus abdominis myocutaneous flap. Br J Surg 1990; 77: 635–637

55. Shepherd J H, Van Dam P A, Jobling T W, Breach N. The use of rectus abdominis myocutaneous flaps following excision of vulvar cancer. Br J Obst Gynaecol 1990; 97: 1020–1025

56. Wang T-N, Whetzel T, Mathes S J, Vasconez L O. A fasciocutaneous flap for vaginal and perineal reconstruction. Plast Reconstr Surg 1987; 80: 95–103

57. Wee J T K, Joseph V T. A new technique of vaginal reconstruction using neurovascular pudendal-thigh flaps: a preliminary report. Plast Reconstr Surg 1989; 83: 701–709

58. Andryjowicz E, Qizilbash A H, DePetrillo A D, O'Connell G J, Taylor M H. Adenocarcinoma in a cecal neovagina — complication of irradiation: report of a case and review of literature. Gynecol Oncol 1985; 21: 235–239

59. Wheeless C R Jr. Neovagina constructed from an omental J flap and a split thickness skin graft. Gynecol Oncol 1989; 35: 224–226

60. Jarrell M A, Malinin T I, Averette H E, Girtanner R E, Harrison C R, Penalver M A. Human dura mater allogarfts in repair of pelvic floor and abdominal wall defects. Obstet Gynecol 1987; 70: 280–285

61. Delmore J E, Turner D A, Gershenson D M, Horbelt D V. Perineal hernia repair using human dura. Obstet Gynecol 1987; 70: 507–608

62. Way S. The use of the "sac" technique in pelvic exenteration. Gynecol Oncol 1974; 2: 476-481

63. Pearse H D. Use of the omental pedicle graft in exenterative surgery. J Urol 1977; 119: 476–477

64. Buchsbaum H J, Christopherson W, Lifshitz S, Bernstein S. Vicryl mesh in pelvic floor reconstruction. Arch Surg 1985; 120: 1389–1391

65. Clarke-Pearson D, Soper J T, Creasman W T. Absorbable synthetic mesh (polyglactin 910) for the formation of a pelvic "lid" after radical pelvic resection. Am J Obstet Gynecol 1988; 158: 158–161

66. Dasmahapatra K S, Swaminathan A P. The use of a biodegradable mesh to prevent radiation-associated small-bowel injury. Arch Surg 1991; 126: 366–369

67. Hoffman M S, Roberts W S, LaPolla J P, Fiorica J V, Cavanagh D. Use of vicryl mesh in the reconstruction of the pelvic floor following exenteration. Gynecol Oncol 1989; 35: 170–171

68. Montz F J, Wheeler J H, Lau L M. Inability of polyglycolic acid mesh to inhibit immediate post-radical pelvic surgery adhesions. Gynecol Oncol 1990; 38: 230–233

69. Pearlman N W, Donohue R E, Wettlaufer J N, Stiegmann G V. Continent ileocolonic urinary reservoirs for filling and lining the post-exenteration pelvis. Am J Surg 1990; 160: 634–637

70. Hatch K D, Shingleton H M, Potter M E, Baker V V. Low rectal resection and anastomosis at the time of pelvic exenteration. Gynecol Oncol 1988; 32: 262–267

71. Wheeless C R Jr, Hempling R E. Rectal J pouch reservoir to decrease the frequency of tenesmus and defecation in low coloproctostomy. Gynecol Oncol 1989; 35: 136–138

72. Shepherd J H, Crowther M E. Complications of gynaecological cancer surgery: a review. J R Soc Med 1986; 79: 289–293
73. Hatch K D, Shingleton H M, Soong S J, Baker V V, Gelder M S. Anterior pelvic exenteration. Gynecol Oncol 1988; 31: 205–216
74. Anthropoulos A P, Manetta A, Larson J E, Podczaski E S, Bartholomew M J, Mortel R. Pelvic exenteration: a morbidity and mortality analysis of a seven-year experience. Gynecol Oncol 1989; 35: 219–223
75. Jakowatz J G, Porudominsky D, Riihimaki D U et al. Complications of pelvic exenteration. Arch Surg 1985; 120: 1261–1265
76. Penalver M, Averette H, Sevin B-U, Lichtinger M, Girtanner R. Gastrointestinal surgery in gynecologic oncology: evaluation of surgical techniques. Gynecol Oncol 1987; 28: 74–82
77. Cavanagh D, Shepherd J H. The place of pelvic exenteration in the primary management of advanced carcinoma of the vulva. Gynecol Oncol 1982; 13: 318–322
78. Reid G C, Morley G W, Schmidt R W, Hopkins M P. The role of pelvic exenteration for sarcomatous malignancies. Obstet Gynecol 1989; 74: 80–84
79. Eisenkop S M, Nalick R H, Teng N N. Modified posterior exenteration for ovarian cancer. Obstet Gynecol 1991; 78: 879–885
80. Terada K, Morley G W. Radical hysterectomy as surgical salvage therapy for gynecologic malignancy. Obstet Gynecol 1987; 70: 913–915

22. Early endometrial carcinoma — no more 'TAH, BSO and cuff'

F. G. Lawton

The ageing of our female population and the potential decline in cervical and ovarian carcinoma with effective screening programmes means that women with endometrial carcinoma will form an increasing workload for the gynaecologist in the future. At present, in the UK endometrial carcinoma is the ninth commonest female cancer with over 3500 cases reported annually.[1] The 5-year relative survival rate for all stages of the disease is 70%, which has traditionally encouraged clinicians to consider it a relatively benign, or at least easily managed, cancer. However, this belief is a consequence of the fact that 75% of women present with disease confined clinically to the endometrium. The 5-year survival rates for stage II–IV endometrial carcinoma (60, 30 and 10% respectively) are very similar to the survival rates seen for cervical and ovarian cancer. In addition, the survival rate has changed little in the last 20 years.[2]

Within the International Federation of Gynecology and Obstetrics (FIGO) stage I disease, subgroups of patients can be identified who will have a far worse 5-year survival than the expected 75%. It will be seen from this chapter that the traditional 'TAH, BSO and cuff' offered to these patients is entirely inappropriate if the true extent of their disease is to be documented. Only after surgical staging can post surgical treatment be tailored appropriately to these patients.

PROGNOSTIC FACTORS IN ENDOMETRIAL CARCINOMA

In common with most other cancers, the most important prognostic factor is the spread of disease from the tissue of origin — the endometrium. Until 1988, FIGO only considered macroscopic extension of the tumour to be important and defined the limits of stages II, III and IV disease to be the endocervix, the true pelvis and beyond, respectively. In addition, within stage I disease, the length of the uterine cavity, measured by preoperative uterine sounding, was deemed prognostically significant.

However, for at least the last 40 years, a number of studies have shown the propensity of even very early endometrial carcinoma to invade the lymphatic system.[3] An important report documenting the experience of Stallworthy's group in Oxford referred to the management of 129 cases of endometrial carcinoma including 104 cases with stage I disease, managed by radical hysterectomy and pelvic lymphadenopathy.[4] Pelvic node metastases were found in 5.5% of well-differentiated tumours and in 26% of poorly differentiated cases. In addition, whilst with myometrial penetration by the tumour of 2 mm or less there were no nodal metastases, when cancer was found within 2 mm of the serosal surface, 24% of patients had positive pelvic nodes.

This study prompted the Gynecologic Oncology Group (GOG) in the USA to examine further the concept of surgical staging in the disease. The final report contained data on 621 cases of stage I endometrial carcinoma.[5] The study found that 22% of patients had extrauterine disease, defined as lymph node metastases, adnexal or intraperitoneal spread, or positive peritoneal cytology. Some 41% of patients had more than superficial myometrial invasion and in 15% of patients, tumour was detected in the capillary-like spaces in the uterine specimen. Univariate analysis confirmed that the two criteria in the FIGO staging system then in force — uterine size and tumour differentiation — were significant factors in predicting pelvic and para-aortic nodal disease. However, the study also identified other factors — depth of myometrial invasion, positive peritoneal cytology and the presence of tumour cells within capillary-like spaces — which also correlated with the incidence of nodal disease. In a multivariate analysis three factors — tumour grade, depth of myometrial invasion and presence of intraperitoneal metastases — were identified as being independently significant with regard to nodal spread.

Using these data, patients at high or low risk of nodal disease could be identified using parameters determined both pre- and intraoperatively (Table 22.1). Patients with well-differentiated cancers showing no myometrial invasion had a zero incidence of pelvic nodal disease. The GOG could identify patients at high and low risk of nodal disease. Pelvic node

Table 22.1   Risk groups for nodal metastases

| | Lymph node metastases | |
	Pelvic %	Para-aortic %
Low-risk		
Grade 1: No myometrial invasion and no intraperitoneal disease	0	0
Moderate-risk		
Inner/middle myometrial invasion		
Grade 2/3 tumour: No intraperitoneal disease		
Only one factor	3	2
Both factors	6	2
High-risk		
Deep myometrial invasion	18	15
Intraperitoneal disease	33	8
Both factors	61	30

disease was not seen in any patient who had a well-differentiated cancer and no myometrial penetration.

The medium-risk group included patients with moderate or poorly differentiated cancers with superficial or middle third myometrial penetration. The frequency of nodal metastases in these patients was 6%. The high-risk group contained patients with intraperitoneal disease and/or deep myometrial invasion. The positive pelvic node rate for patients with deep invasion only was 18% and with intraperitoneal disease 33%. This figure rose to 61% in those patients with both these adverse prognostic factors. In addition, 30% of patients in the high-risk group had positive para-aortic nodes.

OTHER PROGNOSTIC FACTORS

Tumour histology

Approximately 80% of primary endometrial cancers are either pure adeno-carcinomas or adenocarcinomas mixed with metaplastic, benign squamous elements. The age distribution, propensity for myometrial invasion or nodal spread and therefore survival are the same whether or not this squamous differentiation is present.[6] Although the survival for this subgroup of patients approaches 90%,[7] the prognosis for other histological subgroups is much inferior.

Uterine papillary serous carcinoma was first described more than 80 years ago but most early reports failed to emphasize its aggressive nature and poor prognosis. It is usually found at an advanced stage and in older women. Invasion of lymphatic channels in the myometrium is common along with evidence of intraperitoneal spread. A report by Hendrickson et al in 1982[8] was one of the earliest to identify the poor prognosis associated with these cancers. Whilst uterine papillary serous carcinoma was found in only 10% of their 256 cases with clinical stage I disease, these patients had a 50% relapse rate compared with 6% for the other endometrial cancers. Deep myometrial penetration was seen in 63% of the papillary cancers compared with 3% for the other subtypes.

Clear cell endometrial cancer is similar to that which arises in cervix, vagina and ovary but the endometrial variant does not seem to be associated with intrauterine exposure to diethylstilboestrol. Clear cell uterine carcinoma represents about 4% of cases.[9] The 5-year survival is considerably less than 50%.[6,10]

Focal squamous differentiation occurs in about 25% of cases of endometrial adenocarcinoma. The so-called adenoacanthoma contains metaplastic benign squamous cells whilst in the adenosquamous subtype the squamous component is cytologically malignant. The latter type has a greater propensity for myometrial penetration with a higher incidence of nodal metastases and hence a poorer survival.[11]

LYMPH VASCULAR PERMEATION

Lymph vascular space involvement has been regarded, for many years, as an important prognostic factor in early-stage cervical cancer.[12,13] Similarly it is not unreasonable to expect that presence of lymph node metastases should have an effect on prognosis and therefore treatment regimens in endometrial cancer. It has also become apparent that the finding of tumour cells within or adherent to the epithelium of lymphatic or vascular spaces in the endometrium, myometrium or parametrium may also be of prognostic significance in endometrial cancer. Alders et al reported a 26.7% recurrence in death rate in stage I patients with vascular invasion compared with a 9.1% rate without.[14]

Aproximately 15% of patients with clinical stage I disease have lymph vascular invasion.[5] The incidence increases from 7% for well-differentiated tumours to over 30% for grade III cancers and also correlates strongly with the degree of myometrial penetration, the presence of positive peritoneal cytology and spread to lymph nodes. The 5-year survival rate for patients without lymph vascular space involvement is 100% compared with 40% of those with lymph vascular space disease.[15]

PERITONEAL CYTOLOGY

Malignant cells have been found in peritoneal fluid in 12% of patients with stage I disease[5] and 25% of patients with positive peritoneal cytology have positive pelvic nodes compared with only 7% of those without. The corresponding figures for those with para-aortic lymph node metastases are 19 and 4%.

STAGING SYSTEMS FOR ENDOMETRIAL CARCINOMA

The old FIGO staging system arose as a result of the practice of treating most patients with radiotherapy prior to a definitive surgical attempt. Treatment decisions therefore had to be based on the preoperative findings: pelvic examination, endometrial curettage and a sounding of the uterine cavity, since any prognostic information based on subsequent histological examination of the hysterectomy specimens ran the risk of being affected severely by the radiotherapy and could therefore not be considered reliable. A move away from preoperative radiotherapy allowed the impact of the other prognostic factors discussed above to be evaluated closely. Some of these factors — depth of myometrial penetration, peritoneal cytology, intra-abdominal and nodal spread — have been incorporated into the new FIGO staging system.

HIGH-RISK CASES AMONGST PATIENTS WITH CLINICAL FIGO STAGE I DISEASE (Table 22.2)

Around one-fifth of patients with cancer apparently limited to the endo-

Table 22.2 Five-year survival rates for endometrial cancer

Stage	Survival rate %
Histological subtype	
Adenocarcinoma	75.2
Adenosquamous carcinoma	47.5
Papillary carcinoma	51.1
Clear cell carcinoma	35.2
Stage and grade	
Stage IA, Grade 1*	78.7
Stage IA, Grade 3	63
Stage IB, Grade 3	52.7
Stage and depth of myometrial penetration	
Stage 1, less than one-third	82.4
Stage 1, more than one-half	66.8
Stage and peritoneal cytology	
Stage 1, negative washings	82.4
Stage 1, positive washings	66.1

* Old FIGO staging parameters are used.

metrium would have a tumour type other than pure endometroid or adenosquamous cancer.[5,7] Deep myometrial penetration can be expected in 38% of adenosquamous cancers[10] and there will be evidence of extra-uterine spread in the form of positive peritoneal cytology in 12–19%.[5,15] Lymphatic metastases will be present in one-third of cases of papillary cancers.[16] The 5-year survival for stage I patients with nodal disease is in the order of 33–36%.[15,17] Tumour recurrence is five times more likely to develop in those patients with poorly differentiated cancer or with a positive lymph node disease compared with patients with well or moderately differentiated tumours or negative lymph nodes.[18]

Ten per cent of clinical stage I, grade I lesions show deep myometrial penetration.[5] In the GOG study of patients with clinical stage I cancer, pelvic node metastases occurred in only 3% of women with superficially invasive, well-differentiated tumours. Para-aortic nodal metastases occurred in only 1% of these patients. However, this rose to 6% for those patients with deep myometrial penetration, to 14% for patients with moderately differentiated deeply invasive lesions and to 23% for those with poorly differentiated cancers.

A further confounding factor is the discrepancy between the histological diagnosis based on uterine curettings and the final diagnosis after examination of the complete uterine specimen. A preoperative grade I lesion obtained at dilatation and curettage is upgraded at least 20% of the time after complete examination of the hysterectomy specimen.[19] It is clear that in many cases of apparent stage I disease, the surgeon should be prepared to extend the scope of the intended surgical procedure despite the 'reassurance' of preoperative investigation.

It is therefore difficult to support the concept that a 'TAH, BSO and cuff' is the extent of the surgical endeavour necessary for patients with clinical stage I disease. A thorough surgical procedure to stage the patient fully is mandatory in order to plan treatment accurately, to estimate prognosis and to compare data from different centres and, of course, as part of the demands of the FIGO classification.

THE SURGICAL MANAGEMENT OF CLINICAL STAGE I DISEASE — NO MORE 'TAH, BSO AND CUFF'

A surgical approach which attempts to determine all significant surgico-pathological variables will allow individualized patient therapy and thus avoid both under- and overtreatment. Initial surgery, therefore, should consist of an extrafascial total abdominal hysterectomy with bilateral salpingo-oophorectomy. Examination of all abdominopelvic contents will be necessary, with the possibility of pelvic and selective para-aortic lymphadenectomy; therefore a midline suprapubic incision should be used. Since vaginal vault recurrences are likely to be due to early lymphatic spread of disease rather than spread of tumour cells during surgery[20], or because of occult endocervical involvement,[21] no vaginal cuff need be excised.

Immediately after opening the peritoneal cavity, a sample of peritoneal fluid, if present, or a sample after irrigating the peritoneal cavity with saline should be obtained and sent for cytological examination. The diaphragm, liver, omentum and pelvic and para-aortic nodes should all be palpated and any suspicious lesions should be biopsied. As soon as the uterus has been removed, it should be sectioned so that macroscopic myometrial invasion and the presence of endocervical extension can be determined. It is the practice in many hospitals that this is carried out by a pathologist either in theatre or after the specimen has been taken down to the pathology department. Sectioning the uterus with an ordinary surgical scalpel runs the risk of causing distortion of the specimen and may interfere with fixation of the tissue.

If there is any doubt about the spread of tumour, then a frozen section can be examined. Noumoff et al[22] evaluated this technique to assess tumour grade, depth of myometrial invasion and the presence of cervical extension in 60 hysterectomy specimens in patients with stage I endometrial cancer in order to predict which patients would need extended surgical staging. Depth and grade, as established by frozen section, were correct in predicting the need for node sampling in 83.7% of cases.

Patients with adenosquamous, clear cell or papillary cancers and those with tumour spread either to the cervix or adnexa should undergo additional surgical staging regardless of the depth of myometrial penetration or any other intraoperative factors. Patients with poorly differentiated tumours with inner third invasion, moderate to poorly differentiated tumours with middle third invasion and any tumours where there appear to be outer third endometrial spread should also undergo lymphadenectomy.

THE MORBIDITY OF SURGICAL STAGING

The age at presentation of the disease and the high probability of serious age-associated, intercurrent medical conditions may encourage some gynaecologists not even to contemplate extended surgical staging for many of their patients with endometrial cancer. Almost half of the cases of endometrial cancer in the USA occur in women over 65 years of age[23] and it has been shown that nearly two-thirds of patients at this age with gynaecological cancer have important medical conditions which could potentially affect surgical morbidity.[24] In this latter study, surgical staging was carried out in 22 patients aged 70 years and over with endometrial cancer. The mean operating time was 1 hour 25 min (range 1 hour 15 min to 2 hours 5 min). There were no postoperative deaths and only 2 cases of serious postoperative morbidity (pneumonia and deep venous thrombosis). The mean length of postoperative stay was 10.4 days with a range of 7 to 17 days — a figure not statistically different from that of younger women.

Recently, Orr et al[25] have analysed the perioperative morbidity in 168 patients with apparent early-stage endometrial cancer undergoing extended staging in a gynaecological oncology department. Lymphadenectomy was performed in 161 of these patients. An analysis of operative time, blood loss and wound infection rate has shown that there is little additional risk, either short- or long-term, attached to this procedure. Both these studies would suggest that the additional information which can be gained from surgical staging can be obtained safely in the majority of women with endometrial cancer regardless of age or intercurrent medical problems, providing a suitable degree of surgical skill and intra- and postoperative monitoring is available.

The alternative to a planned, extended surgical exploration would be to perform TAH, BSO for all patients who were thought to have clinical stage I disease and then to treat that subgroup with high-risk factors on the basis of histology and myometrial invasion. The rationale for this approach is based on the prevailing opinion that radiotherapy is preferable to radical surgery for patients in this age-group. This assumption, however, is not supported by a number of studies which have shown treatment-related mortality rates of 7–13%, life-threatening complication rates of 14%, fistula rates of 10% and uncompleted radiotherapy because of toxicity in 32% of elderly patients receiving radiotherapy for gynaecological cancer.[26,27] With these complication rates, a blanket policy of radiotherapy for all, especially the elderly, is not tenable.

NON-SURGICAL STAGING TECHNIQUES

Ultrasound, lymphangiography, computed tomography scanning and magnetic resonance imaging, although able to determine depth of myometrial invasion, are unable to identify those patients with the small bulk of disease which may be present in positive para-aortic nodes. In one recent study, the quality of magnetic resonance images was thought adequate for para-aortic node evaluation in only 8% of cases.[28] Importantly, neither the present nor previous FIGO criteria allowed these imaging modalities to influence the stage of the disease.

POSTOPERATIVE THERAPY

There has been only one prospective study to evaluate postoperative pelvic radiotherapy for all patients with FIGO stage I endometrial cancer.[14] After surgery, all patients were treated with 6000 rad to the vaginal vault and were then randomized to receive either 4000 rad to the pelvic lymph nodes or no further therapy. There was a significant reduction in the incidence of vaginal and pelvic recurrences in the group receiving additional pelvic radiation (1.9% compared with 6.9% for the control group, $P < 0.01$), but there was a higher proportion of patients in the treatment group (9.9%) who suffered distant metastatic recurrence compared with controls (5.4%). These results are in keeping with subsequent surgicopathological data from the GOG and emphasize the substantial number of patients with apparent stage I disease who have extrapelvic disease at presentation.[5]

The excellent prognosis for patients with well-differentiated, superficially invasive cancers means that adjuvant radiotherapy is not indicated. For high-risk patients who have negative pelvic and para-aortic nodes, the morbidity of radiotherapy is such that treatment to the whole pelvis is not justified. However, vault radiotherapy will not deliver a high enough dose to the paracervical and parametrial areas, therefore small-field external beam therapy would be indicated. For patients with positive pelvic nodes but negative para-aortic nodes, full-field pelvic and common iliac radiotherapy is required.

Extended-field radiotherapy

The identification of 'low stage but poor prognosis' patients with endometrial cancer — that is, those with para-aortic metastases — provides a major challenge to clinicians. Clearly the identification of nodal metastases is of little importance unless effective treatment can be delivered to the site of disease. When surgery and radiotherapy are employed together, complication rates increase. Laparotomy alone may cause a rise in complication rates because the bowel becomes fixed due to adhesion formation. Lymphadenectomy, in conjunction with radiotherapy, increases the late complication rate.

The majority of data concerning extended-field, para-aortic radiotherapy comes from experience in cervical cancer. Bulky para-aortic nodal disease cannot be cured by radiotherapy and a proportion of patients will be unable to tolerate full-dose therapy. For patients with metastatic endometrial cancer it would therefore seem appropriate to attempt to clear surgically all bulky para-aortic disease in order to allow a chance of cure or long-term, symptom-free survival, with reduced-dose, para-aortic irradiation.

Only small series regarding para-aortic radiotherapy for patients with endometrial cancer have been published.[29–31] Potish et al[30] employed para-aortic irradiation (4500–5075 cGy) as part of the primary treatment following surgery in 22 women. Acute symptoms of radiation therapy occurred in most patients. Nausea, diarrhoea and weight loss were almost universal, although the median weight loss was only 2.3 kg. Chronic effects were minimal with no cases of bowel, bladder, hepatic, renal or spinal cord damage. The 5-year survival for patients with pelvic and para-aortic metastases was 43 and 47% for those with para-aortic disease only. Blythe et al,[31] in a small series of only 6 patients, also reported minimal complications and no serious morbidity or mortality from para-aortic irradiation for a 5-year survival rate of 28.6%.

These studies[24,25,30,31] emphasize that para-aortic node biopsy can be accomplished with minimal extra morbidity when performed by adequately trained clinicians and that radiotherapy can be given safely to the para-aortic area. It would also appear that with appropriate therapy there are patients with para-aortic disease who will enjoy long-term survival and perhaps cure.

CONCLUSIONS

The implications of surgical staging in endometrial cancer

Among patients with clinical stage I endometrial cancer, only 7% will have no risk factors for nodal disease (well-differentiated tumour with no myometrial invasion). The high-risk category (deep myometrial invasion, intraperitoneal disease) will form about 25% of the workload and in these patients the chance of para-aortic nodal disease may be as high as 30%. There can be little argument that node sampling is unnecessary in the former group and mandatory in the latter. Patients in the moderate-risk category (moderate or poor tumour differentiation, inner-middle myometrial penetration) have a 6% chance of nodal metastases and consequently it is the management of this group, nearly 70% of the workload, which is the most contentious.

Some clinicians would be prepared to perform nodal dissection on all these patients, especially if both risk factors were present, whilst others may consider that a 6% chance of nodal disease precludes extended surgery. Nevertheless, especially taking poor histological subtypes into consideration, surgeons should expect that, even disregarding FIGO staging criteria, about 1 in 4 patients with early endometrial cancer will need more than just a 'TAH, BSO and cuff'. Extended surgery, in the form of Wertheim hysterectomy, should not be limited to women with early cervical cancer.

With such extensive data regarding the metastatic potential of the disease, there seems little argument that a similar surgical approach should be necessary for women with early endometrial cancer.

REFERENCES

1. Cancer Research Campaign. Factsheet 8 1988
2. Annual report on the results of treatment in gynaecological cancer, vol 20. Stockholm: FIGO, 1988
3. Boronow R C. Advances in diagnosis, staging and management of cervical and endometrial cancer, stages I and II. Cancer 1990; 65: 648–659
4. Lewis B V, Stallworthy J A, Cowdell R. Adenocarcinoma of the body of the uterus. J Obstet Gynaecol Br Commonwealth 1970; 77: 343–348
5. Creasman W T, Morrow C P, Bundy B N, Homesley H D, Graham J E, Heller P B. Surgical pathologic spread patterns of endometrial cancer. A Gynecologic Oncology group study. Cancer 1987; 60: 2035–2041
6. Christopherson W M. The significance of the pathologic findings in endometrial cancer. Clin Obstet Gynecol 1986; 13: 673–693
7. Hendrickson M, Ross J, Eifel P J, Cox R S, Martinez A, Kempson R. Adenocarcinoma of the endometrium: analysis of 256 cases with carcinoma limited to the uterine corpus. Gynecol Oncol 1982; 13: 373–392
8. Hendrickson M R, Ross J, Eifel P, Martinez A, Kempson R. Uterine papillary serous carcinoma. A highly malignant form of endometrial adenocarcinoma. Am J Surg Pathol 1982; 6: 93–108
9. Kurman P J, Scully R E. Clear cell carcinoma of the endometrium. An analysis of 21 cases. Cancer 1976; 37: 872–882
10. Fanning J, Evans M C, Peters A J, Samuel M, Harmon E R, Bates J S. Endometrial adenocarcinoma histologic subtypes: clinical and pathologic profile. Gynecol Oncol 1989; 32: 288–291
11. Zaino R J, Kurman R, Herbold D et al. The significance of squamous differentiation in endometrial carcinoma. Cancer 1991; 68: 2293–2302
12. Van Nagell J, Donaldson E, Parker J, Van Dyke A H, Wood E G. Prognostic significance of cell type and lesion size in patients with cervical cancer treated by radical surgery. Gynecol Oncol 1977; 5: 142–151
13. Boyce J, Furchter R, Nicastri A, Ambiavagar P-C, Reinis M S, Nelson J H Jr. Prognostic factors in stage I carcinoma of the cervix. Gynecol Oncol 1981; 12: 154–165
14. Aalders J G, Abeler V, Kolstad P, Onsrud M. Postoperative external irradiation and prognostic parameters in stage I endometrial carcinoma. Obstet Gynecol 1980; 56: 419–426
15. Gal D, Recio F O, Zamurovic D, Tancer M L. Lymphvascular space involvement — a prognostic indicator in endometrial adenocarcinoma. Gynecol Oncol 1991; 42: 142–145
16. Schink J C, Rademaker A W, Miller D S, Lurain J R. Tumour size in endometrial cancer. Cancer 1991; 67: 2791–2794
17. Chen S S. Operative treatment in stage I endometrial carcinoma with deep myometrial invasion and/or grade 3 tumour surgically limited to the corpus uteri. Cancer 1989; 63: 1843–1845
18. Lurain J R, Rice B L, Rademaker A W, Pogensee L E, Schink J C, Miller D S. Prognostic factors associated with recurrence in clinical stage I adenocarcinoma of the endometrium. Obstet Gynecol 1991; 78: 63–39
19. Soothill R W, Alcock C J, MacKenzie I Z. Discrepancy between curettage and hysterectomy histology in patients with stage I uterine malignancy. Br J Obstet Gynaecol 1989; 96: 478–481
20. Truskett I D, Constable W C. Management of carcinoma of the corpus uteri. Am J Obstet Gynecol 1968; 101: 689–694
21. Makillop W J, Pringle J F. Stage III endometrial carcinoma. A review of 90 cases. Cancer 1985; 56: 2519–2523

22. Noumoff J S, Menzin A, Mikuta J, Lusk E J, Morgan M, Livolsi V A. The ability to evaluate prognostic variables on frozen section in hysterectomies performed for endometrial carcinoma. Gynecol Oncol 1991; 42: 202–208

23. Baranovsky A, Myers M H. Cancer incidence and survival in patients 65 years of age and older. Cancer 1986; 36: 26–41

24. Lawton F G, Hacker N F. Surgery for invasive gynecologic cancer in the elderly female population. Obstet Gynecol 1990; 76: 287–289

25. Orr J W, Holloway R W, Orr P F, Holiman J L. Surgical staging of uterine cancer: an analysis of perioperative morbidity. Gynecol Oncol 1991; 42: 209–216

26. Kennedy A W, Flagg J S, Webster K D. Gynecologic cancer in the very elderly. Gynecol Oncol 1989; 32: 49–54

27. Grant P T, Jeffrey J F, Fraser R C, Tompkins M G, Filbee J F, Wong O S. Pelvic radiation therapy for gynecologic malignancy in geriatric patients. Gynecol Oncol 1989; 33: 185–188

28. Hricak H, Rubinstein L V, Gherman G M, Karstaedt N. MR imaging evaluation of endometrial carcinoma: results of an NCI cooperative study. Radiology 1991; 179: 829–832

29. Komaki R, Mattingly R F, Hoffman R G, Barber S W, Satre R, Greenberg M. Irradiation of paraaortic lymph node metastases from carcinoma of the cervix or endometrium: preliminary results. Radiology 1983; 147: 245–48

30. Potish R A, Twiggs L B, Adcock L L, Savage J E, Levitt S H, Prem K A. Paraaortic lymph node radiotherapy in cancer of the uterine corpus. Obstet Gynecol 1985; 65: 251–256

31. Blythe J G, Hodel K A, Wahl T P, Baglan R J, Lee F A, Zivnuska F R. Para-aortic node biopsy in cervical and endometrial cancers: does it affect survival? Am J Obstet Gynecol 1986; 155: 306–314

Index

PROGRESS IN OBSTETRICS AND GYNAECOLOGY
Edited by John Studd

All backlist volumes are available.
You can place your order by contacting your local medical bookseller or the Sales Promotion Department,
Robert Stevenson House, 1–3 Baxter's Place, Leith Walk, Edinburgh EH1 3AF, UK
Tel: (031) 556 2424; Telex: 727511 LONGMN G; Fax: (031) 558 1278

Contents of Volume 1

Contents of Volume 2

PROGRESS IN OBSTETRICS AND GYNAECOLOGY

PROGRESS IN OBSTETRICS AND GYNAECOLOGY

PROGRESS IN OBSTETRICS AND GYNAECOLOGY

See front page for *Contents of Volume 9*